Male Reproductive Cancers

CANCER GENETICS

ELAINE OSTRANDER, SERIES EDITOR

Genetics of Colorectal Cancer, edited by *John D. Potter and Noralane M. Lindor,*
2009

For other titles published in this series, go to
www.springer.com/series/7706

William D. Foulkes · Kathleen A. Cooney
Editors

Male Reproductive Cancers

Epidemiology, Pathology and Genetics

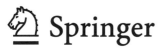 Springer

Editors
William D. Foulkes
Program in Cancer Genetics
Departments of Oncology and
    Human Genetics
McGill University
Montreal, Quebec
Canada
william.foulkes@mcgill.ca

Kathleen A. Cooney
Departments of Internal Medicine
    and Urology
University of Michigan
Ann Arbor, MI
USA
kcooney@umich.edu

ISBN 978-1-4419-0448-5   e-ISBN 978-1-4419-0449-2
DOI 10.1007/978-1-4419-0449-2
Springer New York Dordrecht Heidelberg London

Library of Congress Control Number: 2009930468

Printed on acid-free paper

Springer is part of Springer Science+Business Media (www.springer.com)

Contents

Contributors

Agnes B. Baffoe-Bonnie, MD, MPH, PhD
Merck Research Laboratories, Department of Epidemiology,
North Wales, PA 19454

Louis R Bégin, MD
Chief, Division of Anatomic Pathology, Sacré-Coeur Hospital,
Montreal, QC, Canada, and Department of Pathology,
McGill University, Montreal, QC, Canada

Tarek Bismar, MD
Associate Professor Departments of Pathology & Laboratory Medicine/Oncology/
Biochemistry & Molecular Biology, University of Calgary, Calgary, Alberta,
Canada

Mario Chevrette, PhD
Molecular Biologist and Assistant Professor of Surgery, Division of Urology,
Department of Surgery, McGill University, The Research Institute of the
McGill University Health Center, Montreal, QC, Canada

Michael B. Cook, PhD
Post-doctoral fellow, Hormonal and Reproductive Epidemiology Branch,
Division of Cancer Epidemiology and Genetics, National Cancer Institute,
Bethesda, MD, USA

Kathleen A. Cooney, MD
Professor of Internal Medicine and Urology, Chief,
Division of Hematology/Oncology, University of Michigan,
Ann Arbor, MI, USA

Cezary Cybulski, MD, PhD
Department of Genetics and Pathology, International Hereditary Cancer Center,
Pomeranian Medical University, Pomerania, Poland

Douglas F. Easton, MA, Dip Math Stats, PhD
Cancer Research UK Genetic Epidemiology Unit, Strangeways
Research Laboratory, University of Cambridge, Cambridge, UK

Rosalind A. Eeles, MA, FRCR, FRCP, PhD
Institute of Cancer Research, Cancer Genetics Unit,
Sutton, Surrey, UK

William D. Foulkes, MB, MRCP(UK), PhD
Professor and Director, Program in Cancer Genetics,
Departments of Oncology and Human Genetics,
McGill University, Montreal, QC, Canada

Graham Giles, BSc, MSc, PhD
Professor, Director, Cancer Epidemiology Centre, University of Melbourne,
Carlton, Australia

Julius Gudmundsson, MSc MBA
deCODE genetics, Reykjavik, Iceland

Michelle Guy, PhD
The Institute of Cancer Research, Sutton, Surrey, UK

Laure Humbert, PhD
Research Institute of the McGill University Health Center, McGill University,
Montreal, QC, Canada

Zsofia Kote-Jarai, PhD
The Institute of Cancer Research, Sutton, Surrey, UK

Ethan M. Lange, PhD
Assistant Professor, University of North Carolina at Chapel Hill,
Department of Genetics, Chapel Hill, NC, USA

Jan Lubinski, MD, PhD
Professor, Head, Department of Genetics and Pathomorphology,
Pomeranian Medical University, Pomerania, Poland

Katherine A. McGlynn, PhD, MPH
Investigator, Hormonal and Reproductive Epidemiology Branch,
Division of Cancer Epidemiology and Genetics, National Cancer Institute,
Bethesda, MD, USA

Katherine L. Nathanson, MD
Assistant Professor, Department of Medicine, Division of Medical Genetics,
University of Pennsylvania School of Medicine, Philadelphia, PA, USA

Sabrina Notte, BAA
Program Manager, Program in Cancer Genetics,
Departments of Oncology and Human Genetics,
McGill University, Montreal, QC, Canada

Isaac J. Powell, MD
Clinical Professor, Department of Urology, Wayne State University
School of Medicine, Karmanos Cancer Institute, Detroit, MI, USA

Elizabeth A. Rapley, PhD
Institute of Cancer Research, Cancer Genetics Unit,
Belmont, Sutton, Surrey, UK

Audrey H. Schnell, PhD
Post-doctoral Fellow, Epidemiology & Biostatistics, and Urology,
University of California, San Francisco, San Francisco,
CA, USA

Kári Stefánsson, MD, PhD
CEO, deCODE genetics, Reykjavik, Iceland

John S. Witte, PhD
Professor, Epidemiology & Biostatistics, and Urology, University of California,
San Francisco, San Francisco, CA, USA

Kirk J. Wojno, MD
Adjunct Research Faculty, University of Michigan, Department of Urology,
Ann Arbor, MI, USA;
Director, AmeriPath Institute of Urological Pathology, Warren, MI, USA;
National Director of Urologic Pathology, Palm Beach Gardens, FL, USA

Introduction

The aim of this book is to present a thoughtful, comprehensive, and up-to-date overview of the etiology of two of the most important sites of cancer in the male reproductive tract, namely the prostate gland and the testes. Whereas the clinical presentations and treatment of these two cancers are very different, both cancers have been the focus of a tremendous amount of research over the past several decades. Here, we present reviews that summarize much of this research taking place in the three most important etiological disciplines – epidemiology, pathology, and genetics.

Testicular cancer is relatively uncommon with approximately 8,000 new cases expected in the USA in 2009. The disease is most commonly diagnosed in young men between the ages of 15 and 40 years and typically presents as a mass or enlargement of the testicle. Testicular cancer is more common in men of European descent and less common in African and Asian populations. Clinically, the most striking feature of testicular cancer is the ability to cure men with wide-spread metastatic disease using standard chemotherapy regimens which include cisplatinum and also radiation therapy in some cases.

In contrast, prostate cancer is a disease of advancing age which often presents with changes in urinary function as well as signs and symptoms related to metastatic disease including bone pain, weight loss, and fatigue. In the early 1990s, it was proposed that serum testing for prostate specific antigen or PSA could be utilized in combination with digital rectal examination to detect early asymptomatic cases of prostate cancer. This has led to many studies conducted throughout the world to determine whether early detection and treatment of this common cancer results in improved survival. While these studies are ongoing, many groups have developed varying recommendations with regard to use of strategies for early detection of prostate cancer. Populations that support testing asymptomatic men for prostate cancer generally have more early onset cases, as well as higher rates of localized disease at presentation. Whether or not death rates are concomitantly reduced at population levels will await the results of large randomized trials being conducted currently in the USA and Europe. Like testicular cancer, there are marked geographic and racial differences in prostate cancer incidence throughout the world. African Americans have the highest incidence of prostate cancer in the world while Asian populations generally have a reduced incidence.

Although prostate cancer and testicular cancer have very different clinical presentations and epidemiology, family history is a recognized risk factor for both diseases. This has led to the collection of families with multiple cases of prostate or testicular cancer for use in genetic studies. While the search for definitive high penetrance genes that may serve as susceptibility loci is ongoing, such genes are unlikely to account for more than a very small fraction of all prostate or testicular cancer. Perhaps due to the paucity of highly penetrant alleles, new leads have come from genome-wide association studies. There has also been an explosion of laboratory and bioinformatics approaches that have been applied to tumor tissues resulting in novel observations such as the identification of common gene fusion transcripts in prostate cancer tissue. These innovative strategies can be used to complement ongoing genetic linkage studies to shed additional light onto the molecular basis of cancers of the male reproductive system.

This book is comprised of four distinct parts: Epidemiology, Pathology, Molecular Genetics, and Inherited Susceptibility. Within each section, the chapters are divided by disease. Part A of this book reviews the epidemiology of prostate cancer followed by testicular cancer with an emphasis on clinical and environmental factors associated with these diseases. Part B begins with a describing the various pathological features of prostate cancer that may explain some of the clinical heterogeneity of the disease. This is followed by a complete description of the wide variety of testicular cancers from seminoma to lymphoma as well as a brief section on the use of tumor markers for monitoring disease. Part C focuses on somatic genetic changes in prostate and testicular cancers using new technologies such as comparative genomic hybridization and gene expression profiling. The last section of the book Part D concentrates on the progress made toward understanding inherited susceptibility to prostate cancer and to testicular cancer. The chapters on prostate cancer begin with a comprehensive review of genetic linkage and association studies and their use in identifying susceptibility loci for common diseases such as cancer. This is followed by a review of the special issues relating to studying prostate cancer in specific, unique populations including Icelandic, Polish, Ashkenazi Jewish, and African American men. The chapters on prostate cancer are concluded with a review of approaches used to identify genetic loci that predispose to aggressive forms of prostate cancer. The final chapter focuses on linkage and association studies used to identify testicular cancer susceptibility genes.

Despite the many successes in genetic research over the past several decades, the molecular basis for many common cancers remains elusive. Although it is clear that family history is an important risk factor for both prostate and testicular cancer, it has been difficult to use family based studies to identify susceptibility loci. It is important to consider that what we call "prostate cancer" or "testicular cancer" is likely a group of diseases that may be characterized by a unique set of genetic changes. For example, it has been demonstrated that the there are multiple types of breast cancer characterized by unique "intrinsic" patterns of gene expression, categorizing breast cancers into basal, luminal, HER2 positive tumors. Teams of clinicians, pathologists, and researchers must work closely together to unravel the complex nature of prostate and testicular cancer using advanced technologies and bioinformatics approaches. The resulting potential gain in the understanding of cancer phenotypes as well as the genetic factors that predispose to these cancers has many positive outcomes. Ideally, the most penetrant genes could be used individually to create laboratory tests to characterize cancer risk, and combinations of less penetrant genes could perhaps be pooled to perform a similar function. More importantly, characterization of the key molecular changes in cancer can lead to specific therapies which may target these changes (e.g., the development of the monoclonal antibody trastuzumab for use in treating breast cancers that are express HER2). In addition to a highly collaborative environment, this type of research will necessitate large tissue repositories and clinical registries so that laboratory findings can be quickly translated into clinical practice. International studies will also be required since the epidemiology of both prostate and testicular cancer demonstrates geographical and ethnic differences in incidence and mortality. The future of cancer research will be bright if we continue to support and reward scientists and clinicians for developing successful, large-scale collaborations to unravel the molecular basis for male reproductive cancers.

In this book, we have provided a view of the current state of knowledge regarding testicular cancer and prostate cancer. By broadly covering the epidemiology, pathology, and genetic aspects of these male reproductive cancers, we hope that the reader will be able to begin to consider how information in these three distinct disciplines will coalesce and improve our understanding of these potentially lethal cancers.

Kathleen A. Cooney, MD
William D. Foulkes, MB, PhD

Part A
Epidemiology

Chapter 1
The Epidemiology of Prostate Cancer

Graham Giles

1.1 Introduction

Prostate cancer presents several enduring challenges that continue to defy solution despite extensive research. It has long been known that prostate tumours become increasingly prevalent with age, so much so that their occurrence could be viewed as part of the normal ageing process, as the vast majority of men will develop them if they live long enough (Giles 2003). Importantly, the preponderance of prostate tumours is of low metastatic potential and of slow growth so, although the majority of older men zealously investigated will be found to have microscopically detectable tumours, most men will die with a prostate tumour rather than from one (Bostwick et al. 2004).

In a minority of cases prostate tumours become invasive and potentially lethal. The conundrum here, elegantly articulated by Boccon-Gibod (1996), is how to distinguish "tigers" from "pussycats"; i.e. how to identify at a curable stage the minority of lethal cancers from the majority of non-aggressive tumours. Answers to this question remain elusive. Schnell and Witte (this volume) focus on inherited aspects of susceptibility to aggressive prostate cancer.

Since the late 1980s in many countries the increasingly widespread use of the prostate-specific antigen (PSA) test to screen asymptomatic men for prostate cancer has profoundly altered the definition, diagnosis and treatment of what we know as prostate cancer (Giles 2003). Our inability on the one hand to accurately identify the potentially lethal prostate tumour phenotype(s), and our increasing ability on the other hand to detect what were historically termed "latent" tumours (Yatani et al. 1982), has considerable implications not only for the diagnosis and treatment of prostate cancer but also for research at every level from molecular biology and genetics through to epidemiology and public health (Platz et al. 2004a).

G. Giles
Cancer Epidemiology Centre, The Cancer Council Victoria,
1 Rathdowne Street, Carlton, VIC, 3053, Australia
e-mail: graham.giles@cancervic.org.au

W.D. Foulkes and K.A. Cooney (eds.), *Male Reproductive Cancers:*
Epidemiology, Pathology and Genetics, Cancer Genetics,
DOI 10.1007/978-1-4419-0449-2_1, © Springer Science+Business Media, LLC 2010

1.1.1 Prostate Structure and Function

To better understand some of the problems confronting research on prostate cancer requires some understanding of the prostate's development, structure, and function. The gland is located at the base of the pelvis beneath the urinary bladder and surrounds the urethra. It is said to resemble a walnut and is contained within a fibrous inelastic capsule. The embryonic prostate remains quiescent from birth until puberty during which time it grows under the influence of testosterone to reach its adult weight of 20 g at around 20 years of age (Aumuller 1991). At maturity the prostate has between 30 and 50 branched ducts that are lined with glandular epithelium and which open into the prostatic urethra.

The prostate contributes up to 30% of the volume of semen with its slightly alkaline secretions that contain a number of molecules including prostaglandins, proteolytic enzymes, acid phosphatase, zinc, and citric acid. During sexual arousal, the prostatic secretions are mixed with those (including sperm) from the seminal vesicles to form seminal fluid. The role of the prostatic secretions is to assist in maintaining sperm viability after ejaculation and during transit through the relatively hostile environment of the female reproductive tract (Isaacs 1983).

It was not until the 1980s that McNeal first described the prostate's zonal anatomy (McNeal 1981) and showed the gland to have four distinct anatomical zones. The dorsal aspect, which is accessible via digital rectal examination, is called the peripheral zone and contains about 70% of total volume and 60 to 70% of tumours. The central zone, which includes the ejaculatory ducts, contains 25% of the gland's total volume and is where inflammatory processes such as prostatitis occur. The transitional zone contains only 5% of the gland's volume and 25% of tumours. The anterior zone is fibromuscular and assists in ejaculation.

Full details of the anatomy and pathology of the prostate gland are provided by Bégin and Bismar in their chapter in this volume.

Throughout life the health of the prostate is a balance between cellular proliferation and differentiation and apoptosis. The prostate's development and continued maintenance is strongly influenced by endogenous hormones, particularly androgens but also oestrogens. The action of androgens on the prostate is mediated by the androgen receptor which has a far greater affinity for dihydrotestosterone than for testosterone. Testosterone is converted to dihydrotestosterone by 5 alpha reductase, particularly by the type 2 isoenzyme, and men born with a congenital deficiency of 5 alpha reductase do not develop a normal prostate and are, thus, at low risk of prostate cancer (Randall 1994). Paradoxically, prostate cancer incidence increases contemporaneously with the fall in men's circulating testosterone levels with age. Androgens alone, however, do not explain the full complexity of control mechanisms in the prostate. The proliferative action of androgens (testosterone and dihydrotestosterone) is balanced by other molecules including adrenal androgens (Bosland 2006), oestrogens (Bosland 2005), insulin-like growth factors (IGFs) (Wu et al. 2006a, b; Kambhampati et al. 2005), insulin (Schiel et al. 2006), leptin (Ribeiro et al. 2006) and vitamin D (Weigel 2007). These agents and their complex interactions, especially with the androgen receptor, are not fully understood and continue to attract considerable research interest.

1.1.2 Aspects of Prostate Pathology Relevant to Cancer Epidemiology

As the male's hormonal milieu changes from middle age onwards, the prostate commonly tends to grow in volume, a condition termed benign prostatic hyperplasia (BPH) (Hafez and Hafez 2004). BPH was once considered a risk factor for prostate cancer but this view is no longer held; both BPH and tumours commonly occur in ageing prostates. Due to the inelasticity of the prostate's fibrous outer capsule, in the presence of BPH increasing pressure is placed on the prostatic urethra, producing a range of lower urinary tract symptoms including reduced stream, increased frequency especially at night, increased urgency, incomplete voiding and increased risk of urinary tract infections. Depending on severity and inconvenience, lower urinary tract symptoms bring men to medical attention, and it is in this context that cancer is often incidentally diagnosed (McVary 2006). Transurethral resection of the prostate has commonly been performed to relieve obstructive symptoms of BPH, and a small proportion of prostate tumours are found incidentally on pathological examination of tissue fragments removed during this procedure leading to a degree of over-diagnosis (Bostwick and Chang 1999). As the management of BPH has increasingly become a pharmaceutical rather than a primarily surgical intervention and with the increased use of PSA for cancer early detection, this mode of prostate tumour diagnosis is diminishing.

Prostatic tumours are virtually all adenocarcinomas that arise from the glandular epithelium which lines the prostatic ducts. As described earlier, prostate tumours commonly occur in the peripheral zone of the gland and also tend to be multi-focal with different foci within the same gland often differing in size and morphology. Much research has been spent on identifying tumour markers that would separate the lethal from the indolent tumour phenotypes, but this is still beyond our ability (van Leenders 2007). Currently, a tumour's potential lethality is assessed on the circulating level of PSA in the blood, evidence of spread beyond the capsule and histopathological assessment of needle biopsy cores to estimate tumour volume and grade (Presti 2007).

Prostate tumour aggressiveness is commonly assessed according to the method proposed by Dr. Donald Gleason (Gleason 1992). Using this method, the two largest tumour foci (primary and secondary patterns) are each graded from 1 to 5 according to the histological patterns described by Gleason. The Gleason grades for the two foci, that are rarely more than one grade apart, are added to give a Gleason sum (or score) from 2 to 10. Tumours with Gleason sums below 5 are not considered aggressive. Historically, those tumours with Gleason sums 5 to 7 were considered to be of moderate grade, but in the most recent edition of the TNM Classification of Malignant Tumours (UICC 2002) Gleason sum 7 was added to the poorly differentiated and undifferentiated grade category, formerly Gleason sum 8 to 10. The significance of Gleason sum 7 tumours remains controversial, especially with respect to decisions about treatment. About 30% of cases with a Gleason score sum of 7 have a primary pattern of grade 4 and are considered to be more aggressive than cases having a primary pattern of grade 3. Some consider that any focus of Gleason grade 4 warrants increased clinical suspicion, and this thinking has extended to include any tertiary pattern of grade 5 (Patel et al. 2007). Whatever the clinical importance of these changes, their adoption in epidemiological studies to classify tumours as aggressive/advanced inflates the proportion of cases, so described, and can perturb a study's capacity to detect associations (Platz et al. 2004a). For further information, see additional discussion about the Gleason Grading System in the chapter by Bégin and Bismar.

1.1.3   Prostate Cancer Diagnosis, Screening and Treatment

Prostate cancer has no specific symptoms. In the past, it most commonly presented as was as advanced disease. The diagnosis of prostate cancer is often made during an assessment of symptoms caused by BPH. During diagnostic work up, the prostate's size and the presence of any nodules are assessed by digital rectal examination and ultrasound. The diagnosis of cancer is aided by measuring serum levels of PSA, a protease enzyme produced by the glandular epithelium, some of which permeates into the bloodstream. PSA was originally used clinically to monitor cancer progression after treatment (Kuriyama et al. 1981) but is now commonly used for early detection (Stamey et al. 1987). High serum PSA levels typically indicate the presence of malignancy, but investigations prompted at lower PSA levels lead to the over-diagnosis of many tumours that would probably never have progressed to clinically significant disease during life (Albertsen 2005).

Suspiciously elevated PSA levels are followed up with transrectal-ultrasound-guided, needle biopsies to establish a histopathological diagnosis. Prostate tumours are commonly small and multi-focal, and there is an element of chance in whether the presence of tumour(s) can be adequately sampled by needle biopsy. To reduce the possibility of missing a tumour, the number of needle biopsies taken has increased over time (Shinohara 2006) and the PSA level used as a threshold for biopsy has fallen, especially in the USA (Catalona et al. 2006).

Recognising that PSA testing lacks both specificity and sensitivity, many modifications have been considered to lead to a better cancer test. For example, the PSA molecule is often bound to other serum proteins including protease inhibitors and can be measured in a free or a complexed form. Investigators have noted that there is a lower free/total PSA measurement in men with prostate cancer, and free/total PSA testing has been advocated in the clinical setting in which the total PSA is in the 2.0 to 10 ng/mL range (Hoffman et al. 2000). Others have investigated using age-specific reference ranges and PSA density (PSA/gland volume) and PSA velocity. To date, none of these modifications are in widespread clinical use.

PSA testing for early prostate cancer is performed on a widespread ad hoc basis in many countries. Randomised clinical trials conducted currently are designed to test the efficacy of PSA testing in reducing prostate cancer mortality (Schroder 1994; Gohagan et al. 1994). Because many controls in these trials receive PSA tests as part of their community care, the statistical power of the trials to provide definitive evidence of efficacy has been reduced and this may lengthen them by some years (Beemsterboer et al. 2000).

The WHO has adopted several criteria by which to judge the suitability of a screening program (Wilson and Jungner 1968): the condition considered for screening should be important one, there should be an acceptable treatment for patients with the disease, facilities for diagnosis and treatment should be available, there should be a recognised latent or early symptomatic stage, there should be a suitable test or examination which has few false positives (high specificity) and few false negatives (high sensitivity), the test or examination should be acceptable to the population, the cost, including diagnosis and subsequent treatment, should be economically balanced in relation to expenditure on medical care as a whole. Importantly, the outcome should be measured in terms of mortality reduction rather than improved survival. Prostate cancer screening by PSA testing currently fails to satisfy all these criteria (Denis 1995; Albertsen 1996).

Given the uncertainties that surround its biological heterogeneity and limited evidence of treatment benefits, prostate cancer management is complex (Ali and Hamdy 2007). Men with low-grade, localised cancer and low PSA may opt for watchful waiting with regular repeat PSA tests to monitor the rate of change, PSA velocity. Once PSA velocity reaches a certain rate, decisions may be made with respect to treatment (Lee and D'Amico 2005). Treatments for localised disease include surgery (radical prostatectomy usually with pelvic lymphadenectomy) or external beam radiation therapy. There is also some early success using radioactive seeds implantation to deliver localised radiation (brachytherapy) for men with small and lower-grade tumours (Heysek 2007). Advanced disease is treated by androgen deprivation/blockade which can involve surgical or medical castration. Hormonal therapy is non-curative, and castrate-resistant prostate cancer is typically treated with chemotherapy. External beam radiation may also be used to treat symptomatic bony metastases in the setting of advanced disease.

The principal concern with contemporary approaches to the detection of prostate cancer is over-diagnosis and the considerable effects on quality of life for a substantial proportion of men who are treated unnecessarily (Albertsen 1996; Albertsen et al. 2005). The costs include treatment-related side effects such as impotence, incontinence, and damage to the rectum and bladder neck, and these detriments have to be weighed against the limited evidence of benefit. There are a number of clinical trials that are ongoing in which men with newly diagnosed prostate cancer are randomised to observation or treatment with one of several modalities (e.g. radical prostatectomy or external beam radiation.) These studies are being conducted in different countries with different methods of cancer detection (PSA vs. clinical symptoms) and should begin to provide data to support evidenced-based approaches for detecting and treating prostate cancer (Bill-Axelson et al. 2008; Wilt 2008).

1.2   Descriptive Epidemiology

Prostate cancer is one of the most age-dependent cancers; rare before the age of 50, it increases at an exponential rate thereafter. In the pre-PSA era, prostate cancer incidence was characterised by high rates in North America, especially for American Blacks, intermediate rates in Europe and low rates in Africa and Asia. In Cancer Incidence in Five Continents Volume VI which covers the period 1983 to 1987 (before PSA era), the age-adjusted (standardised to the World population) incidence rates from the U.S. Surveillance Epidemiology and End Results (SEER) program were 62 and 82 per 100,000 American Whites and Blacks, respectively (Parkin et al. 1992). These U.S. rates compared with 52 for Canada, 39 for Australia, 30 for Denmark, 23 for England and Wales, 15 to 17 for the Philippines, 7 to 10 for Japan, 8 for Hong Kong, 4 to 7 for India and 1 to 2 for China. Interestingly, the incidence rates for ethnic groups in the USA were intermediate to those from the countries of origin and the local USA rates; rates for Filipino Americans were 29 to 37, Japanese Americans 33 to 34 and Chinese Americans 20 to 28 per 100,000.

Although international incidence rates for prostate cancer varied substantially in the pre-PSA era, the age-adjusted mortality rates varied to a much smaller degree. Figure 1.1 shows that in Scandinavian countries, among which the zeal for prostate cancer detection differed strongly, it was possible to show that differences in incidence rates in 1983 to 1987 correlated poorly with mortality rates, the latter being closely similar (Tretli et al. 1996). Both incidence and survival in Sweden were almost double that for Denmark, but the mortality rates were virtually identical.

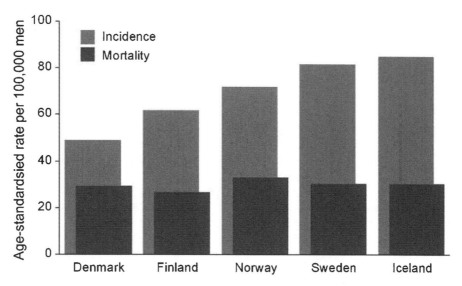

Fig. 1.1 Comparative prostate cancer incidence and mortality rates for Scandinavian countries, 1983 to 1987

Prior to the PSA era, there was already evidence that heightened zeal for early detection had negligible impact on prostate cancer mortality.

Since the advent of PSA and its increasingly widespread use for the early detection of prostate cancer, the incidence of prostate cancer has changed remarkably in many countries. In some populations prostate cancer incidence more than doubled; peaking within a few years of PSA introduction, and then fell, but to a higher level than previously. The extent of the increase can be assessed by comparing incidence rates from Cancer Incidence in Five Continents Volume VIII (Parkin et al. 2002) covering the period 1993 to 1997, with those from volume VI reported earlier. The age-adjusted incidence rates from the U.S. SEER program for 1993 to 1997 were 108 and 185 per 100,000 American Whites and Blacks, respectively. Contemporary rates for other populations were 80 for Canada, 85 to 112 for Australia, 30 for Denmark, 40 for England and Wales, 17 to 22 for the Philippines, 9 to 14 for Japan, 8 for Hong Kong, 2 to 7 for India, and 1 to 3 for China. The incidence rates for ethnic groups in the USA also increased in magnitude but remained intermediate between those from the countries of origin and the local USA rates; rates for Filipino Americans were 82 to 89, Japanese Americans 62 to 65 and Chinese Americans 33 to 79 per 100,000.

An analysis of SEER data demonstrated that the major increase in incidence associated with PSA testing has been for moderate-grade (Gleason sum 5 to 7) tumours, with only modest changes to low- and high-grade disease (Brawley 1997). The increased detection of moderate-grade and localised prostate cancers has increased the apparent survival from prostate cancer, but this is due to the long lead time and length bias associated with these tumours. Depending on screening prevalence, studies have estimated that PSA testing is associated with over-diagnosis ranging from 2% to more than 50% (Zappa et al. 1998; Etzioni et al. 2002; Pashayan et al. 2006; Telesca et al. 2008).

Protagonists for PSA testing have drawn on small changes in mortality from prostate cancer to support its efficacy, but this attribution will only be unequivocally demonstrated by the randomised trials that are still in progress (Schroder 1994; Gohagan et al. 1994). The apparent changes in prostate cancer mortality can at best be described as modest and cannot simply be attributed to PSA testing. They may be due to a range of factors, including the contemporaneous introduction of new therapies (Shahinian et al. 2005; Heysek 2007) and the possible biases surrounding the completion of death certificates and the attribution of cause of death (Feuer et al. 1999).

Figure 1.2 compares trends in age-adjusted mortality rates for the USA, UK, Australia, Denmark, and Japan. The most prominent feature is the rapid rise in mortality that mimicked the rise and subsequent fall in the incidence trends. Apart from the USA, the fall in the mortality rate has yet to reach the level observed before its rapid rise. The mortality rate for prostate cancer in Japan has been steadily increasing from 1950 but is still very low relative to the other countries illustrated, and the rate of increase appears to have been tapering off in recent years.

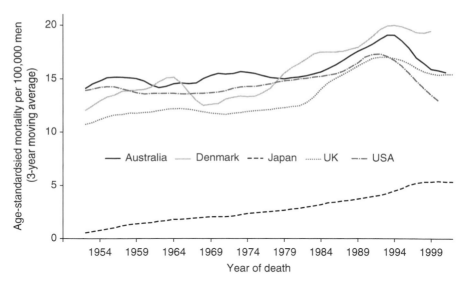

Fig. 1.2 Trends in the age-standardised mortality rate from prostate cancer for selected countries

1.3 The Epidemiological Investigation of Causes

The essential quest for epidemiologists researching prostate cancer is to identify modifiable exposures that are related to the risk of developing "aggressive" prostate cancers that are likely to be fatal (Boyle et al. 2003). Being able to differentiate the small proportion of aggressive cancers from the majority of indolent tumours, in other words separating the "tigers" from the "pussycats", is a necessary step in this search. Epidemiological studies that do not attempt to identify and separately analyse aggressive and/or advanced forms of the disease are fated to produce little of value. A sensitive and specific method of identifying truly aggressive disease would also be of tremendous clinical importance thereby reducing over-diagnosis, unnecessary treatment and unwelcome side effects. Until we have this knowledge, we can do little to prevent life-threatening prostate cancer from occurring.

The principal limitation of past epidemiological studies of prostate cancer has been in combining all diagnoses of prostate cancer as if they are one disease. Given the low metastatic potential of most prostate tumours, their grouping together is destined to produce weak and inconsistent findings and this is reflected in the prostate cancer epidemiology literature (Giles and Ireland 1997). Since the advent of widespread PSA testing, and the subsequent over-diagnosis of tumours that would never have manifested as invasive disease, the problem of disease specificity has worsened in countries such as Australia (Smith and Armstrong 1998). Given this situation, and the lack of good molecular markers of prognosis, epidemiological studies should as a matter of course collect detailed clinical data on case presentation and diagnosis (Platz et al. 2004a) and arrange for centralised histopathology review of diagnostic slides and to retrieve and store archival tissue samples for future molecular pathology analysis as markers become available.

Epidemiological research on prostate cancer has been pursued in numerous case control studies but far fewer prospective cohort studies (Ross and Schottenfeld 1996). Apart from lack of disease specificity already mentioned, case control studies have commonly presented many other problems such as small sample size, inadequate statistical power and poor exposure measurement and have, not surprisingly, produced weak and inconsistent associations with risk (Giles and Ireland 1997). Better evidence has been obtained from a handful of large well-controlled case control studies and a growing number of cohort studies (largely from the U.S.), but these have either been conducted or have come to maturity in the PSA era and have captured incident cases with a different profile of metastatic potential to those from earlier studies. The result of this is that we have probably gained more knowledge about risk factors for early tumourigenesis at the expense of gaining knowledge about risk factors that promote advanced disease.

Apart from the established risk factors of age, race and having a family history of prostate cancer, the evidence for other causes of prostate cancer remains uncertain and this will probably remain the case until the potentially lethal tumour phenotypes are accurately identifiable. Summarised as follows is the best available epidemiological evidence taken predominantly from large, well-designed, prospective, cohort studies highlighting where available risk estimates for aggressive and/or advanced disease. This literature is dominated by reports from North America, particularly from the Health Professionals Follow up Study and a few reports from Europe, Australia and Asia. Currently, none of it is of sufficient quality or strength to provide a solid basis for prevention.

1.3.1   Environmental Factors Not Associated with Prostate Cancer

Prostate cancer incidence does not appear to be associated with cigarette smoking. Contemporary cohort studies such as those of U.S. Health Professionals Follow-Up Study and the Physicians' Health Study have reported estimates of risk close to unity for the incidence of all prostate cancer and either current or past smoking, and modest positive associations with respect to fatal prostate cancer, relative risks (RR) between 1.3 and 2 (Lumey 1996; Lotufo et al. 2000). Similarly, no association has been established between low-to-moderate alcohol consumption and prostate cancer (Breslow and Weed 1998), but the possibility of an association with heavy drinking and the possibility of population subgroups in which alcohol effects might be observed cannot be excluded (Platz et al. 2004b). A protective association with red wine consumption reported from a case control study (Schoonen et al. 2005) has sadly not been confirmed by two subsequent prospective cohort studies (Velicer et al. 2006; Sutcliffe et al. 2007a). Other reviews conclude that vasectomy probably does not increase risk of prostate cancer (Dennis et al. 2002).

Reports of occupational associations with prostate cancer, including military exposures to radiofrequency radiation and herbicides, are weak and inconsistent (Giles 2003). Those that are reported are commonly the result of uncontrolled confounding with social class, e.g. men of higher social status are more likely to seek medical attention and have prostate cancer diagnosed than men of lower education and social status. The probability of detection bias influencing risk estimates has increased in the PSA era. A number of studies have investigated farming practices, and pesticide use in particular, but exposures in this setting have usually been ecological measures and have rarely been determined at the level of the individual (Rafnsson 2007). Note that there is some evidence that Agent Orange, a herbicide known to be contaminated by 2,3,7,8-tetrachlorodibenzo-p-dioxin (TCDD) that was widely used in Vietnam by the U.S. military, is associated with prostate cancer (Chamie et al. 2008). While the data are limited, U.S. veterans who served in Vietnam in the appropriate time period should be aware that prostate cancer is considered to be a service-related illness. Cadmium exposure in the workplace was long suspected to be carcinogenic, but there little evidence of an effect has been established (Navarro Silvera and Rohan 2007). Prostate cancer is unusual amongst malignancies in that there is scant evidence that it is increased after exposure to ionising radiation, including that from the atomic bomb (Preston et al. 2007).

1.3.2 *Environmental Factors Possibly Associated with Prostate Cancer*

Historically, the wide international variation in prostate cancer incidence and the observation that the variation in incidence was most evident for invasive disease, the "latent" form being of similar prevalence regardless of population (Yatani et al. 1982), generated the hypothesis that invasive prostate cancer had environmental causes. The principal environmental suspects have been dietary and nutritional factors and also sexual behaviours and associated infections.

Ecological evidence, such as the low incidence observed for Asian countries and the increased incidence experienced by migrants from Asia to North America (Thomas and Karagas 1987), has long stimulated interest in dietary elements such as soy and phytoestrogens as possible protective factors and was responsible for many early case control studies that centred on lifestyle-related risk factors, particularly diet, and there remains a strong research interest in this topic. Current dietary hypotheses focus on various types of exposure including specific plant foods such as cruciferous vegetables, various phytochemicals such as carotenoids and phytoestrogens, minerals such as zinc and selenium, red meat and its cooking methods, dairy foods, calcium and vitamin D, fats, and energy balance. It must be noted in this context that dietary intakes are notoriously difficult to measure and that the large errors associated with dietary assessment militate against the ability to detect effects of modest-to-small size. Further, the appropriate time frame for any dietary or any other lifestyle factor exposure on prostate cancer risk is not known and measures taken in adult life may have less relevance than earlier ones. Plant-based foods, nutrients and micronutrients have long enjoyed a reputation for being protective against prostate cancer, but this positive view of vegetables and fruit has changed radically following a spate of null reports from good quality cohort studies (Schuurman et al. 1998; Key et al. 2004; Stram et al. 2006). Only a handful of specific foods and related micronutrients remain of current interest.

1.3.2.1 Soy, Other Legumes and Phytoestrogens

Soy and soy products have been promoted as prostate cancer protective, but this view has been based mostly on ecological evidence of low risks in populations, such as those of Asian countries that consume lots of soy. Importantly, these populations also consume small amounts of meat and fat and have low levels of obesity. A meta analysis of two cohort and six case control studies concluded that soy reduced risk of total prostate cancer, the pooled odds ratio (OR) and 95% confidence interval were 0.70 (0.59, 0.83) (Yan and Spitznagel 2005). A large multi-ethnic, case control study in the U.S. found that soy and legumes other than soy were associated with reduced risk of total prostate cancer (Kolonel et al. 2000), and a case control study from the UK showed that men who ate baked beans twice or more weekly were at reduced risk (Key et al. 1997). A recent prospective study from Japan has suggested that intake of soy and its related phytoestrogens while reducing the risk of localised disease some related aspects of the Japanese diet might actually increase the risk of aggressive prostate cancer for Japanese men (Kurahashi et al. 2007).

Any protective effect of soy and other legumes has been attributed to phytoestrogens, two groups of hormone, like diphenolic compounds, isoflavonoids and lignans, produced either directly by plants or by bacterial fermentation of plant compounds in the gut. Phytoestrogens have been shown to inhibit in vivo and in vitro prostate tumour model systems (Griffiths et al. 1998). Although their biological function is not fully understood, they have been reported to inhibit 5 alpha reductase, 17 beta hydroxysteroid dehydrogenase and aromatase enzymes, and to stimulate the synthesis of sex-hormone-binding globulin and of uridine 5' diphospho glucuronosyltransferase (which catalyses the excretion of steroids), suggesting that they may act in part by decreasing the biologically available fraction of androgens. The isoflavanoid genistein is also a potent inhibitor of protein tyrosine kinase that activates various growth factor receptors including the IGF 1 receptor by phosphorylation. Some phytoestrogens have also been shown to act as anti-oestrogens, as weak oestrogens, and as antioxidants (Griffiths et al. 1998).

1.3.2.2 Cruciferous (Brassica) Vegetables

Cruciferous vegetables, which are species of Brassica (the cabbage family), have also been suggested to protect against prostate cancer. A review of 12 studies of Brassica vegetable intakes and prostate cancer risk yielded only six interpretable studies with three statistically significant and one borderline significant reports of reduced risk associated with high consumption (Kristal and Lampe 2002). Since then, an analysis of the European Prospective Investigation of Cancer (EPIC) cohort study (Key et al. 2004) showed that neither fruit and vegetables nor cruciferous vegetables specifically were associated with overall prostate cancer risk. The EPIC study was unable to identify advanced disease at the time of analysis. An analysis of the U.S. Health Professionals Follow-Up Study suggested cruciferous vegetable intake was associated with a reduced risk of localised disease in younger men but no association was observed for advanced disease (Giovannucci et al. 2003). On the other hand, the Prostate, Lung, Colorectal and Ovarian Cancer Screening Trial (Kirsh et al. 2007) has reported an association between cruciferous vegetable intake and risk of advanced prostate cancer (stage III or IV) with an RR of 0.60 (0.36, 0.98) for high compared with low intake. Should cruciferous vegetables truly be associated with reduced risk, this may be because they contain isothiocyanates, particularly sulphoraphane, which may decrease risk of prostate cancer through induction of phase II enzymes, including glutathione S-transferases (Verhoeven et al. 1997). These enzymes are involved in the metabolism of a number of carcinogenic agents. It has been suggested that polymorphic variation in the genes for these enzymes might identify persons at increased risk via some form of gene, environment interaction (Joseph et al. 2004). Future research if having to consider not only tumour phenotypes, but also individual genotypes, will require substantial increases in study size.

1.3.2.3   Carotenoids, Tocopherols and Other Vitamins

Tomato-based foods, particularly tomato sauce, have been reported to be protective against prostate cancer. In addition, dietary intakes and plasma levels of lycopene (a fat-soluble carotenoid found in tomatoes) have also been associated with reduced risk. The evidence for this comes mostly from the U.S. Health Professionals Follow-Up Study and has rarely been duplicated by other studies. In the U.S. Health Professionals Follow-Up Study, high lycopene intake was related to a lower risk of prostate cancer, RR for highest compared with lowest quintiles, 0.84 (0.73, 0.96), the association being stronger for extraprostatic cases, RR 0.65 (0.42, 0.99) (Giovannucci et al. 2002). In the Physicians' Health Study, where prediagnostic plasma lycopene concentrations for 578 cases were compared with those for 1,294 controls, the ORs for all prostate cancers declined with increasing concentrations of plasma lycopene, OR for the highest compared with lowest quintiles 0.75 (0.54, 1.06), but the association was stronger for aggressive prostate cancers, OR 0.56 (0.34, 0.91) (Gann et al. 1999). In a recent report of plasma carotenoid, retinol, and tocopherol concentrations from the EPIC cohort study (Key et al. 2007) none of the micronutrients assayed was significantly associated with total prostate cancer risk, but lycopene and total carotenoid concentrations were inversely associated with the risk of advanced disease. The OR of advanced disease for men in the highest fifth of plasma concentrations compared with men in the lowest fifth was

0.40 (0.19, 0.88) for lycopene and 0.35 (0.17, 0.78) for total carotenoids. Similarly, in the Prostate, Lung, Colorectal, and Ovarian Cancer Screening Trial, little association was found with tomato-based foods or lycopene intake except for suggestive trends of inverse association for men with a family history of prostate cancer (Kirsh et al. 2006b). Lycopene theoretically possesses some advantageous characteristics for a possible chemopreventive agent as it has very high antioxidant capabilities and a propensity to biological concentration in the prostate (Clinton et al. 1996), and the lack of formally established evidence of its beneficial effect has not prevented it being vigorously marketed in pill form by the "health food" industry.

Randomised trials have also examined the possibility of an association between beta carotene supplementation and prostate cancer risk. The Alpha Tocopherol Beta Carotene Cancer Prevention Study found that male smokers who received a 20-mg supplement of beta carotene daily experienced a non-significant increase in risk compared with those not receiving it (Heinonen et al. 1998). The Physicians' Health Study reported that men who took the beta carotene supplements did not have a reduced risk of prostate cancer, but men with low plasma levels of beta carotene who took the supplements had a lower risk than those who did not (Cook et al. 1999). The Beta Carotene and Retinol Efficacy Trial found no association between beta carotene supplementation and prostate cancer risk (Omenn et al. 1996). Supplemental and dietary vitamin E, beta carotene, and vitamin C have also been assessed in regard to prostate cancer risk in the Prostate, Lung, Colorectal, and Ovarian Cancer Screening Trial (Kirsh et al. 2006a). Although no overall association was reported, there was evidence of a protective effect of vitamin E supplement use against advanced prostate cancer only in patients who smoked. Beta carotene supplementation was associated with decreased prostate cancer risk for men with low dietary beta carotene intake, RR 0.52 (0.33, 0.81). There was no association reported for any other carotenoid, including lycopene, or for vitamin C. Serum carotenoid concentrations have also been examined in this trial and high serum concentrations of beta carotene were associated with increased risk for aggressive, clinically relevant prostate cancer, while lycopene and other carotenoids were unrelated to prostate cancer (Peters et al. 2007b). A further analysis of this trial has examined polymorphic variants in the three main isoforms of superoxide dismutase (*SOD*) (Kang et al. 2007). The higher activity *Ala* variant at *SOD2* had been hypothesised to suppress prostate carcinogenesis, but the results suggest that the Ala variant of *SOD2* is associated with an increased risk of prostate cancer, particularly for men with lower dietary intakes or supplements of vitamin E. No association with prostate cancer was observed for polymorphic variants in *SOD3* or *SOD1*.

Dietary and supplemental vitamin E intakes were not associated with prostate cancer risk in the Cancer Prevention Study II Nutrition Cohort (Rodriguez et al. 2004). The AARP Diet and Health Study has reported separately on associations between supplemental and dietary vitamin E intakes and prostate cancer risk (Wright et al. 2007a). Supplemental vitamin E intake was not associated with prostate cancer risk, but dietary gamma tocopherol intake was associated with a reduced risk of advanced prostate cancer, RR comparing highest with lowest quintile 0.68 (0.56, 0.84). In the Alpha Tocopherol Beta Carotene Cancer Prevention Study prediagnostic serum concentrations of alpha tocopherol, but not dietary vitamin E, were associated with lower risk of developing prostate cancer, particularly advanced prostate cancer, the RR for highest compared with lowest quintile of serum alpha tocopherol was 0.80 (0.66, 0.96) which was stronger for the risk of developing advanced disease, RR 0.56 (0.36, 0.85) (Weinstein et al. 2007).

Whatever the future potential of vitamin E/alpha tocopherol might be as a chemopreventive for prostate cancer (Lee et al. 2006), the Alpha Tocopherol Beta Carotene Cancer Prevention Study has given us an object lesson in regard to the unforeseen consequences of administering supra-physiological doses of micronu-trients (Vainio 1999). Men in the beta carotene arm of this trial were observed to have a significantly increased incidence of lung cancer while, incidentally, those in the alpha tocopherol arm had a reduced risk of prostate cancer (Albanes et al. 1996). Multivitamin use is also under suspicion with respect to prostate cancer risk. In the very large AARP Diet and Health Study no association was observed between multivitamin use and risk of localised cancer, but increased risks of advanced prostate cancer, RR 1.32 (1.04, 1.67), and fatal prostate cancer, RR 1.98 (1.07, 3.66), were observed for men who reported using multivitamins more than seven times per week compared with never users (Lawson et al. 2007).

1.3.2.4   Animal-Based Foods, Fats and Related Exposures

In a review of 37 prospective cohort and four intervention studies on dietary risk factors for prostate cancer published between 1966 and 2003, although some stud-ies were limited by small size, poor measurement of dietary exposure and poor control of possible confounders, the authors concluded that they were inconclusive with respect to the role of meat, dairy products and fat, different studies suggesting either an increased risk or no relation with prostate cancer (Dagnelie et al. 2004). This supported an earlier review of the topic (Kolonel 2001).

An analysis of the Health Professionals Follow up Study based on 1,897 total cases, including 249 metastatic prostate cancers, reported intakes of total meat, red meat, and dairy products were not associated with risk of either total or advanced cancer but an increased risk was observed for metastatic disease and red meat con-sumption, RR comparing highest and lowest quintiles 1.6 (1.0, 2.5). This estimate diminished after controlling for saturated and alpha linolenic fatty acids. Similarly, a non-significant association between dairy foods and metastatic cancer, RR 1.4 (0.91, 2.2), was strongly attenuated after controlling for calcium and fatty acid intakes (Michaud et al. 2001).

In a report from the Cancer Prevention Study II Nutrition Cohort that docu-mented 85 and 5,028 cases of incident prostate cancer among 692 Black and 64,856 White men, respectively, no measure of meat consumption was associated with risk of prostate cancer for White men. For Black men, total red meat intake (processed plus unprocessed red meat) was associated with higher risk of prostate cancer, RR comparing highest and lowest quartiles, 2.0 (1.0, 4.2). This increase in risk was mainly associated with cooked processed meats, RR comparing highest and lowest quartiles of consumption of sausages, bacon, and hot dogs, 2.7 (1.3, 5.3) (Rodriguez et al. 2006).

A recent report from the Hawaiian multi-ethnic cohort study after 8 years of follow up analysed 4,404 cases of which 1,278 were advanced or high-grade disease, and found no association between the intake of different types of fat, various meats, and fats from meat with either overall risk or with risk of non-localised or high-grade prostate cancer. Nor was there any difference in risk patterns between any of the four ethnic groups, African Americans, Japanese Americans, Latinos and Whites (Park et al. 2007a). The CLUE II study of Washington County, Maryland, analysed 199 cases, 54 of which were stage III/IV, reported total and red meat consumption was not associated with the risk of prostate cancer but that processed meat was (Rohrmann et al. 2007). The estimates were not statistically significant.

The evidence of an association between prostate cancer risk and red meat consumption seems to be diminishing as the larger prospective cohort studies publish their results, especially those studies which possess sufficient statistical power, assuming they have collected data to control for possible confounders and to perform subgroup analysis based on disease aggressiveness (Park et al. 2007a). Red meat and processed meats still remain under suspicion, however, as adjusting their risk estimates for known confounders does not diminish them to zero. Some propose that the residual association is due to their intake being correlated with particular fats, others with the production of carcinogenic agents formed during cooking, particularly by char grilling (Sinha and Rothman 1999). Meat cooked at high temperatures, particularly by barbequing and grilling, contains heterocyclic amines and polycyclic aromatic hydrocarbons, the formation of which depends on meat type and high, temperature cooking methods, such as barbecuing. One of the most abundant heterocyclic amines in cooked meat is 2 amino 1 methyl 6 phenylimidazo [4,5, b] pyridine (PhIP). The possible influence of meat-cooking methods on the risk of prostate cancer is based on limited evidence and is currently an active area of research. A recent analysis of PhIP DNA adducts in prostatectomy specimens reported grilled meat consumption to be significantly associated with higher adduct levels in tumour cells, and this association was primarily with grilled red meats, particularly hamburger, but not white meats (Tang et al. 2007).

A population-based case control study of 317 cases in New Zealand (Norrish et al. 1999) found that men who consumed well-done beef steak, compared with those who did not, had an increased risk of prostate cancer, OR of 1.7 (1.02, 2.77) but found no association between prostate cancer and heterocyclic amines, including PhIP, OR 1.05 (0.70, 1.59).

These exposures have also been examined in the Prostate, Lung, Colorectal, and Ovarian Cancer Screening Trial using a detailed meat-cooking questionnaire linked to a database for various heterocyclic amines and polycyclic aromatic hydrocarbons (Cross et al. 2005). The analysis was based on a total of 1,338 prostate cancer cases of which 868 were incident cases and 520 were advanced (stage III or IV or a Gleason score of 7 to 10). Total, red or white meat intake was not associated with prostate cancer risk, but the consumption of more than 10 g/day of very-well-done meat, compared with none, was associated with increased risk of incident, but not advanced, disease, RR 1.7 (1.19, 2.40). The only heterocyclic amine to show any association with risk was PhIP, the highest quintile compared with the lowest was associated with an RR of 1.3 (1.01, 1.61). These modest estimates could easily have arisen as a result of multiple testing. The associations were observed only for early disease so, if real, point to these exposures as cancer initiators.

The possible role of fats in the apparent association between red meat and prostate cancer has long been debated and fat, itself, has also been suspected as a risk factor independent of meat. Fatty acids are proposed to modulate prostate cancer risk in several ways: e.g. by affecting serum sex hormone levels; by synthesising eicosanoids (Myers and Ghosh 1999) which affect tumour cell proliferation; by affecting 5 alpha reductase type I activity (Liang and Liao 1992); by forming free radicals from fatty acid peroxidation (Montuschi et al. 2007); by decreasing 1 alpha 25 dihydroxychole-calciferol levels or by increasing IGF 1 levels (Moreno et al. 2006; Yasumaru et al. 2003; Hsi et al. 2002). Regulation of the expression of cyclooxygenase (COX) 2 and lipoxygenase (LOX) enzymes may be brought about by cytokines, pro-antioxidant states, and hormonal factors, the actions of which may be modified by dietary factors such as antioxidants derived from fruit and vegetables. The COX enzyme may be directly inhibited by non-steroidal anti-inflammatory drugs (NSAIDs) (Sooriakumaran and Kaba 2005; Norrish et al. 1998; Zhou and Blackburn 1997).

A review of 29 studies on the association between prostate cancer and total dietary fat and specific fatty acids showed substantial heterogeneity in study design and in fat intake assessment. Although the pooled risk estimate for prostate cancer associated with an increase of 45 g/day in total fat consumption was small (RR of 1.2), heterogeneity between studies was large and the association was not supported by specific fatty acids. The associations with advanced prostate cancer were more homogeneous and suggested a relation with total and saturated fat but none with specific fatty acids. The strongest association was derived from five inconsistent studies of alpha linolenic acid (an omega 3 fatty acid from plants) which increased risk by 1.26 (1.10, 1.45) for every 1.5 g/day increase (Dennis et al. 2004). A review of nine cohort and case control studies that reported on the association between alpha linolenic acid intake or blood levels and prostate cancer came to similar conclusions with a combined RR of 1.70 (1.12–2.58) for high compared with low levels (Brouwer, Katan and Zock 2004). The Health Professionals Follow-Up Study using 2,965 new cases of total prostate cancer, 448 of which were advanced, (Leitzmann et al. 2004b) reported the risk of advanced prostate cancer comparing highest and lowest quintiles of alpha linolenic acid from non-animal sources and from meat and dairy sources to be 2.02 (1.35, 3.03) and 1.53 (0.88, 2.66), respectively. Eicosapentaenoic acid and docosahexaenoic acid intakes were related to lower prostate cancer risk. The RRs for total and advanced prostate cancer from comparisons of extreme quintiles of combined eicosapentaenoic and docosahexaenoic acid intakes were 0.89 (0.77, 1.04) and 0.74 (0.49, 1.08), respectively. Linoleic acid and arachidonic acid intakes were unrelated to the risk of prostate cancer. In an earlier analysis of the Health Professionals Follow-Up Study using 2,482 prostate cancers, of which 617 were diagnosed as advanced prostate cancers including 278 metastatic prostate cancers, eating fish more than three times per week compared with less than twice per month was associated with a reduced risk of prostate cancer, which was strongest for metastatic cancer, RR 0.56 (0.37, 0.86). Intake of marine fatty acids from food showed a similar but weaker association (Augustsson et al. 2003).

The Alpha Tocopherol Beta Carotene Cancer Prevention Study of male smokers found no overall association between serum or dietary alpha linolenic acid or any other unsaturated fatty acid and prostate cancer risk, but high serum linoleic acid was associated with lower risk in men supplemented with alpha tocopherol. High serum myristic acid was associated with an increased risk of prostate cancer (Mannisto et al. 2003). In the Malmo cohort which analysed 817 prostate cancers, 281 of which were advanced, after adjustment for age and energy intake there was no association between intake of any type of fat and risk of total prostate cancer or between fat intake and advanced cancer, but positive associations were observed between risk of prostate cancer and intakes of eicosapentaenoic acid and docosa-hexaenoic acid (Wallstrom et al. 2007).

A case control study from Sweden of 1,378 men with prostate cancer and 782 controls, for whom blood samples were available, reported that eating fatty fish (mostly salmon) once or more per week, compared with never, was associated with reduced risk of prostate cancer, OR 0.57 (0.43, 0.76). The OR comparing the highest with the lowest quartile of marine fatty acids intake was 0.70 (0.51, 0.97). It also reported a significant interaction between fatty fish intake and an SNP in the *COX-2* gene (rs5275: +6365 T/C), but not with the four other SNPs examined. There was a strong inverse association with increasing intake of fatty fish for carriers of the variant allele (OR for once per week or more compared with never was 0.28 (0.18, 0.45), but no association was observed for carriers of the more common allele (Hedelin et al. 2007).

1.3.2.5   Dairy Foods, Calcium and Vitamin D

A meta analysis of reports from cohort studies concluded that high intake of dairy products and calcium may be associated with small increases in risk of prostate cancer; 1.33 (1.00, 1.78) for the highest compared with lowest intake categories of dairy products and 1.46 (0.65, 3.25) for the highest compared with lowest intake categories of calcium (Gao et al. 2005). High intakes of dairy products and calcium have been hypothesised to increase prostate cancer risk by suppressing the production of the active form of vitamin D (1,25,dihydroxyvitamin D) (Giovannucci et al. 1998) which binds to the vitamin D receptor and inhibits prostatic cellular proliferation (Stewart and Weigel 2004). Findings from the Health Professional Follow up Study suggest that calcium intakes exceeding 1,500 mg/day may be associated with a decrease in differentiation in prostate cancer and ultimately with a higher risk of fatal prostate cancer, RR 2.43 (1.32, 4.48), but not with well-differentiated, organ-confined cancers, RR 0.79 (0.50, 1.25) (Giovannucci et al. 2006). On the other hand, a clinical trial that involved calcium supplementation to prevent colorectal cancer showed no evidence of increased risk for prostate cancer (Baron et al. 2005) and not all studies show an association (Park et al. 2007b, c; Torniainen et al. 2007). The strengths and weaknesses of the evidence linking vitamin D with the risk of prostate cancer among others have recently been articulated (Giovannucci 2007). Part of the inconsistency in reports may be due to studies not classifying the prostate cancers according to aggressive/advanced phenotypes. There may also be different associations with risk depending on the prevalent levels of vitamin D and different sources in the study population; comparing an American population (John et al. 2007), for example, with one from Scandinavia (Mitrou et al. 2007) introduces variation in vitamin D status related to that produced by available sun exposure. There may also be differences in risk depending on the time of exposure, and for prostate cancer that might be relatively early in life. There may also be differences in risk associated with polymorphisms in genes belonging to the vitamin D pathway, such as the vitamin D receptor gene and these associations may vary with a subject's age, tumour phenotype and serum vitamin D concentration (Corder et al. 1995; Li et al. 2007; Holick et al. 2007; Mikhak et al. 2007).

1.3.2.6 Trace Elements and Vitamin Supplements

From a review of the epidemiological evidence linking trace elements with risk of malignancy, only zinc and selenium are reported to be associated with prostate cancer (Navarro Silvera and Rohan 2007). Zinc is an essential element for human physiology, particularly that of the prostate gland. The prostate biologically concentrates zinc, levels in the prostate being ten times higher than in other soft tissues (Mawson and Fischer 1952), and more than 10 μg of zinc is secreted per ejaculation (Kerr et al. 1960). Tumour tissue, however, has much lower zinc levels than healthy tissue (Gyorkey et al. 1967). Thus support has grown around the importance of zinc to prostatic health, and consequently vitamin and mineral supplements marketed for men commonly contain zinc. This view is in line with some recent biological models of the role of zinc in prostate health and malignancy (Costello and Franklin 2006). The accumulation of zinc by normal prostate glandular epithelium is an essential aspect of its unique requirement to produce and secrete very large amounts of citrate (Hunt et al. 1992), and in malignancy these normal zinc-accumulating citrate producing epithelial cells are metabolically transformed to citrate oxidising cells that lose the ability to accumulate zinc. A genetic alteration in the expression of the ZIP1 zinc transporter is associated with this metabolic transformation (Franklin and Costello 2007). The use of zinc supplements by older men to prevent prostate cancer is underpinned by this view, but the epidemiological evidence is at best modest and inconsistent (Platz and Helzlsouer 2001). The inconsistency is probably due to a number of factors related to the nature of the small retrospective case control studies which provide the evidence (Kolonel et al. 1988; West et al. 1991; Key et al. 1997; Kristal et al. 1999). Different studies have also measured exposure in different ways some estimating intakes from diet alone, others from supplements, and others from combinations of the two. Few studies have been stratified by disease aggressiveness. The Hawaiian case control study

(Kolonel et al. 1988) reported an increased risk associated with total zinc intake for men 70 years and older, OR 1.7 (1.1, 2.7). The Utah study showed no association with zinc irrespective of disease status (West et al. 1991). The Washington State case control study of 697 cases and 666 controls found a very marginal but dose responsive protective effect associated with supplemental zinc use that did not differ by disease aggressiveness (Kristal et al. 1999). A recent case control study from Italy (Gallus et al. 2007) of 1,294 cases and 1,451 controls, to the contrary, reported an increased risk but only for advanced cancer, OR comparing highest and lowest quintiles of dietary intake 2.02 (1.14, 3.59).

In a study of 115 cases and 227 controls nested in the prospective CLUE II study in Washington County Maryland, moderate-to-high concentrations of zinc in toenails were suggestive of reduced risk but there was no dose response (Platz et al. 2002). The Health Professionals Follow up Study reported that men who took zinc supplements had an increased risk of prostate cancer (Leitzmann et al. 2003); those who consumed more than 100 mg/day of supplemental zinc had an RR for advanced prostate cancer of 2.29 (1.06, 4.95), and those who took zinc supplements for 10 or more years had an RR of 2.37 (1.42, 3.95). The SU.VI.MAX trial reported that men with PSA levels <3 µg/L given supplements (vitamin C, beta carotene, selenium, and zinc) had reduced prostate cancer risk compared with those on placebo, RR 0.52 (0.29, 0.92), but this effect was not observed for men with elevated baseline PSA levels, RR 1.54 (0.87, 2.72) (Meyer et al. 2005). In the AARP Diet and Health Study, for men who reported taking a zinc supplement, taking multivitamins more than daily compared with daily or less was associated with an increased risk of fatal prostate cancer; RR 4.36 (1.83, 10.39), whereas no association with multivitamins was observed for men not taking a zinc supplement, RR 1.13 (0.46, 2.80) (Lawson et al. 2007).

Selenium is an essential trace element for human physiology and forms an important component of several enzymes including glutathione peroxidase. The epidemiological evidence was reviewed in 2001 (Platz and Helzlsouer 2001). A more recent meta analysis of 20 observational studies calculated the pooled standardised mean difference in selenium concentration (in plasma, serum or toenails) between cases and controls to be, 0.23 (0.40, 0.05) indicating a possible inverse association between selenium and risk of prostate cancer. The authors suggested that differences in selenium levels between populations, a possible threshold effect, and the relationship between selenium and the different stages of prostate cancer required further investigation (Brinkman et al. 2006). In the Prostate, Lung, Colorectal, and Ovarian Cancer Screening Trial prediagnostic serum selenium concentrations were not associated with prostate cancer risk, although greater concentrations were associated with reduced prostate cancer risks for men who reported a high intake of vitamin E, in multivitamin users, and for smokers (Peters et al. 2007a). No association was observed between prostate cancer risk and selenium supplementation in the Vitamins and lifestyle (VITAL) study (Peters et al. 2008).

The strongest observational evidence for a protective effect of selenium is from a randomised trial of selenium supplementation for the prevention of skin cancers in which an incidental reduction in the incidence of prostate cancer was observed in the intervention arm (Clark et al. 1996). Selenium supplementation is currently being subjected to trial as a chemopreventive agent. The SELECT study is currently investigating the effect of selenium and vitamin E supplementation on the incidence of prostate cancer (Lippman et al. 2005) while the SU.VI.MAX study is trialling a combination of 120 mg of ascorbic acid, 30 mg of vitamin E, 6 mg of beta carotene, 100 µg of selenium, and 20 mg of zinc, or a placebo (Hercberg et al. 2004).

1.3.2.7 Dietary Patterns

Rather than adopting a reductionist approach, separately examining individual foods and nutrients, it has become fashionable to investigate diet-and-disease relationships in a more integrated way. This has been approached by principal components analysis of the data collected on foods and nutrients to calculate a few orthogonal multivariate components or factors that explain substantive proportions of the variance in the data. Depending on which dietary variable are associated with each of these factors, labels are ascribed to them that are considered to represent them in meaningful terms such as, "meat and potatoes", "fruit and vegetables", "prudent diet", etc. This approach has seldom been applied to prostate cancer, especially in a prospective setting.

In the representative United States Health Examination Epidemiological Follow up Study, principal component analysis was used on responses to a 105-item dietary questionnaire and three distinct patterns were identified: a vegetable and fruit pattern; a red meat and starch pattern characterised by red meats, potatoes, cheese, salty snacks, and desserts; and a Southern pattern characterised by such foods as cornbread, grits, sweet potatoes, okra, beans and rice. Prostate cancer risk was not associated with the vegetable and fruit or red meat and starch patterns, but higher intake of the Southern pattern (by Blacks and non-Blacks) showed a marginally significant reduction in risk comparing upper and lower tertiles, hazards ratio (HR) 0.6 (0.4, 1.1). The association was not attributable to intake of any individual food or nutrient (Tseng et al. 2004).

A small case control study from Canada of 80 cases and 334 controls adopted a similar approach and four dietary patterns were identified: Healthy Living, Traditional Western, Processed and Beverages (Walker et al. 2005). Increased prostate cancer risk was reported in relation to the processed pattern which was correlated with processed meats, red meats, organ meats, refined grains, white bread, onions and tomatoes, vegetable oil and juice, soft drinks and bottled water. The OR for the highest tertile compared to the lowest was 2.75 (1.40, 5.39), with a dose response pattern (trend test $p < 0.0035$).

In the Health Professionals Follow up Study (HPFS), factor analysis identified two major dietary patterns. The first factor corresponded to high intakes of fruits, vegetables, whole grains, fish and poultry and was labelled the prudent pattern. The second factor represented intakes of meat products (red meat and processed meat), refined grains, high fat, and dairy, and was labelled the western pattern. Analysing over 3,000 incident cases of prostate cancer, neither factor was found to be appreciably associated with risk of total prostate cancer or with risk of advanced prostate cancer (Wu et al. 2006b).

1.3.2.8   Energy Balance, Obesity and Physical Activity

The product of dietary energy intake and energy expenditure via metabolic activity and physical activity is termed energy balance. When energy intake exceeds the body's metabolic requirements the excess energy is stored as fat, leading to overweight and obesity. It is increasingly evident that obesity is related to the incidence of prostate cancer, paradoxically reducing the risk of localised disease while increasing that for advanced disease, and that obesity after diagnosis accelerates mortality from prostate cancer (Freedland et al. 2006). Epidemiological reports on these topics are not fully consistent, but some of the differences are likely due to variations in study design, power and physical measurements, many studies relying on self- reported data rather than direct measurements. Dietary energy intake and physical activity are also notoriously difficult to measure with precision in epidemiological studies. Added to this is the failure of some studies to stratify analysis by disease severity and this is important if obesity protects against localised but increases the risk of aggressive disease (Freedland and Platz 2007). Unfortunately, those studies that do stratify analyses by disease severity often vary in their classification of tumour phenotype.

A review of energy intake and prostate cancer risk (Platz 2002) identified 23 analytical epidemiological studies. Of the studies that reported effect estimates comparing top with bottom quantiles, eight case control studies produced a summary OR of 1.3 (1.1, 1.4), while four cohort studies gave a summary OR of 1.0 (0.8, 1.2). The four case control studies that evaluated advanced disease gave a summary OR of 1.6 (1.2, 2.0). None of these studies considered the balance of energy intake with body size and physical activity. The Health Professionals Follow up Study prospectively evaluated the joint associations of energy intake and body size or physical activity with prostate cancer using 2,896 incident prostate cancers of which 339 were metastatic or fatal. There was no association observed between energy intake and total prostate cancer, but there was a positive association between energy intake and metastatic or fatal prostate cancer for men who were leaner, more physically active, younger, and who had a family history of prostate cancer. This suggests that the elevated risk associated with a high energy intake by these men may be attributable to certain metabolic profiles that favour enhanced growth factor production over an increase in adiposity (Platz et al. 2003).

A meta analysis of the associations reported by cohort studies (MacInnis and English 2006) concluded that body mass index (BMI) was weakly associated with prostate cancer risk, particularly for advanced tumours. The overall RR for BMI was 1.05 (1.01, 1.08) per 5 kg/m^2 increment. For studies that reported results by stage of disease, the RRs were stronger for advanced disease, RR 1.12 (1.01, 1.23) per 5 kg/m^2 increment, compared with localised disease, RR 0.96 (0.89, 1.03) per 5 kg/m^2 increment. The NIH, AARP Diet and Health Study examined BMI and adult weight change and prostate cancer risk for 287,760 men who developed 9,986 incident prostate cancers during 5 years of follow up, and 173 prostate cancer deaths (Wright et al. 2007b). BMI was associated with significantly reduced incidence, largely because of localised tumours: the RR comparing men with a BMI of 40 or greater with men who had a BMI of <25 was 0.67 (0.50, 0.89). The risk of dying from prostate cancer increased with increasing BMI, the RR for men with a BMI of 35 or greater compared with men who had a BMI of <25, was 2.12 (1.08, 4.15). Adult weight gain from age 18 years to baseline also was associated positively with fatality but not incidence.

A cohort study in Washington State reported risks separately for non-aggressive and aggressive (regional/distant stage or Gleason sum 7 to 10) prostate cancer (Littman et al. 2007). Compared with men with a BMI of <25 men with a BMI of 30 or greater had a reduced risk of non-aggressive disease, HR 0.69 (0.52, 0.93). Men with a BMI between 25 and 29.9 were at increased risk of aggressive disease, HR 1.4 (1.1, 1.8), but men with a BMI of 30 or greater were not at increased risk of aggressive disease.

The Cancer Prevention Study II Nutrition Cohort has also examined this question and reported that the association between BMI and prostate cancer risk differed by stage and grade (Rodriguez et al. 2007). BMI was reported to be inversely associated with risk of low-grade prostate cancer, RR 0.84 (0.66, 1.06), positively associated with risk of high-grade disease, RR 1.22 (0.96, 1.55) and significantly associated with risk of metastatic or fatal cancer, RR 1.54 (1.06, 2.23). In addition, men who lost >11 pounds between 1982 and 1992 were at a decreased risk of non-metastatic, high-grade, prostate cancer, RR 0.58 (0.42, 0.79). The latter offers some promise of possible success for interventions aimed at reducing obesity.

Body mass index is a problematic measure of obesity as it does not differentiate between adipose mass and lean mass, two major components of body composition having different metabolic, physiological and hormonal associations, lean mass for example being associated with androgens and adipose mass being associated with oestrogens and with the leptin and insulin/IGF pathways (Gade-Andavolu et al. 2006; Giovannucci 2003; Chang et al. 2001; Hsing et al. 2001). It has been argued that insulin and the IGF 1 axis function in an integrated fashion to promote cell growth and survival (Giovannucci 2003). A meta analysis of 19 studies of prostate cancer risk in diabetics found an inverse association, RR 0.84 (0.76, 0.93) especially for cohort studies, RR 0.81 (0.71, 0.92). For studies conducted before PSA screening was introduced as a common procedure the RR was 0.94 (0.85, 1.03), and for studies conducted after this time the RR was 0.73 (0.64, 0.83). These data suggest (in the absence of information on tumour aggressiveness) that diabetes (chronic hyperinsulinaemia) may be protective against early forms of the disease and may promote advanced disease (Kasper and Giovannucci 2006).

Few studies have examined other anthropometric measures such as abdominal obesity and prostate cancer risk, though there is growing recognition of its possible importance. One cohort study that took direct body measurements rather than relying on self-reported data has reported waist circumference to be positively associated with the risk of aggressive disease (MacInnis et al. 2003). This observation may explain at least some of the rise in incidence in low-risk countries as they become westernised, and the rise in incidence for migrants to high-risk countries. The rise in incidence may be due to changes in total dietary energy intake rather than changes in types of food (aside from their energy density). So too, the growing obesity epidemic in other parts of the world is likely to accelerate the incidence trend for clinically significant prostate cancer.

The relationship between physical activity and risk of prostate cancer is important because it is amenable to intervention in efforts to reduce weight and obesity. One review of epidemiological studies of physical activity and prostate cancer concluded that physical activity may have an inverse association with prostate cancer risk, but the evidence was inconsistent and the magnitude of effect was small (Friedenreich and Thune 2001). Another expressed the view that physical activity might affect physiological pathways related to prostate carcinogenesis other than those associated with obesity, such as by modulating testosterone levels and immune function, and by lowering sympathetic nervous system activity thus reducing the production of neurotrophic growth factors (Lee et al. 2001). Physical activity, similar to dietary intakes, is difficult to measure with precision in epidemiological studies. The available evidence is, therefore, not surprising in its inconsistencies. For example, two prospective cohort studies in the United States showed no evidence of an association with physical activity (Putnam et al. 2000; Liu et al. 2000), while another showed that physically inactive men were at increased risk compared with very active men, but this association was limited to Black Americans and was not statistically significant for Caucasians (Clarke and Whittemore 2000) and a cohort study of Norwegians reported an RR of 0.8 (0.62, 1.03) for high compared with low activity (Lund-Nilsen et al. 2000).

In recent years the Netherlands Cohort Study failed to show any effect of physical activity on risk (Zeegers et al. 2005). The Washington State cohort reported that physical activity was not associated with prostate cancer risk overall, but reported some statistically marginal effects for subgroups; e.g. compared with no activity, physical activity at or above the median level was associated with reduced risk for men who were normal weight, HR 0.69 (0.46, 1.0), or who were 65 years or more at diagnosis, HR 0.75 (0.55, 1.0) and who had not had a recent PSA, HR 0.47 (0.28, 0.81). Greater physical activity was associated with an increased risk for men who were obese, HR 1.5 (0.95, 2.4) (Littman et al. 2006). The American Cancer Society Cancer Prevention Study II Nutrition Cohort reported no overall difference in risk of prostate cancer according to level of physical activity, RR 0.90 (0.78, 1.04) but a reduced risk of aggressive prostate cancer for men enjoying >35 metabolic equivalent hours of recreational physical activity per week compared with men who reported no recreational physical activity, RR 0.69 (0.52, 0.92) (Patel et al. 2005). The Health Professionals Follow up Study examined the risk of fatal prostate cancer associated with physical activity and reported no association for total prostate cancer with respect to either total, vigorous or non-vigorous physical activity. For men aged 65 years or older a reduced risk of advanced cancer was observed for men in the highest category of vigorous activity compared with those who did none, RR 0.33 (0.17, 0.62), and for fatal prostate cancer, RR 0.26 (0.11, 0.66).

No associations were observed for younger men. Men with high levels of physical activity were less likely to be diagnosed with poorly differentiated (Gleason sum 7 to 10) cancers (Giovannucci et al. 2005).

The HUNT study from Norway found no association between physical activity and overall risk of prostate cancer but reported that compared with men who reported no activity, the RR for men in the highest category of physical exercise was 0.64 (0.43, 0.95) for advanced prostate cancer and 0.67 (0.48, 0.94) for prostate cancer death (Nilsen et al. 2006).

With respect to the further study of physical activity and prostate cancer, not only is measurement error a problem, researchers should look to the possibility of threshold effects related to the required level of intensity of activity, the timing of physical activity throughout life, the possibility of differential effects for subgroups (e.g. age, ethnic group, disease aggressiveness) and the control of confounders (Lee et al. 2001).

1.3.2.9 Sexual Behaviour and Infections

Because of the prostate's importance to male sexuality and its dependence on an intact supply of testosterone, prostate cancer epidemiology has long been linked with sexual behaviour. The idea that prostate cancer risk might be related to variation in men's androgen milieu and be manifested by differences in sexual activity has been pursued by several studies, a principal focus of which has been a self-reported history of sexually transmitted infections, and behaviours associated with increased risk of infection, such as sexual intercourse with prostitutes, having sexual intercourse without condoms, and having multiple sex partners. Apart from a history of sexually transmitted infections, the most consistent report is that married men are at increased risk compared with the unmarried. The significance of this observation is unclear. It may be that men who never marry differ from married men with respect to testosterone levels, sex drives and risk of sexually transmitted infections. A proportion will also be homosexual, but there is no published research on prostate cancer risk for this population.

A meta analysis of 17 studies reported an elevated RR of prostate cancer for men with a history of sexually transmitted infections, RR 1.4 (1.2, 1.7) especially of syphilis, RR 2.3 (1.3, 3.9). Risk of prostate cancer was also associated with increasing frequency of sexual activity (usually sexual intercourse) RR 1.2 (1.1, 1.3) for an increase of three times per week, but these studies were very heterogeneous ($P < 0.001$). Increasing numbers of sexual partners was also associated with prostate cancer, RR 1.2 (1.1, 1.3) for an increase of 20 partners (Dennis and Dawson 2002). Since then the Health Professionals Follow up Study has published results based on self-reported sexually transmitted infections. Of the 36,033 participants in the analysis, 2,263 were diagnosed with prostate cancer. No association was observed between gonorrhoea, RR 1.04 (0.79, 1.36); or syphilis, RR 1.06 (0.44, 2.59) and prostate cancer or between clinical prostatitis and prostate cancer, RR 1.08 (0.96, 1.20) (Sutcliffe et al. 2006a).

Studies that rely on self-reported behaviours may not provide very reliable evidence, especially when the behaviours are subject to social and moral opprobrium. The search for more objective evidence has led to studies of biological markers of exposure to infections measured either in samples of sera or tissue. An early study implicated human papillomavirus (HPV) infection in prostate carcinogenesis (Dillner et al. 1998), but this has not been confirmed by others (Adami et al. 2003; Rosenblatt et al. 2003). The Scandinavian biobanks have embarked on a range of studies of a range of markers in stored plasma. A study of over 20,000 Finns who developed 165 prostate cancers following the storage of a serum sample was unable to show an association with either Herpes type 2 serology, RR 0.93 (0.44, 1.96); or with type 8 serology, OR 0.74 (0.19, 2.88) (Korodi et al. 2005). A study of Chlamydia trachomatis serology using samples from Scandinavian serum banks that were linked to population-based cancer registries analysed sera for 738 cases of prostate cancer and 2,271 matched controls. An OR of 0.69 (0.51, 0.94) was reported, which was consistent by different serotypes and which demonstrated a consistent dose, response relationship (Anttila et al. 2005).

The Health Professionals Follow up Study has also approached this issue by performing serological analyses for evidence of several sexually transmitted infections. Altogether 691 men with prostate cancer and an equal number of matched controls were analysed for *Chlamydia trachomatis*, Herpes type 8 and HPV subtypes (Sutcliffe et al. 2007b). No associations were observed with *Chlamydia trachomatis*, OR 1.13 (0.65, 1.96), HPV16, OR 0.83 (0.57, 1.23), HPV18, OR 1.04 (0.66, 1.64), and HPV33, OR 1.14 (0.76, 1.72) antibody seropositivity and prostate cancer. An inverse association was reported between HHV8 seropositivity and prostate cancer, OR 0.70 (0.52, 0.95). Another analysis from the Health (HPFS) Follow up Study has examined seropositivity for *Trichomonas vaginalis* in samples from the same 691 pairs used for the previous analysis (Sutcliffe et al. 2006b). It was reported that 13% of cases and 9% of controls were seropositive, OR 1.43 (1.00, 2.03). This association persisted after additional adjustment for having a history of other sexually transmitted infections, and was strongest for men who used aspirin infrequently over the course of their lives, OR 2.05 (1.05, 4.02).

In regard specifically to sexual activity, the literature is inconsistent, with some studies limiting activity to sexual intercourse others including all activities leading to ejaculation. An early observation (Rotkin 1977) suggested that reduced ejaculatory frequency in normal men increased prostate cancer risk by an as yet unknown mechanism. This idea was supported by a later case control study (Fincham et al. 1990) which reported an OR of 4.05 (2.99, 5.48) for men who had had an (undefined) period of interrupted sexual activity. Two studies, a case control study (Giles et al. 2003) and a cohort study (Leitzmann et al. 2004a), have measured total ejaculatory frequency (using the same questionnaire), and both have demonstrated a significant protection effect of about 30% against prostate cancer. The significance of this observation is not clear but may be related to ductal hygiene, frequent ejaculation flushing the ducts, the excretion of carcinogenic compounds from the prostate tissue, long-term circulating androgen levels, or to the prevention of prostatic infections via the urethral lumen. It is feasible that, by excreting zinc, regular ejaculation could help maintain intra-prostatic zinc levels at a safe level in a similar way that blood donation is used to reduce iron overload for people with haemochromatosis.

1.3.3 Host Factors Possibly Associated with Prostate Cancer

The distinct international variation in prostate cancer risk points not only to the influence of environmental factors but also to that of constitutional factors that control the development and maintenance of healthy prostate epithelium. Although there is evidence that migrants from a low-risk population tend to increase their incidence of prostate cancer after moving to a high-risk population, they seldom exceed that of their host population. The longstanding elevated incidence and mortality rates for American Blacks compared with American Whites attest, for example, to a probable constitutional difference in risk (see sub-chapter by Baffoe-Bonnie and Powell).

The host factors which are considered to be related to or to modulate prostate cancer risk include elements of the opposing physiological and metabolic pathways that are responsible for the processes surrounding cellular proliferation, differentiation and apoptosis, and elements of similar pathways that affect the body's ability to respond to the influence of carcinogenic exposures such as obesity, infections and oxidative stress. The integrity and functionality of these pathways is underpinned by variation in the genes that produce the proteins that drive the processes. The main host factors of interest have already been touched on: hormones and growth factors, response to infection and response to exogenous carcinogens. Added to these is the importance of having a family history of prostate cancer and the discovery and characterisation of genetic variants (both rare and common) that can affect risk either singly or via interactions with other genetic variants or with environmental exposures.

1.3.3.1 Sex Steroid Hormones

The prostate's normal growth and function requires androgens. It is generally considered that androgens play a permissive role in prostate carcinogenesis: that their presence is essential for other carcinogenic factors to play their part. Androgen deprivation in almost all forms leads to involution of the prostate, a fall in PSA levels, and apoptosis of prostate cancer and epithelial cells. Prostate cancer has been termed "hormone dependent" because when advanced it is initially responsive to androgens and can be controlled by their reduction/ablation. Given the hormone dependency of advanced disease, it has long been reasoned that androgens might also influence incidence, the so called androgen hypothesis (Ross et al. 1998). Many studies have tested this hypothesis, with contradictory findings (Travis et al. 2007; Wiren et al. 2007), and meta analyses of these studies generally report pooled risk estimates close to unity (Eaton et al. 1999; Roddam et al. 2008). Early cohort study analyses supported the androgen hypothesis as they reported high circulating levels of testosterone and low levels of SHBG to be associated with prostate cancer risk (Gann et al. 1996). These early analyses either failed, or were too small, to take adequately into account tumour heterogeneity, combining all cancers as if they were the same, the majority being localised or non-aggressive. Later larger studies that stratified analyses based on Gleason score or tumour grade have reported that circulating levels of androgens are associated with increased risk of non-aggressive tumours, but reduced risk of aggressive tumours (Stattin et al. 2004a; Platz et al. 2005a; Severi et al. 2006b), consistent with the known function of androgens in maintaining prostate cellular differentiation (Whitacre et al. 2002).

If androgens were responsible for increasing the risk of prostate cancer, why should the incidence of prostate cancer increase rapidly from the fifth decade of age, a time characterised by falling levels of circulating androgens and rising levels of oestrogens? For several years, the potential use of androgen therapy to combat other health effects of male ageing has been deterred by fear of increasing risk of prostate cancer. Some are now arguing that these fears have been unfounded (Purnell et al. 2006; Raynaud 2006). Clearly, the relationship between androgens, ageing and prostate carcinogenesis is complex, and there is very little known about their concentration and interaction with other pathways in the prostate itself (Platz and Giovannucci 2004). Putting their role in the genesis of non-aggressive tumours to one side, the question remains of how, where and at what age androgens might lose their protective influence on cellular differentiation and promote aberrant proliferation. The usual epidemiological study format based on a single blood sample taken at some time in middle life may not be able to address this question appropriately.

Some consider that it is not so much androgens but oestrogens and their metabolites that might be culpable (Bosland 2006; Risbridger et al. 2007). Testosterone can be converted in the prostate to oestrogen by aromatase and oestrogen can be converted in turn to catecholoestrogens, thence to reactive intermediates that can adduct to DNA and cause the generation of reactive oxygen species. Prostate cells are sensitive not only to androgens but also to oestrogen as they express both the alpha and beta forms of the oestrogen receptor (vom Saal et al. 1997). In animal prostate cancer models oestrogen treatment results in increased incidence of prostate cancer. Exposure of the male mouse foetus to a 50% physiologic increase in oestrogen has been shown to induce a sixfold increase in expression of the androgen receptor relative to controls and resulted in the development of an enlarged adult prostate gland (vom Saal et al. 1997). Continuous long-term exposure to a low level of oestrogens in combination with androgen during adulthood also induces prostate enlargement in mice, rats and dogs (Prinsac et al. 2001; Winter et al. 1995). Taken together, these findings suggest that at any time in life (including in utero) an increased exposure to oestrogen can affect prostate cell growth and may thus also impact on prostate growth regulatory dysfunction (Prins et al. 2006; Carruba 2007). Black American women have been shown to have higher serum levels of testosterone (+50%) and oestradiol (+40%) during pregnancy, and this has been hypothesised to influence the higher risk of prostate cancer observed for American

Blacks either by determining subsequent androgen production or target tissue sensitivity (Henderson et al. 1988).

Sex steroid hormones do not exert their influence on the prostate independently; they interact with each other and with other hormonal and growth factor pathways. The vitamin D pathway (Peehl et al. 1994; Schwartz et al. 1997; Blutt and Weigel 1999) and the IGF pathway (Papatsoris et al. 2005; Kambhampati et al. 2005; Meinbach and Lokeshwar 2006; Wu et al. 2006a, b; Peng et al. 2007), for example, are also important for their interactions in controlling cellular proliferation and differentiation.

1.3.3.2   The IGF Axis and Growth Factors

There is mounting evidence that factors surrounding growth and development in intrauterine and early life may have consequences for cancer risk in adulthood (Ekbom 1998). Several studies have examined birth weight and length and risk of prostate cancer, some finding an association (Tibblin et al. 1995; Ekbom et al. 1996; Nilsen et al. 2005; Eriksson et al. 2007), others not (Ekbom et al. 2000; Boland et al. 2003). Of those studies that were able to stratify analysis by disease severity, associations were stronger or solely with risk of advanced or metastatic disease and mortality (Ekbom et al. 1996; Platz et al. 1998; Nilsen et al. 2005; Eriksson et al. 2007). Toxaemia during pregnancy and prolonged gestation are reported to reduce risk of prostate cancer (Ekbom et al. 1996, 2000). IGF 1 may be involved in both normal and abnormal foetal growth, and stimulation of IGF1 synthesis during normal pregnancy may be associated with an increase in growth hormone production by the placenta; thus, maternal and umbilical cord serum IGF 1 and concentrations are lower in preeclampsia and umbilical cord serum IGF1, IGF-binding protein (BP) 1 and IGFBP3 concentrations are associated with low newborn birth weights (Gomez 2006). Birth weight is known to be influenced by IGFs, and it may be that the programming of the IGF axis that occurs in utero will have lifelong consequences (Holt 2002; Gomez 2006).

Height has been shown in several studies to be associated with an increased risk of prostate cancer (MacInnis and English 2006). Attained height is the product of the action of growth hormones and IGFs and the adequacy of nutritional status during puberty and adolescence, especially the availability of energy (Dunger et al. 2006). The subsequent link between height and risk of prostate cancer much later in life is not understood but may be due to taller men having an increased numbers of cells available for malignant transformation (Albanes and Winick 1988) or to the prolonged influence of the IGF axis or more subtle mechanisms (Juul et al. 1994; Giovannucci et al. 2004).

The IGF axis plays a key role in cellular metabolism, differentiation, proliferation, transformation and apoptosis, during normal development and malignant growth. This axis also seems to be essential for prostate cancer bone metastases, angiogenesis and androgen-independent progression (Gennigens et al. 2006). A meta analysis of 21 studies (Renehan et al. 2004) reported elevated concentrations of IGF1 to be associated with an increased risk of prostate cancer, OR comparing 75th and 25th percentiles, 1.49 (1.14, 1.95). In studies published since, a nested case control study within the Physicians' Health Study of 530 cases and 534 controls reported plasma levels of IGF 1 and IGFBP3 to be predictors of advanced-stage prostate cancer, RR 5.1 (2.0, 13.2) for highest compared with lowest quartiles of IGF1 and RR 0.2 (0.1, 0.6) for highest compared with lowest quartiles of IGFBP 3, but not of early-stage prostate cancer. Men with high IGF1 levels and low IGFBP3 levels had an RR for advanced-stage prostate cancer of 9.5 (1.9, 48.4) compared with men with low levels of both (Chan et al. 2002).

In a nested study of 281 cases and 560 controls within a Swedish cohort study, comparing top with bottom quartiles, IGF1 increased prostate cancer risk, OR 1.67 (1.02, 2.71), but this was attenuated after adjustment for IGFBP3 to OR 1.47 (0.81, 2.64). For men with advanced cancer, the OR comparing top with bottom quartiles of IGF1 was 2.87 (1.01, 8.12) (Stattin et al. 2004b). A nested case control study of 462 matched pairs from the Health Professionals Follow up Study reported men with highest compared with lowest quartiles of IGF1 and IGFBP3 concentrations were at increased risk, OR 1.37 (0.92, 2.03) and 1.62 (1.07, 2.46), respectively. No association was reported with regionally invasive or metastatic prostate cancer as the number of cases was small (Platz et al. 2005).

In a case cohort study within the Melbourne Collaborative Cohort Study of 524 cases and a randomly sampled sub-cohort of 1,826 men (Severi et al. 2006a) the risk of prostate cancer was not associated with levels of IGF1 or the molar ratio IGF 1/IGFBP3, but risk increased with levels of IGFBP3, the HR associated with a doubling of IGFBP3 concentration being 1.70 (1.15, 2.52). The HR for the highest quartile compared with the lowest of IGFBP3 was 1.49 (1.11, 2.00). HRs did not differ by tumour aggressiveness or age at diagnosis. A nested case control study within the EPIC cohort study analysed 630 cases and 630 controls and reported the risk of total prostate cancer in the highest compared with the lowest tertiles of serum concentration to be 1.35 (0.99, 1.82) for IGF1, 1.39 (1.02, 1.89) after adjusting for IGFBP3, 1.22 (0.92, 1.64) for IGFBP3, and 1.01 (0.74, 1.37) after adjusting for IGF1 (Allen et al. 2007). There was no significant difference in association by stage of disease, although the association with IGF1 concentration was slightly stronger for advanced, stage disease; the OR for the highest compared with the lowest third being 1.65 (0.88, 3.08) for IGF1 and 1.76 (0.92, 3.40) for IGF1 adjusted for IGFBP3. An analysis of 727 incident prostate cancer cases and 887 matched controls in the Prostate, Lung, Colorectal and Ovarian Cancer Screening Trial showed no clear overall association between IGF1, IGFBP3 and the IGF1 to IGFBP3 molar ratio and prostate cancer risk (Weiss et al. 2007). In men with a BMI of 30 or greater, however, the IGF1 to IGFBP3 molar ratio was associated with increased risk for the highest compared with lowest quartile, OR 2.34 (1.10, 5.01), and was specifically increased for aggressive disease in obese men, OR 2.80 (1.11, 7.08).

IGFs cannot be examined in isolation as they are known to interact with other pathways important to prostate carcinogenesis. In vitro experiments with prostate cancer cell lines demonstrate that the combination of vitamin D and androgens not only synergistically up regulates IGFBP 3 expression, but also inhibits cell growth better than either hormone alone. They also suggest that IGFBP 3 is involved in the anti-proliferative action of high doses of androgens partly through p21 and p27 pathways and that IGFBP3 may contribute significantly to androgen-induced changes in cell growth (Peng et al. 2007).

Vitamin D, 1,25, (OH) D(3) has been shown to promote the action of IGF1 by increasing IGF1 receptors and IGF1 can also elevate 1,25, (OH) D(3) concentrations by stimulating the hydroxylation of 25, (OH) D(3) into the active 1,25, (OH) D(3) hormone. Both growth hormone and IGF1 significantly increase renal 1 alpha hydroxylase expression and serum 1, 25, (OH) D(3) concentrations (Gomez 2006). In prostate cells, 1,25, (OH) D(3) is growth inhibitory for many established cell lines and the role of IGFBPs, especially IGFBP3, can either inhibit or stimulate growth and IGFBP3 expression increases in response to 1,25, (OH) D(3), or its analogues, in established prostate cancer cell lines (Gomez 2006).

1.3.3.3 Inflammation

A role for infection and inflammation in carcinogenesis has long been established for specific cancer types, and interest is growing in this regard for prostate cancer (De Marzo et al. 2007). The prostate gland is prone to infection and inflammation (Palapattu et al. 2005), but whether intraprostatic inflammation contributes to prostate carcinogenesis is unknown. Inflammation is frequently present in prostate biopsies, radical prostatectomy specimens and tissue resected for treatment of benign prostatic hyperplasia. Also, inflammatory infiltrates are often found in and around foci of atrophy that are characterised by an increased proliferative index. These foci called proliferative inflammatory atrophy may be precursors of early prostate cancer or may indicate an intraprostatic environment favourable to cancer development (Platz and De Marzo 2004). Epidemiological studies have indirectly examined the role of chronic inflammation in prostate carcinogenesis through studies of pro-inflammatory and anti-inflammatory factors. When taken together, studies of sexually transmitted infections, clinical prostatitis, and genetic and tissue markers of inflammation and response to infection hint at a link between chronic intraprostatic inflammation and prostate cancer (Roberts et al. 2004; Maclennan et al. 2006; Sciarra et al. 2007).

Circulating markers of inflammation, e.g. C reactive protein, have rarely been studied. A study of 264 cases and 264 controls nested in the CLUE cohort showed no association with prostate cancer and this did not differ by stage or grade, though there was little power to examine this question (Helzlsouer et al. 2006). Another study, the Health Aging and Body Composition study of 2,438 subjects and only 296 incident cancers in total, reported that circulating levels of interleukin, 6 (IL6), and tumour necrosis factor alpha (TNF alpha) were generally more predictive of cancer death than incidence and none were associated with prostate cancer, but it was limited in its statistical power for subgroup analysis and did not consider tumour phenotype (Il'yasova et al. 2005).

A number of studies have shown a protective effect of aspirin and non-steroidal anti-inflammatory drugs (NSAIDs) on prostate cancer risk, particularly for advanced disease (Liu et al. 2006; Cheng et al. 2007). A review of 91 available epidemiological studies of NSAIDs and cancer risk reported that daily intake of NSAIDs, primarily aspirin, produced a significant reduction of 39% in risk of prostate cancer (Harris et al. 2005). Further prospective cohort studies have confirmed this finding (Dasgupta et al. 2006; Jacobs et al. 2007) and others have provided further evidence for the probable causal significance of the association by analysing it with respect to variants in genes for key proteins in inflammatory response pathways such as cyclooxygenase (COX) a key enzymatic mediator in the production of arachidonic acids to prostaglandins and eicosanoids, the type 2 isoform of which is expressed in prostate tumours and the action of which is inhibited by NSAIDs (Sooriakumaran and Kaba 2005). A Swedish study of 1,378 cases and 782 controls reported two SNPs in *COX,2* (+3100 T/G and +8365 C/T), to be associated with decreased risk, ORs of 0.78 (0.64, 0.96) and 0.65 (0.45, 0.94), respectively (Shahedi et al. 2006). A U.S. case control study of NSAIDs and risk of advanced prostate cancer observed an inverse association with NSAIDs use, OR 0.67 (0.52, 0.87), which was modified by a functional polymorphism in the lymphotoxin alpha (LTA) gene (LTA C + 80A). The CC genotype results in higher LTA production and for men with this genotype, the inverse association with prostate cancer risk was stronger, 0.43 (0.28, 0.67), but for men without this genotype, NSAID use was not associated with disease (Liu et al. 2006).

Apart from the specific association with NSAID use, a number of studies have analysed associations between variants in genes that play critical roles in inflammatory pathways and prostate cancer risk, including two putative susceptibility genes identified through family studies, ribonuclease L (*RNASEL*) and macrophage scavenger receptor 1 (*MSR1*), as well as macrophage inhibitory cytokine1 (*MIC1*), interleukins (*IL1B, IL8, IL10*) (Michaud et al. 2006), vascular endothelial growth factor (*VEGF*), prostaglandin endoperoxide synthase 2 (*PTGS2*) (Danforth et al. 2008) intercellular adhesion molecule (*ICAM*), and Toll-like receptors (*TLR4, TLR 1, 6, 10* gene cluster) (Sun et al. 2005, 2007; Zheng et al. 2004; Chen et al. 2007). Some studies, consistent with the complexity of inflammatory processes, suggest that multiple genes may interact to increase prostate risk (Zheng et al. 2006; Sun et al. 2006). In addition to the call for more, well-designed, basic, clinical and epidemiological studies of the role of chronic inflammation in prostate carcinogenesis (Platz and De Marzo 2004), more studies of relevant genetic variants and gene gene/gene environment interaction also seem to be a high priority. For this research to make substantial advances very large studies that include the standardised collection of relevant clinical and pathology data will have to be conducted. Given the hints already in the literature about the risks possibly being limited to advanced disease phenotypes, it is now obligatory that details concerning tumour phenotype be collected. Given the evidence that associations with risk may be restricted not only to a particular disease phenotype, but also to a particular genotype and environmental exposure combination, these data must also be collected to permit subgroup analysis. The latter will demand considerable additional capacity with respect to statistical power and study size.

1.3.3.4 Family History and Genetics

After advancing age, the strongest established risk factor for prostate cancer is having a family history of the disease. Between 10 and 15% of men with prostate cancer have at least one affected first degree relative (Whittemore et al. 1995). Having a first degree relative affected with prostate cancer incurs an overall two- to threefold risk, and this risk increases both with respect to the number of relatives affected and the earlier their age at diagnosis (Zeegers et al. 2003). These observations, that are consistent with the existence of an inherited genetic predisposition, have promoted the historical and burgeoning interest in the genetic epidemiology of prostate cancer and the search for genetic causes, recently comprehensively reviewed (Schaid 2004).

This quest has been pursued using a variety of research designs based on families, twins, case control studies and cohort studies, largely mimicking the approach taken to identifying genetic factors for breast and colorectal cancers (Thompson and Easton 2004). Despite a smattering of promising but premature claims, prostate cancer has failed to reveal similar susceptibility genes, and a consensus is evolving that prostate cancer might be unlike breast and colorectal cancer and may be due to variants in a large number of genes, many of which are of moderate or low penetrance (Singh et al. 2000; Easton et al. 2003; Ostrander et al. 2004; Schaid 2004). Ironically, one of the better established genes for prostate cancer is a breast cancer gene. It has been estimated that 2% of men diagnosed with prostate cancer before age 56 years carry a *BRCA2* mutation (Edwards et al. 2003). Analyses of the pattern of occurrence of affected members in family pedigrees containing multiple cases of prostate cancer have inferred dominant patterns of inheritance, as well as recessive and X-linked patterns (Cui et al. 2001; Conlon et al. 2003). It is, thus, considered that more than one gene when mutated might increase susceptibility to prostate cancer. Twin studies (Lichtenstein et al. 2000; Page et al. 1997; Risch 2001) also support the view that the familial risk of prostate cancer may not be explained by several rare autosomal dominant genes but is much more complex and may involve recessive as well as autosomal traits and multiple genetic interactions (Schaid 2004).

The search for susceptibility genes has been accelerated over the last decade by several linkage studies that have been made increasingly possible and affordable by rapid progress in the accuracy and throughput speed of genotyping technologies. This activity has led to the "discovery" of several chromosomal regions that have been dubbed as putative prostate cancer susceptibility genes regardless of the size of the region or the presence of known genes (Ostrander and Stanford 2000; Langeberg et al. 2007). Unsurprisingly, many of these claims fail attempts at replication by other studies, and the same lack of success has also applied to studies of variants in known (candidate) genes that are genotyped in family and case control designs. There are many reasons for these failures but they are probably mostly due to deficiencies of, and differences in, study design, case ascertainment, study size and data quality. Another problem in this regard is the previously unrecognised biological (and probably genetic) heterogeneity of prostate tumours, the profile of which will differ between populations, between ethnic groups, between men of different family history, with age and over time. Genetic susceptibility to prostate cancer is discussed in detail in the chapters of Lange, and Eeles and colleagues. The molecular genetics of prostate cancer is discussed by Humbert and Chevrette.

Over the last two decades the problem of tumour heterogeneity has been amplified by the over-diagnosis of considerable numbers of very early stage tumours that would not previously have come to light. There is some evidence that men with a family history are more likely than others to seek PSA testing (Cui et al. 2001; Hemminki et al. 2005), and this practice has inflated family histories and adorned family pedigrees with phenocopies (affected cases that do not carry the family's causative variant) the consequence of which is a diminution in our ability to use such families either to discover susceptibility genes or for association studies. Although some hold out hope that a new generation of large-scale multidisciplinary population-based studies will provide answers by investigating gene gene and gene environment interactions (Hsing and Chokkalingam 2006), as with environmental associations, genetic risk associations also appear to differ by disease aggressiveness (Cicek et al. 2004, 2005, 2006; Casey et al. 2006; Christensen et al. 2007; Schaid et al. 2007). This underscores the necessity, repeatedly articulated, of collecting available clinical and tumour details in a standard way and of storing tumour tissue for future molecular pathology classification as it becomes available and technically feasible.

1.4   Conclusions

The established risk factors for prostate cancer are few: advancing age, race and having a family history of prostate cancer. It is becoming clear from those studies which have been able to stratify analyses based on tumour aggressiveness that the risk factors for aggressive and non-aggressive disease (variously defined) may differ.

The Health Professionals Follow up Study recently reviewed its accumulated evidence (Giovannucci et al. 2007) for a number of factors including cigarette smoking history, physical activity, BMI, family history of prostate cancer, race, height, total energy consumption, and intakes of calcium, tomato sauce and alpha linolenic acid. Only African-American ethnic origin, positive family history, higher tomato sauce intake (inversely) and alpha linolenic acid intake had a clear statistically significant association with overall incident prostate cancer. For fatal prostate cancer, recent smoking history, taller height, higher BMI, family history, and high intakes of total energy, calcium and alpha linolenic acid were associated with a statistically significant increased risk and higher vigorous physical activity level was associated with lower risk. In relation to these risk factors, advanced stage at diagnosis was a good surrogate for fatal prostate cancer, but high-grade was not.

This emphasises the importance in this era of over diagnosis due to PSA testing not to lose sight of the main scientific aim; i.e. the quest for markers that will accurately distinguish the "tigers" from the "pussycats". Until this is accomplished, efforts to reveal risk factors (environmental or genetic) for clinically significant disease are likely to be unrewarding. Efforts within cohort studies and family studies to identify aggressive and potentially fatal forms of prostate cancer based on available histopathology, PSA levels and staging are, therefore, to be encouraged as is the routine collection within such studies of archival tissue blocks for future molecular pathology analysis as markers become available. Further, given the relatively low frequency of advanced disease, collaborations that pool information on advanced prostate cancer across cohort studies would enhance statistical power to detect effects of modest size.

Naturally, it would be better to prevent prostate cancer than to treat it. We have some interesting leads from epidemiology, but these require more research before widespread public health initiatives will be possible. To fully explore and to control for the complexity of interrelationships between the several elements involved in prostate carcinogenesis requires very large prospective cohort studies in which blood has been sampled prior to diagnosis. Such studies will be important for identifying which modifiable aspects of lifestyle (diet, alcohol, tobacco, physical activity, etc.) might be targeted for intervention to reduce risk.

Presently, men with a family history of prostate cancer can be given little by way of advice for preventive action. It is likely that one or more genetic mutations associated with an increased risk for prostate cancer will be identified in the near future. Even so, the risks will probably be similar to those for mutations in the first two breast cancer genes and will only be informative for a very small proportion of families. Unfortunately, it is difficult to foresee, when prostate cancer gene mutation carriers are identified in the future, what advice they might be offered – a prophylactic prostatectomy? The issue becomes even more complicated when considering the appropriate advice that might be given to men in a possible future scenario where they may be given a genetic risk profile based on their polymorphism status for several genes. Hopefully, such genetic screening will only occur after its efficacy has been established, when we have a better understanding of tumour heterogeneity and prognosis, and when there are improved treatment options available.

References

Adami HO, Kuper H, Andersson SO et al (2003) Prostate cancer risk and serologic evidence of human papilloma virus infection: a population-based case-control study. Cancer Epidemiol Biomarkers Prev 12(9):872–875

Albanes D, Winick M (1988) Are cell number and cell proliferation risk factors for cancer? J Natl Cancer Inst 80:772–774

Albanes D, Heinonen OP, Taylor PR et al (1996) Alpha-Tocopherol and beta-carotene supplements and lung cancer incidence in the alpha-tocopherol, beta-carotene cancer prevention study: effects of base-line characteristics and study compliance. J Natl Cancer Inst 88(21):1560–1570

Albertsen PC (1996) Screening for prostate cancer is neither appropriate nor cost-effective. Urol Clin North Am 23(4):521–530

Albertsen PC (2005) Is screening for prostate cancer with prostate specific antigen an appropriate public health measure? Acta Oncol 44(3):255–264

Albertsen PC, Hanley JA, Barrows GH et al (2005) Prostate cancer and the Will Rogers phenomenon. J Natl Cancer Inst 97(17):1248–1253

Ali AS, Hamdy FC (2007) The spectrum of prostate cancer care: from curative intent to palliation. Curr Urol Rep 8(3):245–252

Allen NE, Key TJ, Appleby PN et al (2007) Serum insulin-like growth factor (IGF) -I and IGF-binding protein-3 concentrations and prostate cancer risk: results from the European Prospective Investigation into Cancer and Nutrition. Cancer Epidemiol Biomarkers Prev 16(6):1121–1127

Anttila T, Tenkanen L, Lumme S et al (2005) Chlamydial antibodies and risk of prostate cancer. Cancer Epidemiol Biomarkers Prev 14(2):385–389

Augustsson K, Michaud DS, Rimm EB et al (2003) A prospective study of intake of fish and marine fatty acids and prostate cancer. Cancer Epidemiol Biomarkers Prev 12(1):64–67

Aumuller G (1991) Postnatal development of the prostate. Bull Assoc Anat (Nancy) 75:39–42

Baron JA, Beach M, Wallace K et al (2005) Risk of prostate cancer in a randomized clinical trial of calcium supplementation. Cancer Epidemiol Biomarkers Prev 14(3):586–589

Beemsterboer PM, de Koning HJ, Kranse R et al (2000) Prostate specific antigen testing and digital rectal examination before and during a randomized trial of screening for prostate cancer: European randomized study of screening for prostate cancer, Rotterdam. J Urol 164(4):1216–1220

Bill-Axelson A, Holmberg L, Filén F et al (2008) Radical prostatectomy versus watchful waiting in localized prostate cancer: the Scandinavian prostate cancer group-4 randomized trial. J Natl Cancer Inst 100(16):1144–1154

Blutt SE, Weigel NL (1999) Vitamin D and prostate cancer. Proc Soc Exp Biol Med 221:89–98

Boccon-Gibod L (1996) Significant versus insignificant prostate cancer – can we identify the tigers from the pussy cats? J Urol 156(3):1069–1070

Boland LL, Mink PJ, Bushhouse SA et al (2003) Weight and length at birth and risk of early-onset prostate cancer (United States). Cancer Causes Control 14(4):335–338

Bosland MC (2005) The role of estrogens in prostate carcinogenesis: a rationale for chemoprevention. Rev Urol 7(Suppl 3):S4–S10

Bosland MC (2006) Sex steroids and prostate carcinogenesis: integrated, multifactorial working hypothesis. Ann N Y Acad Sci 1089:168–176

Bostwick DG, Chang L (1999) Overdiagnosis of prostatic adenocarcinoma. Semin Urol Oncol 17(4):199–205

Bostwick DG, Burke HB, Djakiew D et al (2004) Human prostate cancer risk factors. Cancer 101(10 Suppl):2371–2490

Boyle P, Severi G, Giles GG (2003) The epidemiology of prostate cancer. Urol Clin North Am 30(2):209–217

Brawley OW (1997) Prostate carcinoma incidence and patient mortality: the effects of screening and early detection. Cancer 80(9):1857–1863

Breslow RA, Weed DL (1998) Review of epidemiologic studies of alcohol and prostate cancer: 1971–1996. Nutr Cancer 30:1–13

Brinkman M, Reulen RC, Kellen E ci al (2006) Are men with low selenium levels at increased risk of prostate cancer? Eur J Cancer 42(15):2463–2471

Brouwer IA, Katan MB, Zock PL (2004) Dietary alpha-linolenic acid is associated with reduced risk of fatal coronary heart disease, but increased prostate cancer risk: a meta-analysis. J Nutr 134(4):919–922

Carruba G (2007) Estrogen and prostate cancer: an eclipsed truth in an androgen-dominated scenario. J Cell Biochem 102(4):899–911

Casey G, Neville PJ, Liu X et al (2006) Podocalyxin variants and risk of prostate cancer and tumor aggressiveness. Hum Mol Genet 15(5):735–741

Catalona WJ, Loeb S, Han M (2006) Viewpoint: expanding prostate cancer screening. Ann Intern Med 144(6):441–443

G. Giles

Chamie K, Devere White RW et al (2008) Agent Orange exposure, Vietnam War veterans, and the risk of prostate cancer. Cancer 113(9):2464–2470

Chan JM, Stampfer MJ, Ma J et al (2002) Insulin-like growth factor-I (IGF-I) and IGF binding protein-3 as predictors of advanced-stage prostate cancer. J Natl Cancer Inst 94(14):1099–1106

Chang S, Hursting SD, Contois JH et al (2001) Leptin and prostate cancer. Prostate 46(1): 62–67

Chen YC, Giovannucci E, Kraft P et al (2007) Association between Toll-like receptor gene cluster (TLR6, TLR1, and TLR10) and prostate cancer. Cancer Epidemiol Biomarkers Prev 16(10):1982–1989

Cheng I, Liu X, Plummer SJ et al (2007) COX2 genetic variation, NSAIDs, and advanced prostate cancer risk. Br J Cancer 97(4):557–561

Christensen GB, Camp NJ, Farnham JM et al (2007) Genome-wide linkage analysis for aggressive prostate cancer in Utah high-risk pedigrees. Prostate 67(6):605–613

Cicek MS, Conti DV, Curran A et al (2004) Association of prostate cancer risk and aggressiveness to androgen pathway genes: SRD5A2, CYP17, and the AR. Prostate 59(1):69–76

Cicek MS, Liu X, Casey G et al (2005) Role of androgen metabolism genes CYP1B1, PSA/KLK3, and CYP11alpha in prostate cancer risk and aggressiveness. Cancer Epidemiol Biomarkers Prev 14(9):2173–2177

Cicek MS, Liu X, Schumacher FR et al (2006) Vitamin D receptor genotypes/haplotypes and prostate cancer risk. Cancer Epidemiol Biomarkers Prev 15(12):2549–2552

Clark LC, Combs GF Jr, Turnbull BW et al (1996) Effects of selenium supplementation for cancer prevention in patients with carcinoma of the skin. A randomized controlled trial. Nutritional Prevention of Cancer Study Group. JAMA 276(24):1957–1963

Clarke G, Whittemore AS (2000) Prostate cancer risk in relation to anthropometry and physical activity: the National Health and Nutrition Examination Survey Epidemiological Follow-Up Study. Cancer Epidemiol Biomarkers Prev 9:875–881

Clinton SK, Emenhiser C, Schwartz SJ et al (1996) Cis-trans lycopene isomers, carotenoids, and retinol in the human prostate cancer. Cancer Epidemiol Biomarkers Prev 5:823–833

Conlon EM, Goode EL, Gibbs M et al (2003) Oligogenic segregation analysis of hereditary prostate cancer pedigrees: evidence for multiple loci affecting age at onset. Int J Cancer 105(5):630–635

Cook NR, Stampfer MJ, Ma J et al (1999) Beta-carotene supplementation for patients with low baseline levels and decreased risks of total and prostate carcinoma. Cancer 86:1783–1792

Corder EH, Friedman GD, Vogelman JH et al (1995) Seasonal variation in Vitamin D, Vitamin D-binding protein, and dehydroepiandrosterone: risk of prostate cancer in black and white men. Cancer Epidemiol Biomarkers Prev 4:655–659

Costello LC, Franklin RB (2006) The clinical relevance of the metabolism of prostate cancer; zinc and tumor suppression: connecting the dots. Mol Cancer 5:17

Cross AJ, Peters U, Kirsh VA et al (2005) A prospective study of meat and meat mutagens and prostate cancer risk. Cancer Res 65(24):11779–11784

Cui J, Staples MP, Hopper JL et al (2001) Segregation analyses of 1,476 population-based Australian families affected by prostate cancer. Am J Hum Genet 68(5):1207–1218

Dagnelie PC, Schuurman AG, Goldbohm RA (2004) Diet, anthropometric measures and prostate cancer risk: a review of prospective cohort and intervention studies. BJU Int 93:1139–1150

Danforth KN, Hayes RB, Rodriguez C et al (2008) Polymorphic variants in PTGS2 and prostate cancer risk: results from two large nested case-control studies. Carcinogenesis 29(3):568–572

Dasgupta K, Di Cesar D, Ghosn J et al (2006) Association between nonsteroidal anti-inflammatory drugs and prostate cancer occurrence. Cancer J 12(2):130–135

De Marzo AM, Platz EA, Sutcliffe S et al (2007) Inflammation in prostate carcinogenesis. Nat Rev Cancer 7(4):256–269

Denis LJ (1995) Prostate cancer screening and prevention: "realities and hope". Urology 46(3 Suppl A):56–61

Dennis LK, Dawson DV (2002) Meta-analysis of measures of sexual activity and prostate cancer. Epidemiology 13(1):72–79

Dennis LK, Dawson DV, Resnick MI (2002) Vasectomy and the risk of prostate cancer: a meta-analysis examining vasectomy status, age at vasectomy, and time since vasectomy. Prostate Cancer Prostatic Dis 5(3):193–203

Dennis LK, Snetselaar LG, Smith BJ et al (2004) Problems with the assessment of dietary fat in prostate cancer studies. Am J Epidemiol 160(5):436–444

Dillner J, Knekt P, Boman J et al (1998) Sero-epidemiological association between human-papillomavirus infection and risk of prostate cancer. Int J Cancer 75:564–567

Dunger DB, Ahmed ML, Ong KK (2006) Early and late weight gain and the timing of puberty. Mol Cell Endocrinol 254–255:140–145

Easton DF, Schaid DJ, Whittemore AS (2003) Where are the prostate cancer genes? A summary of eight genome wide searches. Prostate 57(4):261–269

Eaton NE, Reeves GK, Appleby PN et al (1999) Endogenous sex hormones and prostate cancer: a quantitative review of prospective studies. Br J Cancer 80(7):930–934

Edwards SM, Kote-Jarai Z, Meitz J et al (2003) Two percent of men with early-onset prostate cancer harbor germline mutations in the BRCA2 gene. Am J Hum Genet 72(1):1–12

Ekbom A (1998) Growing evidence that several human cancers may originate in utero. Semin Cancer Biol 8(4):237–244

Ekbom A, Hsieh CC, Lipworth L et al (1996) Perinatal characteristics in relation to incidence of and mortality from prostate cancer. BMJ 313(7053):337–341

Ekbom A, Wuu J, Adami HO et al (2000) Duration of gestation and prostate cancer risk in off-spring. Cancer Epidemiol Biomarkers Prev 9(2):221–223

Eriksson M, Wedel H, Wallander MA et al (2007) The impact of birth weight on prostate cancer incidence and mortality in a population-based study of men born in 1913 and followed up from 50 to 85 years of age. Prostate 67(11):1247–1254

Etzioni R, Penson DF, Legler JM et al (2002) Overdiagnosis due to prostate-specific antigen screening: lessons from U.S. prostate cancer incidence trends. J Natl Cancer Inst 94(13):981–990

Feuer EJ, Merrill RM, Hankey BF (1999) Cancer surveillance series: interpreting trends in prostate cancer – part II: cause of death misclassification and the recent rise and fall in prostate cancer mortality. J Natl Cancer Inst 91(12):1025–1032

Fincham SM, Hill GB, Hanson J et al (1990) Epidemiology of prostatic cancer: a case-control study. Prostate 17(3):189–206

Franklin RB, Costello LC (2007) Zinc as an anti-tumor agent in prostate cancer and in other cancers. Arch Biochem Biophys 463(2):211–217

Freedland SJ, Platz EA (2007) Obesity and prostate cancer: making sense out of apparently conflicting data. Epidemiol Rev 29:88–97

Freedland SJ, Giovannucci E, Platz EA (2006) Are findings from studies of obesity and prostate cancer really in conflict? Cancer Causes Control 17(1):5–9

Friedenreich CM, Thune I (2001) A review of physical activity and prostate cancer risk. Cancer Causes Control 12(5):461–475

Gade-Andavolu R, Cone LA, Shu S et al (2006) Molecular interactions of leptin and prostate cancer. Cancer J 12(3):201–206

Gallus S, Foschi R, Negri E et al (2007) Dietary zinc and prostate cancer risk: a case-control study from Italy. Eur Urol 52(4):1052–1056

Gann PH, Hennekens CH, Ma J et al (1996) Prospective study of sex hormone levels and risk of prostate cancer. J Natl Cancer Inst 88(16):1118–1126

Gann PH, Ma J, Giovannucci E et al (1999) Lower prostate cancer risk in men with elevated plasma lycopene levels: results of a prospective analysis. Cancer Res 59(6):1225–1230

Gao X, LaValley MP, Tucker KL (2005) Prospective studies of dairy product and calcium intakes and prostate cancer risk: a meta-analysis. J Natl Cancer Inst 97(23):1768–1777

Gennigens C, Menetrier-Caux C, Droz JP (2006) Insulin-like growth factor (IGF) family and prostate cancer. Crit Rev Oncol Hematol 58(2):124–145

Giles GG (2003) Epidemiological investigation of prostate cancer. Methods Mol Med 81:1–19

Giles GG, Ireland P (1997) Diet, nutrition and prostate cancer. Int J Cancer 10:13–17

Giles GG, Severi G, English DR et al (2003) Sexual factors and prostate cancer. BJU Int 92(3):211–216

Giovannucci E (2003) Nutrition, insulin, insulin-like growth factors and cancer. Horm Metab Res 35(11–12):694–704

Giovannucci E (2007) Strengths and limitations of current epidemiologic studies: vitamin D as a modifier of colon and prostate cancer risk. Nutr Rev 65(8 Pt 2):S77–S79

Giovannucci E, Rimm EB, Wolk A et al (1998) Calcium and fructose intake in relation to risk of prostate cancer. Cancer Res 58:442–447

Giovannucci E, Rimm EB, Liu Y et al (2002) A prospective study of tomato products, lycopene, and prostate cancer risk. J Natl Cancer Inst 94(5):391–398

Giovannucci E, Rimm EB, Liu Y et al (2003) A prospective study of cruciferous vegetables and prostate cancer. Cancer Epidemiol Biomarkers Prev 12(12):1403–1409

Giovannucci E, Rimm EB, Liu Y et al (2004) Height, predictors of C-peptide and cancer risk in men. Int J Epidemiol 33(1):217–225

Giovannucci EL, Liu Y, Leitzmann MF et al (2005) A prospective study of physical activity and incident and fatal prostate cancer. Arch Intern Med 165(9):1005–1010

Giovannucci E, Liu Y, Rimm EB et al (2006) Prospective study of predictors of vitamin D status and cancer incidence and mortality in men. J Natl Cancer Inst 98(7):451–459

Giovannucci E, Liu Y, Platz EA et al (2007) Risk factors for prostate cancer incidence and progression in the health professionals follow-up study. Int J Cancer 121(7):1571–1578

Gleason DF (1992) Histologic grading of prostate cancer: a perspective. Hum Pathol 23(3):273–279

Gohagan JK, Prorok PC, Kramer BS et al (1994) Prostate cancer screening in the prostate, lung, colorectal and ovarian cancer screening trial of the National Cancer Institute. J Urol 152(5 Pt 2):1905–1909

Gomez JM (2006) The role of insulin-like growth factor I components in the regulation of vitamin D. Curr Pharm Biotechnol 7(2):125–132

Griffiths K, Denis L, Turkes A et al (1998) Possible relationship between dietary factors and pathogenesis of prostate cancer. Int J Urol 5:195–213

Gyorkey F, Min KW, Huff JA et al (1967) Zinc and magnesium in human prostate gland: normal, hyperplastic, and neoplastic. Cancer Res 27(8):1348–1353

Hafez B, Hafez ES (2004) Andropause: endocrinology, erectile dysfunction, and prostate pathophysiology. Arch Androl 50(2):45–68

Harris RE, Beebe-Donk J, Doss H et al (2005) Aspirin, ibuprofen, and other non-steroidal anti-inflammatory drugs in cancer prevention: a critical review of non-selective COX-2 blockade. Oncol Rep 13(4):559–583

Hedelin M, Chang ET, Wiklund F et al (2007) Association of frequent consumption of fatty fish with prostate cancer risk is modified by COX-2 polymorphism. Int J Cancer 120(2):398–405

Heinonen OP, Albanes D, Virtamo J et al (1998) Prostate cancer and supplementation with alpha-tocopherol and betacarotene: incidence and mortality in a controlled trial. J Natl Cancer Inst 90:440–446

Helzlsouer KJ, Erlinger TP, Platz EA (2006) C-reactive protein levels and subsequent cancer outcomes: results from a prospective cohort study. Eur J Cancer 42(6):704–707

Hemminki K, Rawal R, Bermejo JL (2005) Prostate cancer screening, changing age-specific incidence trends and implications on familial risk. Int J Cancer 113(2):312–315

Henderson BE, Bernstein L, Ross RK et al (1988) The early in utero estrogen and testosterone environment of blacks and whites – potential effects on male offspring. Br J Cancer 57:216–218

Hercberg S, Galan P, Preziosi P et al (2004) The SU.VI.MAX Study: a randomized, placebo-controlled trial of the health effects of antioxidant vitamins and minerals. Arch Intern Med 164(21):2335–2342

Heysek RV (2007) Modern brachytherapy for treatment of prostate cancer. Cancer Control 14(3):238–243

Hoffman RM, Clanon DL, Littenberg B et al (2000) Using the Free-to-total Prostate-specific Antigen Ratio to Detect Prostate Cancer in Men with non-specific Elevations of Prostate-specific Antigen Levels. J Gen Intern Med 15(10):739–748

Holick CN, Stanford JL, Kwon EM (2007) Comprehensive association analysis of the vitamin D pathway genes, VDR, CYP27B1, and CYP24A1, in prostate cancer. Cancer Epidemiol Biomarkers Prev 16(10):1990–1999

Holt RI (2002) Fetal programming of the growth hormone-insulin-like growth factor axis. Trends Endocrinol Metab 13(9):392–397

Hsi LC, Wilson LC, Eling TE (2002) Opposing effects of 15-lipoxygenase-1 and -2 metabolites on MAPK signaling in prostate. Alteration in peroxisome proliferator-activated receptor gamma. J Biol Chem 277(43):40549–40556

Hsing AW, Chokkalingam AP (2006) Prostate cancer epidemiology. Front Biosci 11:1388–1413

Hsing AW, Chua S Jr, Gao YT et al (2001) Prostate cancer risk and serum levels of insulin and leptin: a population-based study. J Natl Cancer Inst 93(10):783–789

Hunt CD, Johnson PE, Herbel J et al (1992) Effects of dietary zinc depletion on seminal volume and zinc loss, serum testosterone concentrations, and sperm morphology in young men. Am J Clin Nutr 56(1):148–157

Il'yasova D, Colbert LH, Harris TB et al (2005) Circulating levels of inflammatory markers and cancer risk in the health aging and body composition cohort. Cancer Epidemiol Biomarkers Prev 14(10):2413–2418

Isaacs JT (1983) Prostatic structure and function in relation to the etiology of prostate cancer. Prostate 4:351–366

Jacobs EJ, Thun MJ, Bain EB et al (2007) A large cohort study of long-term daily use of adult-strength aspirin and cancer incidence. J Natl Cancer Inst 99(8):608–615

John EM, Koo J, Schwartz GG (2007) Sun exposure and prostate cancer risk: evidence for a protective effect of early-life exposure. Cancer Epidemiol Biomarkers Prev 16(6):1283–1286

Joseph MA, Moysich KB, Freudenheim JL et al (2004) Cruciferous vegetables, genetic polymorphisms in glutathione S-transferases M1 and T1, and prostate cancer risk. Nutr Cancer 50(2):206–213

Juul A, Bang P, Hertel NT et al (1994) Serum insulin-like growth factor-I in 1030 healthy children, adolescents, and adults: relation to age, sex, stage of puberty, testicular size, and body mass index. J Clin Endocrinol Metab 78:744–752

Kambhampati S, Ray G, Sengupta K et al (2005) Growth factors involved in prostate carcinogenesis. Front Biosci 10:1355–1367

Kang D, Lee KM, Park SK et al (2007) Functional variant of manganese superoxide dismutase (SOD2 V16A) polymorphism is associated with prostate cancer risk in the prostate, lung, colorectal, and ovarian cancer study. Cancer Epidemiol Biomarkers Prev 16(8):1581–1586

Kasper JS, Giovannucci E (2006) A meta-analysis of diabetes mellitus and the risk of prostate cancer. Cancer Epidemiol Biomarkers Prev 15(11):2056–2062

Kerr WK, Keresteci G, Ayohb HM (1960) The distribution of zinc within the human prostate. Cancer 13:550–554

Key TJ, Silcocks PB, Davey GK et al (1997) A case-control study of diet and prostate cancer. Br J Cancer 76:678–687

Key TJ, Allen N, Appleby P et al (2004) Fruits and vegetables and prostate cancer: no association among 1104 cases in a prospective study of 130544 men in the European Prospective Investigation into Cancer and Nutrition (EPIC). Int J Cancer 109(1):119–124

Key TJ, Appleby PN, Allen NE et al (2007) Plasma carotenoids, retinol, and tocopherols and the risk of prostate cancer in the European Prospective Investigation into Cancer and Nutrition study. Am J Clin Nutr 86(3):672–681

Kirsh VA, Hayes RB, Mayne ST et al (2006a) Supplemental and dietary vitamin E, beta-carotene, and vitamin C intakes and prostate cancer risk. J Natl Cancer Inst 98(4):245–254

Kirsh VA, Mayne ST, Peters U et al (2006b) A prospective study of lycopene and tomato product intake and risk of prostate cancer. Cancer Epidemiol Biomarkers Prev 15(1):92–98

Kirsh VA, Peters U, Mayne ST et al (2007) Prostate, Lung, Colorectal and Ovarian Cancer Screening Trial. Prospective study of fruit and vegetable intake and risk of prostate cancer. J Natl Cancer Inst 99(15):1200–1209

Kolonel LN (2001) Fat, meat, and prostate cancer. Epidemiol Rev 23(1):72–81

Kolonel LN, Yoshizawa CN, Hankin JH (1988) Diet and prostatic cancer: a case-control study in Hawaii. Am J Epidemiol 127:999–1012

Kolonel LN, Hankin JH, Whittemore AS et al (2000) Vegetables, fruits, legumes and prostate cancer: a multiethnic case-control study. Cancer Epidemiol Biomarkers Prev 9(8):795–804

Korodi Z, Wang X, Tedeschi R (2005) No serological evidence of association between prostate cancer and infection with herpes simplex virus type 2 or human herpesvirus type 8: a nested case-control study. J Infect Dis 191(12):2008–2011

Kristal AR, Lampe JW (2002) Brassica vegetables and prostate cancer risk: a review of the epidemiological evidence. Nutr Cancer 42(1):1–9

Kristal AR, Stanford JL, Cohen JH et al (1999) Vitamin and mineral supplement use is associated with reduced risk of prostate cancer. Cancer Epidemiol Biomarkers Prev 8:887–892

Kurahashi N, Iwasaki M, Sasazuki S (2007) Soy product and isoflavone consumption in relation to prostate cancer in Japanese men. Cancer Epidemiol Biomarkers Prev 16(3):538–545

Kuriyama M, Wang MC, Lee CI et al (1981) Use of human prostate-specific antigen in monitoring prostate cancer. Cancer Res 41(10):3874–3876

Langeberg WJ, Isaacs WB, Stanford JL (2007) Genetic etiology of hereditary prostate cancer. Front Biosci 12:4101–4110

Lawson KA, Wright ME, Subar A et al (2007) Multivitamin use and risk of prostate cancer in the National Institutes of Health – AARP Diet and Health Study. J Natl Cancer Inst 99(10):754–764

Lee AK, D'Amico AV (2005) Utility of prostate-specific antigen kinetics in addition to clinical factors in the selection of patients for salvage local therapy. J Clin Oncol 23(32): 8192–8197

Lee IM, Sesso HD, Chen JJ et al (2001) Does physical activity play a role in the prevention of prostate cancer? Epidemiol Rev 23(1):132–137

Lee IM, Gaziano JM, Buring JE (2006) Vitamin E in the prevention of prostate cancer: where are we today? J Natl Cancer Inst 98(4):225–227

Leitzmann MF, Stampfer MJ, Wu K et al (2003) Zinc supplement use and risk of prostate cancer. J Natl Cancer Inst 95(13):1004–1007

Leitzmann MF, Platz EA, Stampfer MJ et al (2004a) Ejaculation frequency and subsequent risk of prostate cancer. JAMA 291(13):1578–1586

Leitzmann MF, Stampfer MJ, Michaud DS et al (2004b) Dietary intake of n-3 and n-6 fatty acids and the risk of prostate cancer. Am J Clin Nutr 80(1):204–216

Li H, Stampfer MJ, Hollis JB et al (2007) A prospective study of plasma vitamin D metabolites, vitamin D receptor polymorphisms, and prostate cancer. PLoS Med 4(3):e103

Liang T, Liao S (1992) Inhibition of steroid 5 alpha reductase by specific aliphatic unsaturated fatty acids. Biochem J 285:557–562

Lichtenstein P, Holm NV, Verkasalo PK et al (2000) Environmental and heritable factors in the causation of cancer – analyses of cohorts of twins from Sweden, Denmark, and Finland. N Engl J Med 343(2):78–85

Lippman SM, Goodman PJ, Klein EA et al (2005) Designing the Selenium and Vitamin E Cancer Prevention Trial (SELECT). J Natl Cancer Inst 97(2):94–102

Littman AJ, Kristal AR, White E (2006) Recreational physical activity and prostate cancer risk (United States). Cancer Causes Control 17(6):831–841

Littman AJ, White E, Kristal AR (2007) Anthropometrics and prostate cancer risk. Am J Epidemiol 165(11):1271–1279

Liu SE, Lee IM, Linson P et al (2000) A prospective study of physical activity and risk of prostate cancer in US physicians. Int J Epidemiol 29:29–35

Liu X, Plummer SJ, Nock NL et al (2006) Non steroidal anti inflammatory drugs and decreased risk of advanced prostate cancer: modification by lymphotoxin alpha. Am J Epidemiol 164(10):984–989

Lotufo PA, Lee IM, Ajani UA et al (2000) Cigarette smoking and risk of prostate cancer in the Physicians' Health Study. Int J Cancer 87:141–144

Lumey LH (1996) Prostate cancer and smoking: a review of case-control and cohort studies. Prostate 29:249–260

Lund-Nilsen TI, Johnsen R, Vatten LJ (2000) Socio-economic and lifestyle factors associated with the risk of prostate cancer. Br J Cancer 82:1358–1363

MacInnis RJ, English DR (2006) Body size and composition and prostate cancer risk: systematic review and meta-regression analysis. Cancer Causes Control 17(8):989–1003

MacInnis RJ, English DR, Gertig DM et al (2003) Body size and composition and prostate cancer risk. Cancer Epidemiol Biomarkers Prev 12(12):1417–1421

MacLennan GT, Eisenberg R, Fleshman RL et al (2006) The influence of chronic inflammation in prostatic carcinogenesis: a 5-year follow up study. J Urol 176(3):1012–1016

Mannisto S, Pietinen P, Virtanen MJ et al (2003) Fatty acids and risk of prostate cancer in a nested case-control study in male smokers. Cancer Epidemiol Biomarkers Prev 12(12): 1422–1428

Mawson CA, Fischer MI (1952) Occurrence of zinc in human prostate gland. Canad J Med Sci 30:336–339

McNeal JE (1981) The zonal anatomy of the prostate. Prostate 2:35–49

McVary KT (2006) BPH: epidemiology and comorbidities. Am J Manag Care 12:S122–S128

Meinbach DS, Lokeshwar BL (2006) Insulin-like growth factors and their binding proteins in prostate cancer: cause or consequence? Urol Oncol 24(4):294–306

Meyer F, Galan P, Douville P et al (2005) Antioxidant vitamin and mineral supplementation and prostate cancer prevention in the SU.VI.MAX trial. Int J Cancer 116:182–186

Michaud DS, Augustsson K, Rimm EB et al (2001) A prospective study on intake of animal products and risk of prostate cancer. Cancer Causes Control 12(6):557–567

Michaud DS, Daugherty SE, Berndt SI (2006) Genetic polymorphisms of interleukin-1B (IL-1B), IL-6, IL-8, and IL-10 and risk of prostate cancer. Cancer Res 66(8):4525–4530

Mikhak B, Hunter DJ, Spiegelman D et al (2007) Vitamin D receptor (VDR) gene polymorphisms and haplotypes, interactions with plasma 25-hydroxyvitamin D and 1, 25-dihydroxyvitamin D, and prostate cancer risk. Prostate 67(9):911–923

Mitrou PN, Albanes D, Weinstein SJ et al (2007) A prospective study of dietary calcium, dairy products and prostate cancer risk (Finland). Int J Cancer 120(11):2466–2473

Montuschi P, Barnes P, Roberts LJ 2nd (2007) Insights into oxidative stress: the isoprostanes. Curr Med Chem 14(6):703–717

Moreno J, Krishnan AV, Peehl DM et al (2006) Mechanisms of vitamin D-mediated growth inhibition in prostate cancer cells: inhibition of the prostaglandin pathway. Anticancer Res 26(4A):2525–2530

Myers CE, Ghosh J (1999) Lipoxygenase inhibition in prostate cancer. Eur Urol 35(5–6):395–398

Navarro Silvera SA, Rohan TE (2007) Trace elements and cancer risk: a review of the epidemiologic evidence. Cancer Causes Control 18(1):7–27

Nilsen TI, Romundstad PR, Troisi R et al (2005) Birth size and subsequent risk for prostate cancer: a prospective population-based study in Norway. Int J Cancer 113(6):1002–1004

Nilsen TI, Romundstad PR, Vatten LJ (2006) Recreational physical activity and risk of prostate cancer: a prospective population-based study in Norway (the HUNT study). Int J Cancer 119(12):2943–2947

Norrish AE, Jackson RT, McRae CU (1998) Non-steroidal anti-inflammatory drugs and prostate cancer progression. Int J Cancer 77:511–515

Norrish AE, Ferguson LR, Knize MG et al (1999) Heterocyclic amine content of cooked meat and risk of prostate cancer. J Natl Cancer Inst 91:2038–2044

Omenn GS, Goodman GE, Thornquist MD et al (1996) Risk factors for lung cancer and for intervention effects in CARET, the Beta-Carotene and Retinol Efficacy Trial. J Natl Cancer Inst 88:1550–1559

Ostrander EA, Stanford JL (2000) Genetics of prostate cancer: too many loci, too few genes. Am J Hum Genet 67:1367–1375

Ostrander EA, Markianos K, Stanford JL (2004) Finding prostate cancer susceptibility genes. Annu Rev Genomics Hum Genet 5:151–175

Page WF, Braun MM, Partin AW et al (1997) Heredity and prostate cancer: a study of World War II veteran twins. Prostate 33(4):240–245

Palapattu GS, Sutcliffe S, Bastian PJ et al (2005) Prostate carcinogenesis and inflammation: emerging insights. Carcinogenesis 26(7):1170–1181

Papatsoris AG, Karamouzis MV, Papavassiliou AG (2005) Novel insights into the implication of the IGF-1 network in prostate cancer. Trends Mol Med 11(2):52–55

Park SY, Murphy SP, Wilkens LR et al (2007a) Fat and meat intake and prostate cancer risk: the multiethnic cohort study. Int J Cancer 121(6):1339–1345

Park SY, Murphy SP, Wilkens LR et al (2007b) Calcium, vitamin D, and dairy product intake and prostate cancer risk: the Multiethnic Cohort Study. Am J Epidemiol 166:1259–1269

Park Y, Mitrou PN, Kipnis V et al (2007c) Calcium, dairy foods, and risk of incident and fatal prostate cancer: the NIH-AARP Diet and Health Study. Am J Epidemiol 166:1270–1279

Parkin DM, Muir C, Waterhouse J et al (eds) (1992) Cancer incidence in five continents, vol 6. IARC, Lyon

Parkin DM, Whelan SL, Ferlay J et al (eds) (2002) Cancer incidence in five continents, vol 8. IARC, Lyon

Pashayan N, Powles J, Brown C et al (2006) Excess cases of prostate cancer and estimated over-diagnosis associated with PSA testing in East Anglia. Br J Cancer 95(3):401–405

Patel AV, Rodriguez C, Jacobs EJ et al (2005) Recreational physical activity and risk of prostate cancer in a large cohort of U.S. men. Cancer Epidemiol Biomarkers Prev 14(1):275–279

Patel AA, Chen MH, Renshaw AA et al (2007) PSA failure following definitive treatment of prostate cancer having biopsy Gleason score 7 with tertiary grade 5. JAMA 298(13):1533–1538

Peehl DM, Skowronski RJ, Leung GK et al (1994) Antiproliferative effects of 1, 25-dihydroxyvitamin D3 on primary cultures of human prostatic cells. Cancer Res 54:805–810

Peng L, Wang J, Malloy PJ et al (2007) The role of insulin-like growth factor binding protein-3 in the growth inhibitory actions of androgens in LNCaP human prostate cancer cells. Int J Cancer 122(3):558–566

Peters U, Foster CB, Chatterjee N et al (2007a) Serum selenium and risk of prostate cancer-a nested case-control study. Am J Clin Nutr 85(1):209–217

Peters U, Leitzmann MF, Chatterjee N et al (2007b) Serum lycopene, other carotenoids, and prostate cancer risk: a nested case-control study in the prostate, lung, colorectal, and ovarian cancer screening trial. Cancer Epidemiol Biomarkers Prev 16(5):962–968

Peters U, Littman AJ, Kristal AR et al (2008) Vitamin E and selenium supplementation and risk of prostate cancer in the Vitamins and lifestyle (VITAL) study cohort. Cancer Causes Control 19(1):75–87

Platz EA (2002) Energy imbalance and prostate cancer. J Nutr 132(11 Suppl):3471S–3481S

Platz EA, De Marzo AM (2004) Epidemiology of inflammation and prostate cancer. J Urol 171(2 Pt 2):S36–S40

Platz EA, Giovannucci E (2004) The epidemiology of sex steroid hormones and their signaling and metabolic pathways in the etiology of prostate cancer. J Steroid Biochem Mol Biol 92(4):237–253

Platz EA, Helzlsouer KJ (2001) Selenium, zinc, and prostate cancer. Epidemiol Rev 23(1):93–101

Platz EA, Giovannucci E, Rimm EB et al (1998) Retrospective analysis of birth weight and prostate cancer in the Health Professionals Follow-up Study. Am J Epidemiol 147(12):1140–1144

Platz EA, Helzlsouer KJ, Hoffman SC et al (2002) Prediagnostic toenail cadmium and zinc and subsequent prostate cancer risk. Prostate 52(4):288–296

Platz EA, Leitzmann MF, Michaud DS et al (2003) Interrelation of energy intake, body size, and physical activity with prostate cancer in a large prospective cohort study. Cancer Res 63(23):8542–8548

Platz EA, De Marzo AM, Giovannucci E (2004a) Prostate cancer association studies: pitfalls and solutions to cancer misclassification in the PSA era. J Cell Biochem 91(3):553–571

Platz EA, Leitzmann MF, Rimm EB et al (2004b) Alcohol intake, drinking patterns, and risk of prostate cancer in a large prospective cohort study. Am J Epidemiol 159(5):444–453

Platz EA, Leitzmann MF, Rifai N et al (2005a) Sex steroid hormones and the androgen receptor gene CAG repeat and subsequent risk of prostate cancer in the prostate-specific antigen era. Cancer Epidemiol Biomarkers Prev 14(5):1262–1269

Platz EA, Pollak MN, Leitzmann MF et al (2005b) Plasma insulin-like growth factor-1 and binding protein-3 and subsequent risk of prostate cancer in the PSA era. Cancer Causes Control 16(3):255–262

Presti JC Jr (2007) Prostate biopsy strategies. Nat Clin Pract Urol 4(9):505–511

Preston DL, Ron E, Tokuoka S et al (2007) Solid cancer incidence in atomic bomb survivors: 1958–1998. Radiat Res 168(1):1–64

Prins GS, Huang L, Birch L et al (2006) The role of estrogens in normal and abnormal development of the prostate gland. Ann N Y Acad Sci 1089:1–13

Prinsac GS, Birch L, Habermann H et al (2001) Influence of neonatal estrogens on rat prostate development. Reprod Fertil Dev 13(4):241–252

Purnell JQ, Bland LB, Garzotto M et al (2006) Effects of transdermal estrogen on levels of lipids, lipase activity, and inflammatory markers in men with prostate cancer. J Lipid Res 47(2):349–355

Putnam SD, Cerhan JR, Parker AS et al (2000) Lifestyle and anthropometric risk factors for prostate cancer in a cohort of Iowa men. Ann Epidemiol 10(6):361–369

Rafnsson V (2007) Farming and prostate cancer. Occup Environ Med 64(3):143

Randall VA (1994) Role of 5 alpha-reductase in health and disease. Baillieres Clin Endocrinol Metab 8(2):405–431

Raynaud JP (2006) Prostate cancer risk in testosterone-treated men. J Steroid Biochem Mol Biol 102(1–5):261–266

Renehan AG, Zwahlen M, Minder C et al (2004) Insulin-like growth factor (IGF)-I, IGF binding protein-3, and cancer risk: systematic review and meta-regression analysis. Lancet 363(9418):1346–1353

Ribeiro R, Lopes C, Medeiros R (2006) The link between obesity and prostate cancer: the leptin pathway and therapeutic perspectives. Prostate Cancer Prostatic Dis 9(1):19–24

Risbridger GP, Ellem SJ, McPherson SJ (2007) Estrogen action on the prostate gland: a critical mix of endocrine and paracrine signaling. J Mol Endocrinol 39(3):183–188

Risch N (2001) The genetic epidemiology of cancer: interpreting family and twin studies and their implications for molecular genetic approaches. Cancer Epidemiol Biomarkers Prev 10(7):733–741

Roberts RO, Bergstralh EJ, Bass SE et al (2004) Prostatitis as a risk factor for prostate cancer. Epidemiology 15(1):93–99

Roddam AW, Severi G, English DR, Giles GG, The Endogenous Hormones and Prostate Cancer Collaborative Group (2008) Endogenous sex hormones and prostate cancer: a collaborative analysis of eighteen prospective studies. J Natl Cancer Inst 100(3):170–183

Rodriguez C, Jacobs EJ, Mondul AM et al (2004) Vitamin E supplements and risk of prostate cancer in U.S. men. Cancer Epidemiol Biomarkers Prev 13(3):378–382

Rodriguez C, McCullough ML, Mondul AM et al (2006) Meat consumption among Black and White men and risk of prostate cancer in the Cancer Prevention Study II Nutrition Cohort. Cancer Epidemiol Biomarkers Prev 15(2):211–216

Rodriguez C, Freedland SJ, Deka A et al (2007) Body mass index, weight change, and risk of prostate cancer in the Cancer Prevention Study II Nutrition Cohort. Cancer Epidemiol Biomarkers Prev 16(1):63–69

Rohrmann S, Platz EA, Kavanaugh CJ et al (2007) Meat and dairy consumption and subsequent risk of prostate cancer in a US cohort study. Cancer Causes Control 18(1):41–50

Rosenblatt KA, Carter JJ, Iwasaki LM et al (2003) Serologic evidence of human papillomavirus 16 and 18 infections and risk of prostate cancer. Cancer Epidemiol Biomarkers Prev 12(8):763–768

Ross RK, Schottenfeld D (1996) Prostate cancer. In: Schottenfeld D, Fraumeni JF Jr (eds) Cancer epidemiology and prevention. Oxford University Press, Oxford, pp 1180–1206

Ross RK, Pike MC, Coetzee GA et al (1998) Androgen metabolism and prostate cancer: establishing a model of genetic susceptibility. Cancer Res 58:4497–4504

Rotkin ID (1977) Studies in the epidemiology of prostatic cancer: expanded sampling. Cancer Treat Rep 61(2):173–180

Schaid DJ (2004) The complex genetic epidemiology of prostate cancer. Hum Mol Genet 13(Spec No 1):R103–R121

Schaid DJ, Stanford JL, McDonnell SK et al (2007) Genome-wide linkage scan of prostate cancer Gleason score and confirmation of chromosome 19q. Hum Genet 121(6):729–735

Schiel R, Beltschikow W, Steiner T et al (2006) Diabetes, insulin, and risk of cancer. Methods Find Exp Clin Pharmacol 28(3):169–175

Schoonen WM, Salinas CA, Kiemeney LA et al (2005) Alcohol consumption and risk of prostate cancer in middle-aged men. Int J Cancer 113(1):133–140

Schroder FH (1994) The European screening study for prostate cancer. Can J Oncol 4(Suppl 1):102–105

Schuurman AG, Goldbohm RA, Dorant E et al (1998) Vegetable and fruit consumption and prostate cancer risk: a cohort study in The Netherlands. Cancer Epidemiol Biomarkers Prev 7(8):673–680

Schwartz GG, Wang MH, Zang M (1997) 1 alpha, 25- dihydroxyvitamin D (calcitriol) inhibits the invasiveness of human prostate cancer cells. Cancer Epidemiol Biomarkers Prev 6:727–732

Sciarra A, Di Silverio F, Salciccia S et al (2007) Inflammation and chronic prostatic diseases: evidence for a link? Eur Urol 52(4):964–972

Severi G, Morris HA, MacInnis RJ et al (2006a) Circulating insulin-like growth factor-I and binding protein-3 and risk of prostate cancer. Cancer Epidemiol Biomarkers Prev 15(6):1137–1141

Severi G, Morris HA, MacInnis RJ et al (2006b) Circulating steroid hormones and the risk of prostate cancer. Cancer Epidemiol Biomarkers Prev 15(1):86–91

Shahedi K, Lindström S, Zheng SL et al (2006) Genetic variation in the COX-2 gene and the association with prostate cancer risk. Int J Cancer 119(3):668–672

Shahinian VB, Kuo YF, Freeman JL et al (2005) Increasing use of gonadotropin-releasing hormone agonists for the treatment of localized prostate carcinoma. Cancer 103(8):1615–1624

Shinohara K (2006) Improving cancer detection by prostate biopsy: the role of core number and site. Nat Clin Pract Urol 3(10):526–527

Singh R, Eeles RA, Durocher F et al (2000) High risk genes predisposing to prostate cancer development-do they exist? Prostate Cancer Prostatic Dis 3(4):241–247

Sinha R, Rothman N (1999) Role of well-done, grilled red meat, heterocyclic amines (HCAs) in the etiology of human cancer. Cancer Lett 143(2):189–194

Smith DP, Armstrong BK (1998) Prostate-specific antigen testing in Australia and association with prostate cancer incidence in New South Wales. Med J Aust 169:17–20

Sooriakumaran P, Kaba R (2005) The risks and benefits of cyclo-oxygenase-2 inhibitors in prostate cancer: a review. Int J Surg 3(4):278–285

Stamey TA, Yang N, Hay AR et al (1987) Prostate-specific antigen as a serum marker for adenocarcinoma of the prostate. N Engl J Med 317(15):909–916

Stattin P, Lumme S, Tenkanen L et al (2004a) High levels of circulating testosterone are not associated with increased prostate cancer risk: a pooled prospective study. Int J Cancer 108(3):418–424

Stattin P, Rinaldi S, Biessy C et al (2004b) High levels of circulating insulin-like growth factor-I increase prostate cancer risk: a prospective study in a population-based non screened cohort. J Clin Oncol 22(15):3104–3112

Stewart LV, Weigel NL (2004) Vitamin D and prostate cancer. Exp Biol Med (Maywood) 229:277–284

Stram DO, Hankin JH, Wilkens LR et al (2006) Prostate cancer incidence and intake of fruits, vegetables and related micronutrients: the multiethnic cohort study (United States). Cancer Causes Control 17(9):1193–1207

Sun J, Wiklund F, Zheng SL et al (2005) Sequence variants in Toll-like receptor gene cluster (TLR6-TLR1-TLR10) and prostate cancer risk. J Natl Cancer Inst 97(7):525–532

Sun J, Wiklund F, Hsu FC et al (2006) Interactions of sequence variants in interleukin-1 receptor-associated kinase4 and the toll-like receptor 6-1-10 gene cluster increase prostate cancer risk. Cancer Epidemiol Biomarkers Prev 15(3):480–485

Sun J, Turner A, Xu J et al (2007) Genetic variability in inflammation pathways and prostate cancer risk. Urol Oncol 25(3):250–259

Sutcliffe S, Giovannucci E, Alderete JF et al (2006a) Plasma antibodies against Trichomonas vaginalis and subsequent risk of prostate cancer. Cancer Epidemiol Biomarkers Prev 15(5):939–945

Sutcliffe S, Giovannucci E, De Marzo AM et al (2006b) Gonorrhea, syphilis, clinical prostatitis, and the risk of prostate cancer. Cancer Epidemiol Biomarkers Prev 15(11):2160–2166

Sutcliffe S, Giovannucci E, Gaydos CA et al (2007a) Plasma antibodies against Chlamydia trachomatis, human papillomavirus, and human herpesvirus type 8 in relation to prostate cancer: a prospective study. Cancer Epidemiol Biomarkers Prev 16(8):1573–1580

Sutcliffe S, Giovannucci E, Leitzmann MF (2007b) A prospective cohort study of red wine consumption and risk of prostate cancer. Int J Cancer 120(7):1529–1535

Tang D, Liu JJ, Rundle A, Neslund-Dudas C et al (2007) Grilled meat consumption and PhIP-DNA adducts in prostate carcinogenesis. Cancer Epidemiol Biomarkers Prev 16(4):803–808

Telesca D, Etzioni R, Gulati R (2008) Estimating lead time and overdiagnosis associated with PSA screening from prostate cancer incidence trends. Biometrics 64(1):10–19

Thomas DB, Karagas MR (1987) Cancer in first and second generation Americans. Cancer Res 47:5771–5776

Thompson D, Easton D (2004) The genetic epidemiology of breast cancer genes. J Mammary Gland Biol Neoplasia 9(3):221–236

Tibblin G, Eriksson M, Cnattingius S et al (1995) High birthweight as a predictor of prostate cancer risk. Epidemiology 6(4):423–424

Torniainen S, Maria Hedelin M, Autio V et al (2007) Lactase persistence, dietary intake of milk, and the risk for prostate cancer in Sweden and Finland. Cancer Epidemiol Biomarkers Prev 16(5):956–961

Travis RC, Key TJ, Allen NE et al (2007) Serum androgens and prostate cancer among 643 cases and 643 controls in the European Prospective Investigation into Cancer and Nutrition. Int J Cancer 121(6):1331–1338

Tretli S, Engeland A, Haldorsen T et al (1996) Prostate cancer – look to Denmark? J Natl Cancer Inst 88(2):128

Tseng M, Breslow RA, DeVellis RF et al (2004) Dietary patterns and prostate cancer risk in the National Health and Nutrition Examination Survey Epidemiological Follow-up Study cohort. Cancer Epidemiol Biomarkers Prev 13(1):71–77

UICC (International Union Against Cancer) (2002) TNM Classification of malignant tumours, 6th edn. Sobin LH, Wittekind Ch (eds) Wiley, New York

Vainio H (1999) Chemoprevention of cancer: a controversial and instructive story. Br Med Bull 55(3):593–599

van Leenders G (2007) Despite extensive efforts, the validation of prognostic tissue markers in prostate cancer has not yet resulted in the widespread implementation of novel diagnostic tests. Eur Urol 52(1):125

Velicer CM, Kristal A, White E (2006) Alcohol use and the risk of prostate cancer: results from the VITAL cohort study. Nutr Cancer 56(1):50–56

Verhoeven DT, Verhagen H, Goldbohm RA et al (1997) Review of mechanisms underlying anti-carcinogenesis by brassica vegetables. Chem Biol Interact 103:79–129

vom Saal FS, Timms BG, Montano MM et al (1997) Prostate enlargement in mice due to fetal exposure to low doses of estradiol or diethylstilbestrol and opposite effects at high doses. Proc Natl Acad Sci USA 94:2056–2061

Walker M, Aronson KJ, King W et al (2005) Dietary patterns and risk of prostate cancer in Ontario, Canada. Int J Cancer 116(4):592–598

Wallstrom P, Bjartell A, Gullberg B et al (2007) A prospective study on dietary fat and incidence of prostate cancer (Malmö, Sweden). Cancer Causes Control 18(10):1107–1121

Weigel NL (2007) Interactions between vitamin D and androgen receptor signaling in prostate cancer cells. Nutr Rev 65(8 Pt 2):S116–S117

Weinstein SJ, Wright ME, Lawson KA (2007) Serum and dietary vitamin E in relation to prostate cancer risk. Cancer Epidemiol Biomarkers Prev 16(6):1253–1259

Weiss JM, Huang WY, Rinaldi S et al (2007) IGF-1 and IGFBP-3: Risk of prostate cancer among men in the Prostate, Lung, Colorectal and Ovarian Cancer Screening Trial. Int J Cancer 121(10):2267–2273

West DW, Slattery ML, Robison LM et al (1991) Adult dietary intake and prostate cancer risk in Utah: a case-control study with special emphasis on aggressive tumors. Cancer Causes Control 2:85–94

Whitacre DC, Chauhan S, Davis T et al (2002) Androgen induction of in vitro prostate cell differentiation. Cell Growth Differ 13:1–11

Whittemore AS, Wu AH, Kolonel LN et al (1995) Family history and prostate cancer risk in black, white, and Asian men in the United States and Canada. Am J Epidemiol 141(8):732–740

Wilson JM, Jungner YG (1968) Principles and practice of mass screening for disease. Bol Oficina Sanit Panam 65(4):281–393

Wilt TJ (2008) SPCG-4: a needed START to PIVOTal data to promote and protect evidence-based prostate cancer care. J Natl Cancer Inst 100(16):1123–1125

Winter ML, Bosland MC, Wade DR et al (1995) Induction of benign prostatic hyperplasia in intact dogs by near-physiological levels of 5 alpha-dihydrotestosterone and 17 beta-estradiol. Prostate 26(6):325–333

Wiren S, Stocks T, Rinaldi S et al (2007) Androgens and prostate cancer risk: a prospective study. Prostate 67(11):1230–1237

Wright ME, Weinstein S, Lawson KA et al (2007a) Supplemental and dietary vitamin E intakes and risk of prostate cancer in a large prospective study. Cancer Epidemiol Biomarkers Prev 16(6):1128–1135

Wright ME, Chang SC, Schatzkin A et al (2007b) Prospective study of adiposity and weight change in relation to prostate cancer incidence and mortality. Cancer 109(4):675–684

Wu JD, Haugk K, Woodke L et al (2006a) Interaction of IGF signaling and the androgen receptor in prostate cancer progression. J Cell Biochem 99(2):392–401

Wu K, Hu FB, Willett WC (2006b) Dietary patterns and risk of prostate cancer in U.S. men. Cancer Epidemiol Biomarkers Prev 15(1):167–171

Yan L, Spitznagel EL (2005) Meta-analysis of soy food and risk of prostate cancer in men. Int J Cancer 117(4):667–669

Yasumaru M, Tsuji S, Tsujii M et al (2003) Inhibition of angiotensin II activity enhanced the antitumor effect of cyclooxygenase-2 inhibitors via insulin-like growth factor I receptor pathway. Cancer Res 63(20):6726–6734

Yatani R, Chigusa I, Akazaki K et al (1982) Geographic pathology of latent prostatic carcinoma. Int J Cancer 29:611–616

Zappa M, Ciatto S, Bonardi R et al (1998) Overdiagnosis of prostate carcinoma by screening: an estimate based on the results of the Florence Screening Pilot Study. Ann Oncol 9(12):1297–1300

Zeegers MP, Jellema A, Ostrer H (2003) Empiric risk of prostate carcinoma for relatives of patients with prostate carcinoma: a meta-analysis. Cancer 97(8):1894–1903

Zeegers MP, Dirx MJ, van den Brandt PA (2005) Physical activity and the risk of prostate cancer in the Netherlands cohort study, results after 9.3 years of follow-up. Cancer Epidemiol Biomarkers Prev 14(6):1490–1495

Zheng SL, Augustsson-Bälter K, Chang B et al (2004) Sequence variants of toll-like receptor 4 are associated with prostate cancer risk: results from the Cancer Prostate in Sweden Study. Cancer Res 64(8):2918–2922

Zheng SL, Liu W, Wiklund F et al (2006) A comprehensive association study for genes in inflammation pathway provides support for their roles in prostate cancer risk in the CAPS study. Prostate 66(14):1556–1564

Zhou JR, Blackburn GL (1997) Bridging animal and human studies: what are the missing segments in dietary fat and prostate cancer? Am J Clin Nutr 66:1572S–1580S

Chapter 2
The Epidemiology of Testicular Cancer

Katherine A. McGlynn and Michael B. Cook

2.1 Introduction

Testicular cancer is a rare tumor among the general population, but is the most common type of cancer among young men in many countries. The vast majority of testicular cancers are germ cell tumors. As a result, the terms "testicular cancer" and "testicular germ cell tumors" (TGCT) are often used interchangeably. Globally, the incidence of TGCT is highest among men of northern European ancestry and lowest among men of Asian and African descent. Incidence rates of TGCT have been increasing around the world for at least 50 years, but mortality rates, at least in developed countries, have been declining. While reasons for the decreases in mortality are related to improvements in therapeutic regimes introduced in the late 1970s, reasons for the increase in incidence are less well understood. An accumulating body of evidence suggests, however, that TGCT arises in fetal life. As the great majority of TGCTs arise among men between the ages of 15 and 44 years, this chapter will focus on the etiology of the tumors in this age group.

2.2 Histology and Precursor Lesions

Approximately 98% of all primary testicular cancers arise from germ cells. The remaining 2% include stromal tumors such as Leydig cell (~0.2%) and Sertoli cell tumors (~0.1%), as well as other more rare or poorly defined histologic types. Among testicular germ cell tumors (TGCTs), approximately 55% are classic seminomas, 44% are nonseminomas (embryonal carcinoma, teratoma, yolk sac tumor, choriocarcinoma), and 1% are spermatocytic seminomas.

K.A. McGlynn (✉)
Hormonal and Reproductive Epidemiology Branch, Division of Cancer Epidemiology and
Genetics, National Cancer Institute, NIH, DHHS, 6120 Executive Boulevard, Suite 550,
Bethesda, MD, [20852] 7234, USA
e-mail: mcglynnk@mail.nih.gov

W.D. Foulkes and K.A. Cooney (eds.), *Male Reproductive Cancers:*
Epidemiology, Pathology and Genetics, Cancer Genetics,
DOI 10.1007/978-1-4419-0449-2_2, © Springer Science+Business Media, LLC 2010

In 1972, Skakkebaek first proposed that testicular carcinoma in situ (CIS) was the precursor lesion for TGCT (Skakkebaek 1972). It is now generally accepted that CIS (also known as intratubular germ cell neoplasia, unclassified type or IGCNU) gives rise to all seminomas and nonseminomas of adolescents and young adults, but not to infantile nonseminomas or spermatocytic seminomas (Oosterhuis and Looijenga 2005). CIS cells have many features in common with primordial germ cells and early gonocytes, suggesting that CIS arises at a very early stage of development in cells that failed to differentiate properly (Rajpert-De Meyts et al. 1998). In contrast to the tumors of adolescents and young adults, infantile nonseminomas appear to arise directly from primordial germ cells or gonocytes (Almstrup et al. 2006) Spermatocytic seminomas, which largely occur in older men, appear to arise from premeiotic germ cells (Stoop et al. 2001). Both infantile nonseminomas and the spermatocytic seminomas of older men are thought to be etiologically distinct from the TGCTs that occur in young men and adolescents. For a detailed discussion of the pathology of testes cancer, see the chapter by Wojno and Bégin in this volume.

2.3   Incidence and Mortality

2.3.1   Incidence: Age Patterns

Unlike most types of cancer, the incidence of TGCT peaks in young adulthood. Eighty-four percent of TGCT occurs among men between the ages of 15 and 44 years, 15% occurs in men aged 45 years and older, while only 1% occurs in boys less than 15 years of age (Fig. 2.1). The incidence of nonseminoma peaks at approximately age 25 years, while the incidence of seminoma peaks 10 years later, at age 35 years. Among very young boys (0–4 years), nonseminomas are the sole histologic type of TGCT. In the U.S. SEER registries between 1973 and 2004, 67% of the nonseminomas in this young age group were yolk sac tumors, 17% were embryonal carcinomas, and 13% were teratomas (surveillance Epidemiology and End Results 2006).

2.3.2   Incidence: Racial and Geographic Patterns

In 2002, the global age-standardized incidence rate of testicular cancer was 1.5 per 100,000 men (Ferlay et al. 2004). In comparison, the age-standardized incidence rate of lung cancer, the most common tumor among men, was 35.5 per 100,000. In general, the incidence of testicular cancer is better correlated with ethnic/racial group than with geographic location. For example, the highest rates of testicular cancer in the world are in seen in populations of northern European ancestry, regardless of where they reside (Fig. 2.2). Scandinavian men, in particular Danish and Norwegian men, have rates five

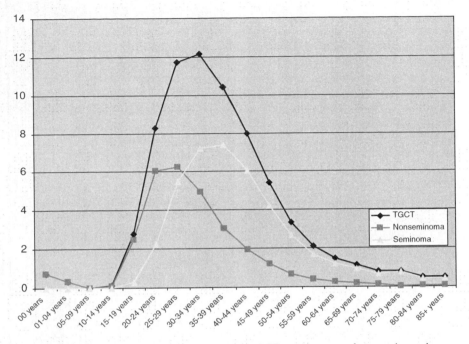

Fig. 2.1 Incidence of testicular germ cell tumors (TGCT), seminoma, and nonseminoma by age. SEER-9 registries, 1973–2005

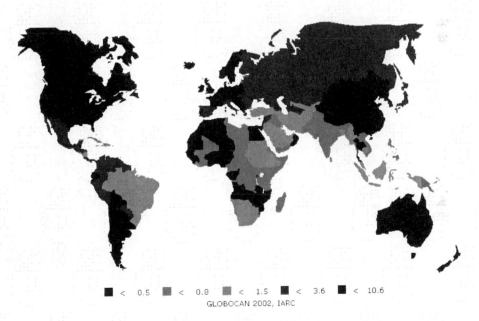

Fig. 2.2 Testis age-standardized incidence rate per 100,000

to ten times higher than men of African and Asian descent. In the great majority of countries with multiethnic populations, the incidence of TGCT among white men is appreciably higher than the incidence among men of other races and ethnicities. For example, in the United States, the incidence of TGCT between 1973 and 2004 among white men was 5.46 per 100,000. In contrast, the incidence among black men was 0.95 per 100,000, while the incidence among men of Native American or Asian ancestry was 2.05 per 100,000 (Shah et al. 2007). Similarly, in a comparison of incidence rates among South Africans, men of European ancestry had significantly higher rates than men of African ancestry (Coovadia 1978). One notable exception to this general pattern, however, is found in New Zealand where the incidence among Maori men (10.6 per 100,000 in 2002) is three times higher than the incidence among non-Maori men (3.5 per 100,000) (New Zealand Health Information Service 2006).

In addition to experiencing high absolute rates, men of European ancestry have seen the greatest increase in incidence over the last 50–70 years. An example occurs in the United States where testicular cancer incidence increased in white American men by 52% between 1973 and 1998. Similar increases in incidence among men of European heritage have been seen in Ontario (Weir et al. 1999), Norway (Wanderas et al. 1995), Denmark, Sweden, the former East Germany, Poland (Bergstrom et al. 1996), and Australia (Stone et al. 1991). Northern European rates began to increase among men born after 1920 (Bergstrom et al. 1996). Data from the Connecticut Tumor Registry mirror this observation among white American men, whose rates began to increase by the mid-1950s (Zheng et al. 1996). Recent reports suggest that incidence of TGCT, particularly of nonseminoma, may have begun to stabilize in some high-risk populations (McGlynn et al. 2003). In contrast, rates among African-American men, a low-risk population, appear to have begun increasing in the 1990s (McGlynn et al. 2005a).

In almost all populations studied, the increase in incidence has been found to be more consistent with a birth-cohort effect than with a calendar period effect (Bergstrom et al. 1996; Ekbom and Akre 1998; McGlynn et al. 2003). Dating back to at least the 1930s, incidence has generally increased with successive birth cohorts. A notable exception to the increase occurred among the cohort of men born in Denmark, Norway, and Sweden during the years surrounding World War II (1939–1945). The cohort-specific dip in risk has suggested that war-related deprivations were responsible (Moller 1989). In contrast, the cohort of men born in Poland, the former East Germany, and Finland, countries that, arguably, were even more affected by wartime deprivations, saw a continued increase in risk during the war years (Ekbom and Akre 1998). The overall pattern of increasing incidence only among specific ethnic and/or racial groups argues that there has either been an ethnic-specific change in a risk factor or that there has been a global change in a risk factor that only affects genetically susceptible ethnic groups. At this time, however, the factor or factors responsible for the increase in rates remain unidentified.

2.3.3 Mortality

The prognosis of TGCT since the late 1970s in developed countries has been very favorable, with a survival rate between 90 and 95% (Boyle 2004). Prior to that time, the survival rate was approximately 10%. The great improvement in a short period of time was largely due to the introduction of cisplatin-based therapy (Einhorn and Donohue 1977) and the appreciation of the combined management of disease (Peckham et al. 1979). As a result of these developments, mortality from TGCT has declined dramatically in most developed countries; examples being Denmark (Osterlind 1986), England and Wales (Power et al. 2001), Scotland (Boyle et al. 1987), Canada (Bertuccio et al. 2007), and the United States (Bertuccio et al. 2007). In contrast, mortality from TGCT remains elevated in countries where state-of-the-art therapy is unavailable; examples being many countries of Central and South America (Bertuccio et al. 2007), as well as countries of Southern and Eastern Europe (Bray et al. 2006).

2.3.4 Migrant Patterns

The majority of migrant studies of testicular cancer have found that first-generation migrants (i.e., foreign-born men of foreign-born parents) retain the risk of their home country, regardless of whether they migrate from low-risk to high-risk, or high-risk to low-risk, countries (Graham and Gibson 1972; McCredie et al. 1994; Swerdlow et al. 1995; Parkin and Iscovich 1997; Hemminki and Li 2002a; Ekbom et al. 2003). These findings support the hypothesis that TGCT risk is determined in early life, but do not distinguish between genetic and environmental effects. Studies of second-generation migrants (i.e., native-born men of foreign-born parents) have been limited by rather small numbers. In general, however, the studies have reported that second-generation men have risks similar to their parents' home countries (Graham and Gibson 1972; Parkin and Iscovich 1997; Hemminki and Li 2002a). The interpretation of the risks in second-generation men, however, is uncertain as many immigrant families retain customs from the parents' home country.

2.4 Associated Medical Conditions

A number of pre-existing medical conditions have been associated with the development of TGCT. These conditions include prior diagnosis of TGCT in the contralateral gonad (Coupland et al. 1999; Fossa et al. 2005), cryptorchism (Dieckmann and Pichlmeier 2004) impaired spermatogenesis, inguinal hernia (Gallagher et al. 1995; Coupland et al. 2004), hydrocele (Gallagher et al. 1995; Moller et al. 1996), prior testicular biopsy (Swerdlow et al. 1997b; Moller et al. 1998), atopy (Swerdlow et al. 1987b), testicular atrophy (Haughey et al. 1989; Oliver 1990; Moller et al. 1996), and microlithiasis (Ikinger et al. 1982). In 2001, Skakkebaek and colleagues proposed the existence of a Testicular Dysgenesis Syndrome (TDS) that included TGCT, impaired spermatogenesis, cryptorchism, and hypospadias (Skakkebaek et al. 2001). The proposal was based on reports that the four conditions appear to share some common risk factors, may originate during fetal life, and may have increased in incidence during the past several decades. At the current time, the existence of the syndrome remains largely hypothetical, though it has provided a good theoretical framework for ongoing research.

2.4.1 Cryptorchism

Cryptorchism, or undescended testis, is the antecedent medical condition most closely associated with TGCT (Osterlind et al. 1991; Colls et al. 1996; Wanderas et al. 1997; McMaster et al. 2006). The relative risk of TGCT among men with a prior diagnosis of cryptorchism has been estimated in various populations to be between 2.5 (Schottenfeld et al. 1980) and 17.0 (Coldman et al. 1982). A recent meta-analysis of 20 case-control studies, however, estimated the overall relative risk to be 4.8 (95%CI: 4.0–5.7) (Dieckmann and Pichlmeier 2004). Nevertheless, only 10% of testicular cancers develop in men with cryptorchism (United Kingdom Testicular Cancer Andy Group 1994a). Whether cryptorchism itself predisposes to cancer or whether the two outcomes share common risk factors is not well understood. Evidence suggesting that the two conditions may simply share a common etiology is that 10–25% of men with unilateral cryptorchism develop TGCT in the contralateral gonad (Batata et al. 1982). In addition, both conditions have been associated in some studies with common risk factors such as low birth weight, premature birth, and the presence of other gonadal anomalies (Moller and Skakkebaek 1996). Several reports have noted no ethnic discrepancy in the incidence of cryptorchism among newborns, despite that fact that the rate of TGCT is five times as great in European-American men as in African-American men (Berkowitz et al. 1995; McGlynn et al. 2005a) In addition, Kallmann Syndrome, a condition of congenital hypogonadotropic hypogonadism, is characterized by cryptorchism, but not by testicular cancer (Ginsburg 1997). Arguing, however, that the condition of cryptorchism is itself risk-producing is the observation in some studies that orchiopexy (i.e., surgical repair of cryp-torchism) prior to 10 years of age substantially reduces the risk of TGCT (United Kingdom Testicular Cancer Study Group 1994a; Pettersson et al. 2007b). In whatever way the two outcomes are related, it is clear that cryptorchism itself cannot explain the increase in TGCT. Although the prevalence of cryptorchism has been reported by some studies to have increased between the 1950s and the 1980s, the proportion of testicular cancer patients with cryptorchism appears to have remained constant at approximately 10% (Chilvers and Pike 1989).

2.4.2   Subfertility

Prospective studies have demonstrated that subfertility precedes diagnosis of, and likely transformation to, TGCT (Lass et al. 1998; Petersen et al. 1999; Jacobsen et al. 2000; Raman et al. 2005). Whether temporal trends in subfertility are correlated with trends in TGCT, however, has been a matter of some controversy. A meta-analysis of 61 studies of sperm counts concluded in 1992 that there had been a global decline in semen quality over the previous 50 years (Carlsen et al. 1992). The study's conclusions and methodology were the subject of some debate, however (Olsen et al. 1995; Fisch and Goluboff 1996; Fisch et al. 1996; Lerchl and Nieschlag 1996; Becker and Berhane 1997; Swan et al. 1997). Subsequent research on the topic has proven inconclusive, with some studies reporting significant decreases in sperm count, some studies reporting no decreases, and some reporting increases (Safe 2000). While the accumulated research has been unable to reach consensus on whether sperm counts are declining, it has amply demonstrated that there is great diversity in sperm counts, both geographically and temporally.

2.4.3   Microlithiasis

Testicular microlithiasis is characterized by multiple microcalcifications found within the seminiferous tubules. This asymptomatic, nonprogressive disease was first linked to testicular cancer by Ikinger et al. (1982) and has subsequently been found to be present in 2.4–5.6% of asymptomatic men (Peterson et al. 2001; Serter et al. 2006). Interestingly, the prevalence of testicular microlithiasis is higher in African American (14.1%) than white men (4.3%) (Peterson et al. 2001), which is the converse trend of testicular cancer risk in these ethnic groups (McGlynn et al. 2003).

There have been many reports of concomitant presentation of testicular microlithiasis and testicular cancer (Cast et al. 2000; Bach et al. 2001; Lam et al. 2007), while numerous case reports have described patients who have received a diagnosis of testicular cancer subsequent to that of microlithiasis (Pourbagher et al. 2005). Some prospective studies, however, have not found an increased testicular cancer risk in men with microlithiasis (Ganem et al. 1999; Bennett et al. 2001; Lam et al. 2007); others have (Derogee et al. 2001; Otite et al. 2001; von Eckardstein et al. 2001). Testicular CIS, the precursor lesion of TGCT, has also been shown to be associated with microlithiasis (Lenz et al. 1996; von Eckardstein et al. 2001; Holm et al. 2003). However, the extent, location, and laterality of testicular microlithiasis have been shown not to correlate with the presence or absence of testicular cancer (Backus et al. 1994). Testicular microlithiasis likely represents a condition which has a shared etiology with testicular cancer and may be a marker of general testicular dysgenesis, given its reported associations with cryptorchidism (Renshaw 1998), subfertility (von Eckardstein et al. 2001), and other benign conditions (Nistal et al. 2006). For a further discussion of microlithiasis and testes cancer risk, see the chapter by Rapley in this volume.

2.5   Perinatal Risk Factors

In recent years, the theory that TGCT is initiated in very early life has spurred a great deal of interest in perinatal factors. While a number of associations have been examined, factors that have received particular attention include birth weight, gestational age, maternal age, maternal smoking, maternal parity, birth order, and sibship size.

2.5.1   Birth Weight and Gestational Age

Low birth weight has been reported to be associated with TGCT risk by a number of studies (Depue et al. 1983; Brown et al. 1986; Akre et al. 1996; Moller and Skakkebaek 1997; Ahlgren et al. 2007). A recent meta-analysis, however, found only modest statistical support for the relationship, estimating the overall odds ratio to be 1.28 (95%CI = 0.99–1.65) (Richiardi et al. 2007). High birth weight has also been associated with TGCT in at least one study (Richiardi et al. 2002), although the majority of studies have not supported a relationship (Richiardi et al. 2007) A factor closely related to low birth weight, decreased gestational age, has also been associated with increased TGCT risk (Gershman and Stolley 1988; Richiardi et al. 2002; Coupland et al. 2004). Disentangling the effects of birth weight and gestational age, however, has proven to be challenging, particularly as gestational age is often imprecisely recorded (Klebanoff 2007). A combination of birth weight and gestational age, size-for-gestational-age, may be a better measure of risk than either factor alone (Richiardi et al. 2002).

2.5.2   Maternal Age

Maternal age has been reported to be both inversely (Dieckmann et al. 2001; Coupland et al. 2004; Aschim et al. 2006) and directly (Moller and Skakkebaek 1997; Sabroe and Olsen 1998; Wanderas et al. 1998; English et al. 2003) associated with risk. In addition, several studies have reported no association (Swerdlow et al. 1982; Weir et al. 2000). The results, however, are not necessarily contradictory as it is conceivable there is a U-shaped relationship between maternal age and TGCT risk, such that risk is increased in association with both younger (<20) and older (≥30) maternal age.

2.5.3   Maternal Parity, Birth Order, Sibship Size

Low maternal parity and low birth order have been associated with increased TGCT risk in some (Swerdlow et al. 1987a; Prener et al. 1992; Sabroe and Olsen 1998; Westergaard et al. 1998; Richiardi et al. 2004), but not all (Dieckmann et al. 2001;

Richiardi et al. 2002; Coupland et al. 2004; Aschim et al. 2006) studies. Studies that have reported finding a link between TGCT and low birth order estimate a risk of two-thirds for sons born third or later, compared to first-born sons. The causal link between low maternal parity and TGCT risk has been speculated to be due to higher maternal estrogen levels in primiparous mothers (Sharpe 2003) but other explanations, such as late exposure to a common infectious agent or a different psychosocial environment, are also possible.

Sibship size has also been considered in relation to TGCT risk and is likely to be a proxy for other exposures distinct from those related to birth order. A large Swedish study, investigating sibship size and risk of all solid tumors, found a risk ratio of 0.71 (95%CI: 0.62–0.82) for testicular cancer for five or more siblings versus none (Altieri and Hemminki 2007). Some previous studies have found similar associations (Morrison 1976b; Swerdlow et al. 1987a; Richiardi et al. 2004) while others have not (Prener et al. 1992; Moller and Skakkebaek 1996; Dieckmann et al. 2001). The high correlation between sibship size and birth order makes the independent effect of each difficult to distinguish, but a large stratified analysis indicated that both variables are independent risk factors (Richiardi et al. 2004). The estrogen hypothesis does not fully explain the association of TGCT risk with sibship size, and does not account for parental subfertility, which has been proposed to be the causal factor of this relationship (Swerdlow et al. 1987a). Lastly, a decline over time in the association of sibship size and TGCT risk may be due to decreasing sensitivity of sibship size as a proxy for fertility, which may have resulted from increased reproductive control offered by technological advances and increased accessibility to contraception and assisted reproductive techniques (Richiardi et al. 2004).

2.5.4 Maternal Smoking

An examination of parallel trends in rates of testicular cancer and female lung and bladder cancers led Clemmesen (1997) to hypothesize that maternal cigarette smoking was a risk factor for TGCT. Clemmesen also suggested that the maternal smoking hypothesis was consistent with the dip in TGCT risk among men born during World War II in Denmark (Moller 1989). Using a similar ecologic design, Pettersson et al. (2004) found a correlation between the prevalence of smoking among young women and testicular cancer incidence in Sweden, Norway, and Denmark, though not in Finland. In contrast to the ecologic studies, the maternal smoking hypothesis has not been supported by retrospective studies (Henderson et al. 1979; Brown et al. 1986; Swerdlow et al. 1987a; Moller 1996; Weir et al. 2000; Coupland et al. 2004; McGlynn et al. 2006; Pettersson et al. 2007a). It seems unlikely, therefore, that maternal smoking is a risk factor for TGCT. It remains possible, however, that lung cancer in mothers and testicular cancer in sons cluster in families due to a common genetic mechanism rather than to a common environmental exposure.

2.5.5   Other Perinatal Factors

A number of other perinatal factors have occasionally been associated with risk for testicular cancer. These factors for which there is some evidence of association include hormonae use during pregnancy (Depue et al. 1983; Weir et al. 2000), bleeding during pregnancy (Brown et al. 1986; Weir et al. 2000), maternal body weight (Depue et al. 1983; Aschim et al. 2005), maternal socioeconomic status (Moller and Skakkebaek 1996), breech presentation (Coupland et al. 2004), twin birth (Dieckmann et al. 2001; Hemminki and Li 2002b), and trisomy 21 (Down syndrome) (Aschim et al. 2006; Patja et al. 2006). The evidence for hyperemesis gravidarum (Coupland et al. 2004; Aschim et al. 2006), Cesarean section (Moller and Skakkebaek 1997), and having been breastfed (Coupland et al. 2004) is unclear. At present, there is little evidence that paternal age (English et al. 2003; Richiardi et al. 2004), birth length (English et al. 2003; Aschim et al. 2006), pre-eclampsia (Richiardi et al. 2002), circumcision (Swerdlow et al. 1987b), varicocele (Gallagher et al. 1995; Moller et al. 1996), and neonatal jaundice (Richiardi et al. 2002) are associated with TGCT.

2.6   Maternal Endogenous Hormones

Indirect evidence suggests that the intrauterine hormonal milieu may affect the risk of TGCT. For example, excessive nausea early in pregnancy, reported by some studies to increase the risk of TGCT (Petridou et al. 1997), is believed to be due to increased estrogen levels. Similarly, the increased risk reported among first-born sons and dizygotic twins may be related to higher maternal estrogen levels in these pregnancies (Bernstein et al. 1986). Maternal obesity, a condition consistent with decreased sex-hormone-binding globulin (SHBG) levels and increased free estrogen levels, has also been associated with TGCT risk (Henderson et al. 1988b). Because of these associations, the "estrogen hypothesis" of TGCT was formally introduced in 1993 (Sharpe and Skakkebaek 1993). A complementary hypothesis has suggested that high maternal estrogen levels may not be as culpable as low maternal testosterone levels (Henderson et al. 1988a). This hypothesis was based on the observation that African-American women had higher testosterone levels in pregnancy than white American women (Henderson et al. 1988a). The direct evidence to support the maternal hormone hypotheses, however, has not been great due to the difficulty in examining the relationship between maternal hormone levels and risk of cancer among children 30 years later. Several studies, however, have examined maternal hormone levels in relationship to cryptorchism (Burton et al. 1987; Bernstein et al. 1988; Key et al. 1996; McGlynn et al. 2005b). The results of these studies, in general, have not supported either the maternal estrogen or the maternal androgen hypothesis.

2.7 Maternal Exogenous Hormones

Diethylstilbestrol (DES), a nonsteroidal estrogen first synthesized in 1938, is several times more potent than the endogenous estrogen, 17β-estradiol. In 1947, the U.S. Food and Drug Administration approved the use of DES in pregnant women to prevent threatened or recurrent abortion. Although it was known by 1953 that DES was ineffective for this purpose (Dieckmann et al. 1953), prescription of DES continued in the U.S. until 1971 and in Europe until 1978. In the U.S., an estimated five to ten million persons were exposed either during pregnancy or while in utero (Noller and Fish 1974).

In mice, in utero DES exposure results in numerous testicular defects including cryptorchism, inflammation, hyperplasia, and adenocarcinoma of the rete testis (Newbold et al. 1985). In humans, several case reports have noted the occurrence of testicular cancer in sons of DES-exposed mothers (Loughlin et al. 1980), and a multicenter study reported a nonsignificant threefold risk of TGCT based on seven cases in the exposed group and two cases in the nonexposed group (Strohsnitter et al. 2001). Other researchers have reported conflicting results (Depue et al. 1983; Moss et al. 1986; Gershman and Stolley 1988) and reviews of the literature have concluded, in general, that the supporting data are equivocal (Giusti et al. 1995). Other disorders of the male reproductive tract, such as hypospadias, cryptorchism, and impaired fertility, have also not been strongly linked to DES exposure (Storgaard et al. 2006). The Danish experience of low exposure to DES in the 1950s, yet greatly increasing TGCT rates, argues that DES alone is unlikely to explain the increase in incidence (Buetow 1995).

2.8 Endocrine-Disrupting Chemicals

Arguably the most hotly debated topic in testicular cancer, at present, is whether there is an association with endocrine-disrupting chemicals (EDCs) (Golden et al. 1998). EDCs have been defined as exogenous agents that interfere with the production, release, transport, metabolism, binding, action, or elimination of the natural hormones in the body responsible for the maintenance of homeostasis and the regulation of developmental processes (Kavlock et al. 1996). EDCs include compounds that are estrogenic (e.g., isoflavones, phthalates, o,p'-DDT, o,p'-DDE, bisphenol A, alkylphenols, some PCBs), antiestrogenic (e.g., dibenzo-p-dioxin, tributyltin, some PCBs), antiandrogenic (e.g., vincolzolin, p,p'-DDE, methoxychlor, dibenzo-p-dioxin, flutamide, linuron, natural pyrethrin, tris (4-chlorophenyl)-methanol), and antigestagenic (e.g., carbamate) (Pflieger-Bruss et al. 2004). Of these chemicals, groups that have received particular attention in regard to male reproductive disorders are the persistent organochlorine pesticides (POPs) (e.g., aldrin, dieldrin, endrin, dichlorodiphenyltrichloroethane (DDT), dichlorodiphenyldichloroethylene (DDE)) and the polychlorinated biphenyls (PCBs).

POPs and PCBs act as either weak estrogens or antiandrogens by binding to the estrogen and androgen receptors (Toppari et al. 1996). While the early focus of attention was on the ability of these compounds to act as weak estrogens, subsequent reports highlighted the capability of some compounds to act as antiandrogens. As noted by Kelce et al. (1995), p,p'-DDE, a persistent metabolite of DDT, is a potent androgen receptor antagonist. Consistent with this finding is the observation that most of the EDC effects noted in animals have affected the males of experimental animal species rather than the females.

None of the EDCs appear to bind to sex-hormone-binding globulin, and thus, may be capable of increasing total estrogen activity. As DES was hundreds to thousands of times more potent than any known EDC, it has been argued that it would be unlikely to see outcomes associated with the EDCs that were not associated with DES (Golden et al. 1998). However, it can also be argued that the net combined estrogenic effects of EDCs may exceed those of DES. In support of an effect independent of the estrogen and androgen receptors, it was recently reported that two organochlorine pesticides, toxaphene and chlordane, were capable of binding to the estrogen-related receptor α-1 orphan receptor and modulating aromatase activity (Yang and Chen 1999). If EDC exposure is capable of producing the postulated spectrum of effects seen among the TDS disorders, it seems likely that the exposure would have to be early in gestational life (Parker 1997).

Thus far, only one epidemiologic study of EDCs and TGCT has been reported (Hardell et al. 2003). In an examination of 58 TGCT cases and 61 controls and their respective mothers ($n = 35$ case mothers, 22 control mothers) in Sweden, Hardell et al. found that cases had significantly higher levels of cis-Nonachlor than did controls. Mothers of cases had significantly higher levels of cis-nonachlor, as well as trans-nonachlor, hexachlorobenzene and the sum of polychlorinated biphenyl congeners. When the mothers' levels were examined separately by the histology of the sons' tumors (seminoma, nonseminoma), all four of the noted results remained significant in the nonseminoma group, but not in the seminoma group (Hardell et al. 2004). Whether histologic differences truly exist, however, is uncertain as there were small numbers of tumors in each group after stratification.

In addition to the one TGCT study, several, mostly small, studies of EDCs and cryptorchism and/or hypospadias have been reported from around the world. One study of cryptorchism reported that hexachlorobenzene was significantly associated with risk (Hosie et al. 2000), though the finding was not supported by two subsequent studies (Waliszewski et al. 2005; Pierik et al. 2007) Heptachloroepoxide has been associated with risk in one study (Hosie et al. 2000), but not in another (Pierik et al. 2007). In addition, trans-Nonachlor (Damgaard et al. 2006), but not β hexachlorocyclohexane (Waliszewski et al. 2005; Pierik et al. 2007) has been associated with risk of cryptorchism. Little support for an association of DDT or DDE with risk of cryptorchism and hypospadias has been offered by four studies (Longnecker et al. 2002; Flores-Luevano et al. 2003; Bhatia et al. 2005; Waliszewski et al. 2005). In sum, the evidence to support a link between EDCs and testicular cancer or cryptorchism in humans is equivocal. Larger studies of both outcomes will be required to determine whether an association exists.

2.9   Postnatal Risk Factors

2.9.1   Anthropometry

A number of studies have examined associations between body mass index (BMI) and/or height and TGCT. While two studies found an inverse relationship with BMI (Petridou et al. 1997; Akre et al. 2000) and one study found a direct relationship (Garner et al. 2003) most studies have reported no association (Whittemore et al. 1984; Davies et al. 1990; Thune and Lund 1994; United Kingdom Testicular Cancer Study Group 1994a; Gallagher et al. 1995; Srivastava and Kreiger 2000; Dieckmann and Pichlmeier 2002; Rasmussen et al. 2003; Richiardi et al. 2003; Bjorge et al. 2006; McGlynn et al. 2007). Height, in contrast, has been positively associated with risk in the majority of studies in which it has been examined. Of at least 13 studies reported in the English language literature, seven reported significant positive associations (Gallagher et al. 1995; Akre et al. 2000; Dieckmann and Pichlmeier 2002; Rasmussen et al. 2003; Richiardi et al. 2003; Bjorge et al. 2006; McGlynn et al. 2007). An additional two studies reported nonsignificant positive associations (Swerdlow et al. 1989; United Kingdom Testicular Cancer Study Group 1994a), while four studies reported no association (Whittemore et al. 1984; Davies et al. 1990; Thune and Lund 1994; Petridou et al. 1997). Overall, the bulk of the evidence suggests that taller men are at increased risk of TGCT. As height is a complex trait determined by both genetic and environmental influences, the reason that height is related to TGCT remains to be elucidated. It has been suggested, however, that the association may be related to childhood nutrition (Gallagher et al. 1995), age at puberty (Akre et al. 2000), and/or individual variation in the insulin-like growth factor I system (Zavos et al. 2004).

2.9.2   Age at Puberty

While younger age at puberty has been reported to increase TGCT risk (Moss et al. 1986; United Kingdom Testicular Cancer Study Group 1994a), most studies have found, conversely, that older age at puberty decreases risk (Swerdlow et al. 1989; United Kingdom Testicular Cancer Study Group 1994a; Gallagher et al. 1995; Moller and Skakkebaek 1996; Weir et al. 1998; Coupland et al. 1999). As later age at puberty tends to result in greater height, the associations of puberty and height with TGCT risk are not likely to be mediated by a common pathway.

2.9.3   Nutrition

A nutritional etiology of TGCT has not been examined extensively; however associations have been reported for diets high in fat and total calories (Armstrong and Doll 1975; Sigurdson et al. 1999), and high in consumption of dairy foods, particularly milk and cheese (Decarli and La Vecchia 1986; Davies et al. 1996; Ganmaa et al. 2002; Garner et al. 2003). It has been suggested that the dairy food-TGCT association might arise from naturally occurring or synthetic hormones in dairy products (Ganmaa et al. 2002). No relationship, however has been found between dietary phytoestrogen intake and TGCT (Walcott et al. 2002). It is also possible that an association between dairy food consumption and TGCT might appear to exist because populations with the highest risks of TGCT, northern Europeans, are the populations least likely to suffer from lactose intolerance. The association between taller stature and TGCT, suggests that any association with diet is likely to be with diet in early life.

2.9.4   Endogenous Hormones in Men

The suggestion that exogenous endocrine modulators may affect risk of TGCT raises the question of whether endogenous hormones might also affect risk. This has been a difficult question to address because of the retrospective nature of most TGCT studies. Several studies, however, have compared endogenous hormone levels of men prior to orchiectomy with levels in control men (Petersen et al. 1999). In general, these studies have found that men with TGCT have higher follicle-stimulating hormone (FSH) levels and somewhat lower testosterone levels than do control men. Studies in cryptorchid men have reported a similar hormonal milieu (Lee et al. 1998). The associations of reduced body muscle mass and reduced frequency of baldness among men with TGCT have also suggested that testosterone levels in TGCT patients may be in the lower end of the spectrum (Petridou et al. 1997; Walcott et al. 2002). Similarly, evidence that severe acne during adolescence may be inversely related to TGCT, has suggested that higher testosterone levels are protective (Depue et al. 1983; Walcott et al. 2002). The observations of high FSH and low testosterone have suggested that TGCT arises in a state of "gonadotropin overdrive" in which the testes have lost the ability to respond to gonadotropins (Oliver 1990). Arguing the importance of hypersecretion of gonadotropins in TGCT is the observation that men with low levels of gonadotropins (e.g., men with hypogonadotropic hypogonadism) rarely develop TGCT despite their high rate of cryptorchism.

2.9.5   Physical Activity

Two case-control studies have reported that childhood physical activity is inversely associated with development of TGCT (United Kingdom Testicular Cancer Study Group 1994b; Gallagher et al. 1995). The United Kingdom Testicular Cancer Study Group (1994b) found that participating in various sports at age 16, 20 years, or 1 year prior to diagnosis was protective. An inverse relationship between recreational activity and TGCT risk was also reported by a Canadian study (Gallagher et al. 1995). Three further studies found no association with TGCT (Paffenbarger et al. 1987; Dosemeci et al. 1993; Thune and Lund 1994), although two of these studies had fewer than 50 cases (Paffenbarger et al. 1987; Thune and Lund 1994) and the third study based physical activity solely on adult occupational history (Dosemeci et al. 1993) and may, therefore, have missed the exposure time window of importance for TGCT risk. Only one study has reported that physical activity and TGCT risk are positively associated (Srivastava and Kreiger 2000). Analyzing data from 212 cases, the study found that moderate and strenuous recreational activity levels during the midteens approximately doubled risk of TGCT. Overall, however, the evidence suggests that increased childhood physical activity and TGCT risk are inversely associated.

2.9.6   Socioeconomic Status and Urban/Rural Residence

Early studies indicated that higher socioeconomic status was associated with an increased risk of testicular cancer (Ross et al. 1979; Depue et al. 1983; Office of Population Censuses and Surveys (OPCS) 1993), while more current studies are indicative of no association (Moller and Skakkebaek 1996; Coupland et al. 2004). These observations may be explained by a recent study from Finland which suggests that testicular cancer rates of different socioeconomic classes are converging, causing the association of socioeconomic status and testicular cancer to diminish (Pukkala and Weiderpass 2002).

Evidence that TGCT risk shares an association with urban/rural residence is conflicting. Some studies have reported that rural residence significantly increases TGCT risk (Lipworth and Dayan 1969; Talerman et al. 1974), while other studies have found only nonsignificantly increased risk estimates for rural residence (Graham et al. 1977; United Kingdom Testicular Cancer Study Group 1994b; Petridou et al. 1997). Conversely, some studies have found no association with urban/rural dwelling (Sonneveld et al. 1999; Toledano et al. 2001) and two studies found higher TGCT risk in urban populations (Moller 1997; Huyghe et al. 2003). Although various methodologies for assigning urban/rural status have been employed by these studies, there remains a lack of consensus on whether residence is associated with risk. Quantitation of more specific exposures associated with these locales may be a better strategy to further elucidate any potential relationship.

2.9.7   Occupation

While there have been many analyses of occupation in relation to testicular cancer, no single profession has yet been unanimously endorsed as a risk factor. Occupational groups suggested to be at increased risk of TGCT, at least by some studies, are firefighters (Stang et al. 2003; Bates 2007) metal workers (Rhomberg et al. 1995; Pollan et al. 2001), leather workers (Marshall et al. 1990), and aircraft technicians (Foley et al. 1995; Ryder et al. 1997) Agricultural workers (Moller 1997; Hardell et al. 1998) have also been reported to be at increased risk, possibly due to pesticide exposure (Fleming et al. 1999; Guo et al. 2005). Positive associations have also been found with unionized carpenters (Dement et al. 2003), paper mill maintenance employees (Andersson et al. 2003), and writers (Knight et al. 1996). A reduced risk among concrete workers has also been observed (Knutsson et al. 2000).

Occupational exposure to extreme temperatures (Zhang et al. 1995) has been associated with increased testicular cancer risk. The evidence remains unclear whether exposure to dimethylformamide (Ducatman et al. 1986; Levin et al. 1987; Calvert et al. 1990; International Agency for Research on Cancer 1999) or magnetic fields (Floderus et al. 1999; Baumgardt-Elms et al. 2002) increases risk. Occupational exposure to cellular or cordless telephones (Hardell et al. 2007), ionizing radiation (Sont et al. 2001), PVC plastics (Westberg et al. 2005), or diesel or gasoline exhaust fumes (Guo et al. 2004) does not appear to alter risk. In general, white collar workers have been found to be at higher risk of TGCT than blue collar workers; thus, observed occupational associations may be confounded by socioeconomic status (Van den Eeden et al. 1991). In summary, although some occupations and their generic hazards have been associated with TGCT risk, the evidence has been too inconsistent and sparse to identify any specific exposure of importance.

2.9.8   Viruses

An infectious etiology of testicular cancer was first suggested based on epidemiologic similarities with Hodgkin disease (Newell et al. 1984). Using paralytic polio as a model, the authors hypothesized that viral infections in late childhood or adolescence might induce adverse tissue responses that would lead to these cancers in young adulthood. Further support for a viral etiology has been the observation that men infected with human immunodeficiency virus (HIV) have an increased risk of testicular cancer (Logothetis et al. 1985; Gabutti et al. 1995; Lyter et al. 1995; Goedert et al. 1998; Frisch et al. 2001) and that other cancers over-represented in HIV(+) individuals are linked to viral infections (e.g., Kaposi sarcoma and human herpes virus 8 (HHV-8); non-Hodgkin lymphoma and Epstein-Barr virus (EBV)). While a number of studies have examined viral antibody titers in TGCT, few have had adequate power to test the hypotheses (Algood et al. 1988; Mueller et al. 1988; Akre et al. 1999). Though infection with the mumps virus is known to cause orchitis in 20–30% of postpubertal males and sterility in a smaller subset, a relationship with testicular cancer has not been clearly demonstrated (Brown et al. 1987; Mueller et al. 1988). Candidate viruses implicated by several studies are EBV and cytomegalovirus (CMV) (Algood et al. 1988; Mueller et al. 1988; Akre et al. 1999). Both viruses are members of the herpes family and are known to cause p53 overexpression, a common finding in TGCT (Muganda et al. 1994). In addition, both viruses have been demonstrated to have oncogenic potential (Morris et al. 1995) and CMV infection during pregnancy, in several case reports, has been associated with cryptorchism. Conversely, at least one study reported that mononucleosis, a manifestation of EBV infection, had an inverse association with TGCT risk (Moss et al. 1986).

One of the more intriguing findings in TGCT has been the observation that many TGCTs express endogenous retroviruses. Human endogenous retroviruses (HERVs), with similarities to exogenous retroviruses known to cause disease in animals, constitute approximately 0.1–0.6% of the human genome (Leib-Mosch et al. 1990). Although most HERVs are defective due to multiple stop codons, recent research indicates that some members of the class II HERV family retain some of their original retroviral functions. For example, HERV sequences are expressed in several tissues and cell lines (Lower et al. 1996) and some encode particles released from teratocarcinoma cell lines (Lower et al. 1993). In addition antibodies specific for the HERV-K10 *gag* and *env* proteins have been identified in patients with seminomas (Sauter et al. 1995). HERV-K transcripts have now been detected in most types of testicular germ cell tumors, as well as in CIS and in the gonocytes of dysgenetic gonads (Herbst et al. 1998). The reason that HERV-K is turned on and the significance of HERV-K expression in TGCT are not understood. It may simply be an epiphenomenon, as suggested by the stimulation of HERV expression by female steroid hormones in a breast cancer cell line (Ono et al. 1987). Immunodeficiency of the host does not appear to be adequate to induce HERV-K10 expression, however, as HIV(+) men are no more likely to have HERV-K antibodies than HIV(−) men (Goedert et al. 1999). As has been demonstrated with other TGCT tumor markers (i.e., human chorionic gonadotropin and alphafetoprotein), HERV-K expression resolves on excision of the tumor. Whether the 60% of TGCT patients who have antibodies to HERV-K10 (Goedert et al. 1999) have different risk factor patterns than the TGCT patients who do not have antibodies has not been previously examined.

2.9.9 Other Factors

Increased TGCT risk has also been reported in association with testicular trauma (Brown et al. 1987; Haughey et al. 1989; Coupland et al. 1999). Some early evidence that increased scrotal temperatures, perhaps due to tight outer- or underwear, might be related to risk (Haughey et al. 1989), has not received wide support by most studies (Brown et al. 1987; Karagas et al. 1989; United Kingdom Testicular Cancer Study Group 1994a). It remains unclear whether testicular torsion (Chilvers et al. 1987; Moller et al. 1996) or having had a history of at least one sexually transmitted disease (United Kingdom Testicular Cancer Study Group 1994b; Moller and Skakkebaek 1999; Husson and Herrinton 2003) are risk factors for TGCT.

2.10   Histologic Difference in Risk Factors

A number of studies have examined whether there are differences in risk factors between seminomas and nonseminomas. As noted by Moller and colleagues (1993), it is unlikely that substantial differences in risk factors exist between tumors of various histologies because of the similarity in incidence trends. In addition, mixed tumors composed of both seminoma and nonseminoma elements are not uncommon. The majority of risk factor analyses stratified by histologic group also appear to support a shared etiopathogenesis for seminomas and nonseminomas (Moss et al. 1986; Pike et al. 1987; Prener et al. 1992, 1996; Moller and Skakkebaek 1997; Hardell et al. 1998; Sabroe and Olsen 1998; Weir et al. 2000). Nevertheless, there is some evidence that certain factors may be more strongly associated with one histologic type or the other. Several studies have reported that cryptorchidism (Morrison 1976a; Stone et al. 1991; Prener et al. 1996; Coupland et al. 1999), low birth weight (Wanderas et al. 1998; English et al. 2003), and low birth order (Sabroe and Olsen 1998; Richiardi et al. 2004) are factors predominantly associated with an increased risk of seminoma. Moreover, participation in specific sporting activities (Coupland et al. 1999) and long gestational duration (Richiardi et al. 2002) may be more protective against seminoma (Coupland et al. 1999). Risk factors primarily associated with an increased risk of nonseminoma include testicular trauma (Stone et al. 1991; Coupland et al. 1999), history of at least one sexually transmitted disease (Coupland et al. 1999), younger age at shaving initiation (McGlynn et al. 2007), and short gestational duration (Richiardi et al. 2002). In addition, later puberty may have a stronger protective effect against nonseminoma than seminoma (Moss et al. 1986; Moller and Skakkebaek 1996; Coupland et al. 1999). The literature as a whole, however, is not congruent for any one of these histologic dissimilarities.

2.11   Family and Twin Studies

Study of familial clustering of testicular cancer has been somewhat limited by the relative rarity of the disease. Nevertheless, it has been reported that in comparison with men in the general population, the risk of testicular cancer is eightfold higher in brothers and fourfold higher in sons of affected men (Dieckmann and Pichlmeier 1997; Hemminki and Li 2004; Hemminki and Chen 2006). In order for an environmental exposure to fully account for such an observation, the exposure would have to be perfectly shared among siblings and to increase risk by more than tenfold (Khoury et al. 1988). The higher familial risk among brothers of cases, compared to fathers, is consistent with that a recessive mode of inheritance or a susceptibility locus on the X gene. Evidence supporting a recessive model was reported from a segregation analysis of 978 Scandinavian testicular cancer patients and their families, although a dominant model could not be conclusively ruled out (Heimdal et al. 1997). A similar inference was derived from an analysis of bilateral disease

(Nicholson and Harland 1995). Both studies estimated a risk of disease among homozygotes at 45%. Less evidence for a dominant mode of inheritance, however, may simply reflect that paternal transmission may have been significantly hampered in earlier generations. Prior to the introduction of cisplatin as a chemotherapeutic agent in the late 1970s (Einhorn and Donohue 1977) the poor prognosis for metastatic disease made it likely that affected individuals would not live long enough to reproduce. In addition, reduced fertility is associated both with the cancer itself and with its treatment (1994a). Regardless of whether a greater risk is associated with an affected brother or an affected father, a relative risk of 6–10 is consistent with the involvement of predisposing genes (Hopper and Carlin 1992).

Compared to the general population, it has been reported that testicular cancer risk is increased among twins (Dieckmann et al. 2001; Hemminki and Li 2002b). The standardized incidence ratio of risk in men with an affected cotwin is estimated to be 37.5 (95%CI: 12.3–115.6), which is dramatically higher than the eightfold risk cited for men with an affected brother (Swerdlow et al. 1997a). When comparing monozygous vs. dizygous twins, studies have consistently reported that the risk of TGCT, particularly of seminoma, is higher in dizygous twins (Braun et al. 1995; Swerdlow et al. 1997a; Hemminki and Chen 2005). Such a finding argues against a genetic etiology and may support the "estrogen hypothesis" as maternal estrogen levels may be higher in dizygous births due to the existence of two placentae (Sharpe 2003). Alternatively, it has been suggested that hypersecretion of FSH could be linked to TGCT in sons as mothers of dizygotic twins have a genetic tendency to hypersecrete which may be a heritable trait (Lambalk and Boomsma 1998). In support of this postulate, it has been demonstrated that some men undergoing surgery for testicular cancer have higher FSH levels than unaffected men (Satge et al. 1997). In addition, men with Down syndrome (Satge et al. 1997), a condition associated with testicular cancer (Patja et al. 2006), have higher FSH levels, as do their mothers (van Montfrans et al. 1999). For a detailed discussion of the contribution of genetic factors to the etiology of testicular cancer, see the chapter in this volume by Rapley.

Despite the evidence that testicular cancer clusters in families, it is likely that the risk is largely mediated by environmental exposures. Firstly, familial occurrence of testicular cancer is very rare with the number of diagnoses made in first-degree relatives of index cases constituting just 1–2.8% of the total (Heimdal et al. 1996; Westergaard et al. 1996; Dieckmann and Pichlmeier 1997; Hemminki and Czene 2002; Hemminki and Li 2004). Secondly, testicular cancer risks are higher in brothers whose ages differ by fewer than 5 years (SIR = 10.81; 95%CI: 7.29–15.45) than in brothers whose ages differ by 5 years or greater (SIR = 6.69; 95%CI: 4.19–10.15) (Hemminki and Li 2004). Thirdly, testicular cancer was reported to have the highest proportion of childhood environmental effects in a familial study of all main cancers (Czene et al. 2002), although part of this estimate may be a consequence of the inability of the model to account for nonadditive (recessive) genetic effects. These studies emphasize the environmental component of testicular cancer pathogenesis and underscore the need to identify such factors, lest they confound the heritable estimates of risk derived from family and linkage studies.

In addition to supporting clustering of testicular cancers, family studies have also reported associations with several other tumors. Record linkage studies of family data from Sweden and Norway have found significant clustering of parental lung cancer with testicular cancer in sons (Stone et al. 1991; Zheng et al. 1996; Petridou et al. 1997; Ekbom and Akre 1998; Pharris-Ciurej et al. 1999), though studies from Denmark have not found similar associations (Kroman et al. 1996; Westergaard et al. 1996). However, one of the Swedish studies noted that although TGCT was significantly associated with parental lung cancer, the association was stronger for late-onset TGCT, which argues against a prenatal exposure (Hemminki and Chen 2006). The extent to which the family clusters can be attributed to smoking is uncertain. For example, a study from the U.K. reported a borderline significantly increased risk of lung cancer among mothers of testicular cancer patients (OR = 5.0, 95%CI = 0.9–29.6), but found no association between maternal smoking and risk of TGCT among the same individuals (Swerdlow et al. 1987a). Perhaps even more telling is the result of a recent study in the U.S. that examined cancer in the families of nonsmoking lung cancer probands. The study found that there was a significantly increased risk of testicular cancer among the relatives of the non-smoking lung cancer cases (Gorlova et al. 2007). This result may suggest that the lung cancer-testicular cancer association is due to common genetic susceptibility rather than to smoking. If this is the case, it presents opportunities for identifying susceptibility genes that may not have been previously considered. Evidence of an increased incidence of breast cancer in mothers of testicular cancer patients (Moss et al. 1986; Anderson et al. 2000; Hemminki and Li 2004) has been reported by some, but not all studies (Kroman et al. 1996; Bromen et al. 2004). Testicular cancer has also been reported to be associated with leukemia, distal colon and kidney cancers, melanoma and connective tissues tumors in a report from the Swedish Family-Cancer Database (Hemminki and Chen 2006).

As with other familial cancer syndromes, there is evidence that both the age of onset and the laterality of the tumor differ in familial vs. sporadic cases. Forman et al. (1992) found that testicular cases with a family history had a significantly earlier age of onset (29 years) when compared with cases who reported no family history (32.5 years). The same researchers also found that the incidence of bilateral disease was 7.3% in the familial cases versus 2.6% in the nonfamilial cases.

2.12   Cancer Risks Among Testicular Cancer Survivors

Testicular cancer survivors have been reported to be at increased risk of developing second cancers, the highest risk of which is a metachronous tumor of the contralateral testis (Fossa et al. 2005; McMaster et al. 2006). Regarding extratesticular malignancies following testicular cancer, an analysis of 14,984 two-month testicular cancer survivors found increased risks for cancers of the rectum, bladder, thyroid, kidney, pancreas, and acute nonlymphocytic leukemia, the latter three of which were also increased in those who did not receive radiotherapy (McMaster et al. 2006).

An analysis of European cancer registries, which included 29,511 testicular cancer patients, presented similar results (Richiardi et al. 2006). Increased risks, which the authors postulate may have arisen from shared risk factors with TGCT, included esophageal, lung, gall bladder, and bile duct cancers (Richiardi et al. 2006). Increased risks for myeloid and nonlymphoid leukemias were considered a consequence of leukemogenic toxicity, while observed excesses of pancreatic, urinary tract, connective- and soft-tissue sarcoma, and certain gastrointestinal malignancies were thought to pertain to radiotherapy (Richiardi et al. 2006).

The largest study conducted to date, which partially overlaps both geographically and temporally with both the previously discussed studies (McMaster et al. 2006; Richiardi et al. 2006), included 40,576 one-year testicular cancer survivors (Travis et al. 2005). Increased risks were observed for cancers of the stomach, pancreas, pleura, bladder, colon, esophagus, and lung, although there was evidence that the increased risk was associated with radiotherapy, chemotherapy, and combined therapy of the initial testicular cancer (Travis et al. 2005).

New malignancies following testicular cancer may vary by histology of the initial cancer, although many of these second tumor differences are likely the result of the specific therapeutic regimens for the first tumor. In an analysis of SEER data, increased risk of pancreatic cancer following seminoma and increased risk of kidney cancer following nonseminoma were observed, and these excesses remained after exclusion of patients who received radiotherapy (McMaster et al. 2006). An analysis of combined European cancer registry data, however, found risks differed by histology for larynx, small intestine, soft-tissue sarcoma, bladder, myeloid leukemia, brain and nervous system cancers (Richiardi et al. 2006). Lastly, compared to nonseminoma patients, seminoma patients have been found to have an increased risk of metachronous contralateral testicular cancer, an observation considered to be unrelated to radiotherapy (Fossa et al. 2005).

2.13 Conclusions

Despite the increasing rates of testicular germ cell tumors seen during much of the twentieth century, TGCT etiology remains poorly understood. Large geographic and ethnic discrepancies in rates argue that both environmental and genetic factors may contribute to causing testicular TGCT. The association with perinatal risk factors and congenital anomalies, as well as young age of onset, suggests that the tumor may originate in utero. The challenge in testicular cancer epidemiology will be to obtain accurate information about events surrounding the perinatal period of adults. A second challenge will be determining, if the tumor is initiated in utero, whether life style choices, such as diet and physical activity, can decrease the risk of developing the tumor.

References

Ahlgren M, Wohlfahrt J, Olsen LW, Sorensen TI, Melbye M (2007) Birth weight and risk of cancer. Cancer 110:412–419

Akre O, Ekbom A, Hsieh CC, Trichopoulos D, Adami HO (1996) Testicular nonseminoma and seminoma in relation to perinatal characteristics. J Natl Cancer Inst 88:883–889

Akre O, Lipworth L, Tretli S, Linde A, Engstrand L, Adami HO, Melbye M, Andersen A, Ekbom A (1999) Epstein-Barr virus and cytomegalovirus in relation to testicular-cancer risk: a nested case-control study. Int J Cancer 82:1–5

Akre O, Ekbom A, Sparen P, Tretli S (2000) Body size and testicular cancer. J Natl Cancer Inst 92:1093–1096

Algood CB, Newell GR, Johnson DE (1988) Viral etiology of testicular tumors. J Urol 139:308–310

Almstrup K, Sonne SB, Hoei-Hansen CE, Ottesen AM, Nielsen JE, Skakkebaek NE, Leffers H, Rajpert-De Meyts E (2006) From embryonic stem cells to testicular germ cell cancer – should we be concerned? Int J Androl 29:211–218

Altieri A, Hemminki K (2007) Number of siblings and the risk of solid tumours: a nation-wide study. Br J Cancer 96:1755–1759

Anderson H, Bladstrom A, Olsson H, Moller TR (2000) Familial breast and ovarian cancer: a Swedish population-based register study. Am J Epidemiol 152:1154–1163

Andersson E, Nilsson R, Toren K (2003) Testicular cancer among Swedish pulp and paper workers. Am J Ind Med 43:642–646

Armstrong B, Doll R (1975) Environmental factors and cancer incidence and mortality in different countries, with special reference to dietary practices. Int J Cancer 15:617–631

Aschim EL, Grotmol T, Tretli S, Haugen TB (2005) Is there an association between maternal weight and the risk of testicular cancer? An epidemiologic study of Norwegian data with emphasis on World War II. Int J Cancer 116:327–330

Aschim EL, Haugen TB, Tretli S, Daltveit AK, Grotmol T (2006) Risk factors for testicular cancer – differences between pure non-seminoma and mixed seminoma/non-seminoma? Int J Androl 29:458–467

Bach AM, Hann LE, Hadar O, Shi W, Yoo HH, Giess CS, Sheinfeld J, Thaler H (2001) Testicular microlithiasis: what is its association with testicular cancer? Radiology 220:70–75

Backus ML, Mack LA, Middleton WD, King BF, Winter TC 3rd, True LD (1994) Testicular microlithiasis: imaging appearances and pathologic correlation. Radiology 192:781–785

Batata MA, Chu FC, Hilaris BS, Whitmore WF, Golbey RB (1982) Testicular cancer in cryptorchids. Cancer 49:1023–1030

Bates MN (2007) Registry-based case-control study of cancer in California firefighters. Am J Ind Med 50:339–344

Baumgardt-Elms C, Ahrens W, Bromen K, Boikat U, Stang A, Jahn I, Stegmaier C, Jockel KH (2002) Testicular cancer and electromagnetic fields (EMF) in the workplace: results of a population-based case-control study in Germany. Cancer Causes Control 13:895–902

Becker S, Berhane K (1997) A meta-analysis of 61 sperm count studies revisited. Fertil Steril 67:1103–1108

Bennett HF, Middleton WD, Bullock AD, Teefey SA (2001) Testicular microlithiasis: US follow-up. Radiology 218:359–363

Bergstrom R, Adami HO, Mohner M, Zatonski W, Storm H, Ekbom A, Tretli S, Teppo L, Akre O, Hakulinen T (1996) Increase in testicular cancer incidence in six European countries: a birth cohort phenomenon. J Natl Cancer Inst 88:727–733

Berkowitz GS, Lapinski RH, Godbold JH, Dolgin SE, Holzman IR (1995) Maternal and neonatal risk factors for cryptorchidism. Epidemiology 6:127–131

Bernstein L, Depue RH, Ross RK, Judd HL, Pike MC, Henderson BE (1986) Higher maternal levels of free estradiol in first compared to second pregnancy: early gestational differences. J Natl Cancer Inst 76:1035–1039

Bernstein L, Pike MC, Depue RH, Ross RK, Moore JW, Henderson BE (1988) Maternal hormone levels in early gestation of cryptorchid males: a case-control study. Br J Cancer 58:379–381

Bertuccio P, Malvezzi M, Chatenoud L, Bosetti C, Negri E, Levi F, La Vecchia C (2007) Testicular cancer mortality in the Americas, 1980–2003. Cancer 109:776–779

Bhatia R, Shiau R, Petreas M, Weintraub JM, Farhang L, Eskenazi B (2005) Organochlorine pesticides and male genital anomalies in the child health and development studies. Environ Health Perspect 113:220–224

Bjorge T, Tretli S, Lie AK, Engeland A (2006) The impact of height and body mass index on the risk of testicular cancer in 600,000 Norwegian men. Cancer Causes Control 17:983–987

Boyle P (2004) Testicular cancer: the challenge for cancer control. Lancet Oncol 5:56–61

Boyle P, Kaye SB, Robertson AG (1987) Changes in testicular cancer in Scotland. Eur J Cancer Clin Oncol 23:827–830

Braun MM, Ahlbom A, Floderus B, Brinton LA, Hoover RN (1995) Effect of twinship on incidence of cancer of the testis, breast, and other sites (Sweden). Cancer Causes Control 6:519–524

Bray F, Ferlay J, Devesa SS, McGlynn KA, Moller H (2006) Interpreting the international trends in testicular seminoma and nonseminoma incidence. Nat Clin Pract Urol 3:532–543

Bromen K, Stang A, Baumgardt-Elms C, Stegmaier C, Ahrens W, Metz KA, Jockel KH (2004) Testicular, other genital, and breast cancers in first-degree relatives of testicular cancer patients and controls. Cancer Epidemiol Biomarkers Prev 13:1316–1324

Brown LM, Pottern LM, Hoover RN (1986) Prenatal and perinatal risk factors for testicular cancer. Cancer Res 46:4812–4816

Brown LM, Pottern LM, Hoover RN (1987) Testicular cancer in young men: the search for causes of the epidemic increase in the United States. J Epidemiol Community Health 41:349–354

Buetow SA (1995) Epidemiology of testicular cancer. Epidemiol Rev 17:433–449

Burton MH, Davies TW, Raggatt PR (1987) Undescended testis and hormone levels in early pregnancy. J Epidemiol Community Health 41:127–129

Calvert GM, Fajen JM, Hills BW, Halperin WE (1990) Testicular cancer, dimethylformamide, and leather tanneries. Lancet 336:1253–1254

Carlsen E, Giwercman A, Keiding N, Skakkebaek NE (1992) Evidence for decreasing quality of semen during past 50 years. BMJ 305:609–613

Cast JE, Nelson WM, Early AS, Biyani S, Cooksey G, Warnock NG, Breen DJ (2000) Testicular microlithiasis: prevalence and tumor risk in a population referred for scrotal sonography. AJR Am J Roentgenol 175:1703–1706

Chilvers CED, Pike MC (1989) Epidemiology of undescended testis. In: Oliver RTD, Blandy JP, Hope-Stone HF (eds) Urological and genital cancer. Blackwell, Oxford, pp 306–321

Chilvers CE, Pike MC, Peckham MJ (1987) Torsion of the testis: a new risk factor for testicular cancer. Br J Cancer 55:105–106

Clemmesen J (1997) Is pregnancy smoking causal to testis cancer in sons? A hypothesis. Acta Oncol 36:59–63

Coldman AJ, Elwood JM, Gallagher RP (1982) Sports activities and risk of testicular cancer. Br J Cancer 46:749–756

Colls BM, Harvey VJ, Skelton L, Thompson PI, Frampton CM (1996) Bilateral germ cell testicular tumors in New Zealand: experience in Auckland and Christchurch 1978–1994. J Clin Oncol 14:2061–2065

Coovadia YM (1978) Primary testicular tumours among White, Black and Indian patients. S Afr Med J 54:351–352

Coupland CA, Chilvers CE, Davey G, Pike MC, Oliver RT, Forman D (1999) Risk factors for testicular germ cell tumours by histological tumour type. United Kingdom Testicular Cancer Study Group. Br J Cancer 80:1859–1863

Coupland CA, Forman D, Chilvers CE, Davey G, Pike MC, Oliver RT (2004) Maternal risk factors for testicular cancer: a population-based case-control study (UK). Cancer Causes Control 15:277–283

Czene K, Lichtenstein P, Hemminki K (2002) Environmental and heritable causes of cancer among 9.6 million individuals in the Swedish Family-Cancer Database. Int J Cancer 99:260–266

Damgaard IN, Skakkebaek NE, Toppari J, Virtanen HE, Shen H, Schramm KW, Petersen JH, Jensen TK, Main KM (2006) Persistent pesticides in human breast milk and cryptorchidism. Environ Health Perspect 114:1133–1138

Davies TW, Prener A, Engholm G (1990) Body size and cancer of the testis. Acta Oncol 29:287–290

Davies TW, Palmer CR, Ruja E, Lipscombe JM (1996) Adolescent milk, dairy product and fruit consumption and testicular cancer. Br J Cancer 74:657–660

Decarli A, La Vecchia C (1986) Environmental factors and cancer mortality in Italy: correlational exercise. Oncology 43:116–126

Dement J, Pompeii L, Lipkus IM, Samsa GP (2003) Cancer incidence among union carpenters in New Jersey. J Occup Environ Med 45:1059–1067

Depue RH, Pike MC, Henderson BE (1983) Estrogen exposure during gestation and risk of testicular cancer. J Natl Cancer Inst 71:1151–1155

Derogee M, Bevers RF, Prins HJ, Jonges TG, Elbers FH, Boon TA (2001) Testicular microlithiasis, a premalignant condition: prevalence, histopathologic findings, and relation to testicular tumor. Urology 57:1133–1137

Dieckmann KP, Pichlmeier U (1997) The prevalence of familial testicular cancer: an analysis of two patient populations and a review of the literature. Cancer 80:1954–1960

Dieckmann KP, Pichlmeier U (2002) Is risk of testicular cancer related to body size? Eur Urol 42:564–569

Dieckmann KP, Pichlmeier U (2004) Clinical epidemiology of testicular germ cell tumors. World J Urol 22:2–14

Dieckmann WJ, Davis ME, Rynkiewicz LM, Pottinger RE (1953) Does the administration of diethylstilbestrol during pregnancy have therapeutic value? Am J Obstet Gynecol 66:1062–1081

Dieckmann KP, Endsin G, Pichlmeier U (2001) How valid is the prenatal estrogen excess hypothesis of testicular germ cell cancer? A case control study on hormone-related factors. Eur Urol 40:677–683 discussion 684

Dosemeci M, Hayes RB, Vetter R, Hoover RN, Tucker M, Engin K, Unsal M, Blair A (1993) Occupational physical activity, socioeconomic status, and risks of 15 cancer sites in Turkey. Cancer Causes Control 4:313–321

Ducatman AM, Conwill DE, Crawl J (1986) Germ cell tumors of the testicle among aircraft repairmen. J Urol 136:834–836

Einhorn LH, Donohue J (1977) Cis-diamminedichloroplatinum, vinblastine, and bleomycin combination chemotherapy in disseminated testicular cancer. Ann Intern Med 87:293–298

Ekbom A, Akre O (1998) Increasing incidence of testicular cancer – birth cohort effects. APMIS 106:225–229 discussion 229–231

Ekbom A, Richiardi L, Akre O, Montgomery SM, Sparen P (2003) Age at immigration and duration of stay in relation to risk for testicular cancer among Finnish immigrants in Sweden. J Natl Cancer Inst 95:1238–1240

English PB, Goldberg DE, Wolff C, Smith D (2003) Parental and birth characteristics in relation to testicular cancer risk among males born between 1960 and 1995 in California (United States). Cancer Causes Control 14:815–825

Ferlay J, Bray F, Pisani P, Parkin DM (2004) GLOBOCAN 2002: cancer incidence, mortality and prevalence worldwide. IARC CancerBase No. 5. version 2.0 ed. IARC, Lyon

Fisch H, Goluboff ET (1996) Geographic variations in sperm counts: a potential cause of bias in studies of semen quality. Fertil Steril 65:1044–1046

Fisch H, Goluboff ET, Olson JH, Feldshuh J, Broder SJ, Barad DH (1996) Semen analyses in 1,283 men from the United States over a 25-year period: no decline in quality. Fertil Steril 65:1009–1014

Fleming LE, Bean JA, Rudolph M, Hamilton K (1999) Cancer incidence in a cohort of licensed pesticide applicators in Florida. J Occup Environ Med 41:279–288

Floderus B, Stenlund C, Persson T (1999) Occupational magnetic field exposure and site-specific cancer incidence: a Swedish cohort study. Cancer Causes Control 10:323–332

Flores-Luevano S, Farias P, Hernandez M, Romano-Riquer P, Weber JP, Dewailly E, Cuevas-Alpuche J, Romieu I (2003) [DDT/DDE concentrations and risk of hypospadias. Pilot case-control study]. Salud Publica Mex 45:431–438

Foley S, Middleton S, Stitson D, Mahoney M (1995) The incidence of testicular cancer in Royal Air Force personnel. Br J Urol 76:495–496

Forman D, Oliver RT, Brett AR, Marsh SG, Moses JH, Bodmer JG, Chilvers CE, Pike MC (1992) Familial testicular cancer: a report of the UK family register, estimation of risk and an HLA class 1 sib-pair analysis. Br J Cancer 65:255–262

Fossa SD, Chen J, Schonfeld SJ, McGlynn KA, McMaster ML, Gail MH, Travis LB (2005) Risk of contralateral testicular cancer: a population-based study of 29,515 U.S. men. J Natl Cancer Inst 97:1056–1066

Frisch M, Biggar RJ, Engels EA, Goedert JJ (2001) Association of cancer with AIDS-related immunosuppression in adults. JAMA 285:1736–1745

Gabutti G, Vercelli M, De Rosa MG, Orengo MA, Casella C, Garrone E, Orlandini C, Piersantelli N, Torresin A, Rizzo F et al (1995) AIDS related neoplasms in Genoa, Italy. Eur J Epidemiol 11:609–614

Gallagher RP, Huchcroft S, Phillips N, Hill GB, Coldman AJ, Coppin C, Lee T (1995) Physical activity, medical history, and risk of testicular cancer (Alberta and British Columbia, Canada). Cancer Causes Control 6:398–406

Ganem JP, Workman KR, Shaban SF (1999) Testicular microlithiasis is associated with testicular pathology. Urology 53:209–213

Ganmaa D, Li XM, Wang J, Qin LQ, Wang PY, Sato A (2002) Incidence and mortality of testicular and prostatic cancers in relation to world dietary practices. Int J Cancer 98:262–267

Garner MJ, Birkett NJ, Johnson KC, Shatenstein B, Ghadirian P, Krewski D (2003) Dietary risk factors for testicular carcinoma. Int J Cancer 106:934–941

Gershman ST, Stolley PD (1988) A case-control study of testicular cancer using Connecticut tumour registry data. Int J Epidemiol 17:738–742

Ginsburg J (1997) Unanswered questions in carcinoma of the testis. Lancet 349:1785–1786

Giusti RM, Iwamoto K, Hatch EE (1995) Diethylstilbestrol revisited: a review of the long-term health effects. Ann Intern Med 122:778–788

Goedert JJ, Cote TR, Virgo P, Scoppa SM, Kingma DW, Gail MH, Jaffe ES, Biggar RJ (1998) Spectrum of AIDS-associated malignant disorders. Lancet 351:1833–1839

Goedert JJ, Sauter ME, Jacobson LP, Vessella RL, Hilgartner MW, Leitman SF, Fraser MC, Mueller-Lantzsch NG (1999) High prevalence of antibodies against HERV-K10 in patients with testicular cancer but not with AIDS. Cancer Epidemiol Biomarkers Prev 8:293–296

Golden RJ, Noller KL, Titus-Ernstoff L, Kaufman RH, Mittendorf R, Stillman R, Reese EA (1998) Environmental endocrine modulators and human health: an assessment of the biological evidence. Crit Rev Toxicol 28:109–227

Gorlova OY, Weng SF, Zhang Y, Amos CI, Spitz MR (2007) Aggregation of cancer among relatives of never-smoking lung cancer patients. Int J Cancer 121:111–118

Graham S, Gibson RW (1972) Social epidemiology of cancer of the testis. Cancer 29:1242–1249

Graham S, Gibson R, West D, Swanson M, Burnett W, Dayal H (1977) Epidemiology of cancer of the testis in upstate New York. J Natl Cancer Inst 58:1255–1261

Guo J, Kauppinen T, Kyyronen P, Heikkila P, Lindbohm ML, Pukkala E (2004) Risk of esophageal, ovarian, testicular, kidney and bladder cancers and leukemia among Finnish workers exposed to diesel or gasoline engine exhaust. Int J Cancer 111:286–292

Guo J, Pukkala E, Kyyronen P, Lindbohm ML, Heikkila P, Kauppinen T (2005) Testicular cancer, occupation and exposure to chemical agents among Finnish men in 1971–1995. Cancer Causes Control 16:97–103

Hardell L, Nasman A, Ohlson CG, Fredrikson M (1998) Case-control study on risk factors for testicular cancer. Int J Oncol 13:1299–1303

Hardell L, Van Bavel B, Lindstrom G, Carlberg M, Dreifaldt AC, Wijkstrom H, Starkhammar H, Eriksson M, Hallquist A, Kolmert T (2003) Increased concentrations of polychlorinated biphenyls, hexachlorobenzene, and chlordanes in mothers of men with testicular cancer. Environ Health Perspect 111:930–934

Hardell L, Van Bavel B, Lindstrom G, Carlberg M, Eriksson M, Dreifaldt AC, Wijkstrom H, Starkhammar H, Hallquist A, Kolmert T (2004) Concentrations of polychlorinated biphenyls in blood and the risk for testicular cancer. Int J Androl 27:282–290

Hardell L, Carlberg M, Ohlson CG, Westberg H, Eriksson M, Hansson Mild K (2007) Use of cellular and cordless telephones and risk of testicular cancer. Int J Androl 30:115–122

Haughey BP, Graham S, Brasure J, Zielezny M, Sufrin G, Burnett WS (1989) The epidemiology of testicular cancer in upstate New York. Am J Epidemiol 130:25–36

Heimdal K, Olsson H, Tretli S, Flodgren P, Borresen AL, Fossa SD (1996) Familial testicular cancer in Norway and southern Sweden. Br J Cancer 73:964–969

Heimdal K, Olsson H, Tretli S, Fossa SD, Borresen AL, Bishop DT (1997) A segregation analysis of testicular cancer based on Norwegian and Swedish families. Br J Cancer 75: 1084–1087

Hemminki K, Chen B (2005) Are twins at risk of cancer: results from the Swedish family-cancer database. Twin Res Hum Genet 8:509–514

Hemminki K, Chen B (2006) Familial risks in testicular cancer as aetiological clues. Int J Androl 29:205–210

Hemminki K, Czene K (2002) Attributable risks of familial cancer from the Family-Cancer Database. Cancer Epidemiol Biomarkers Prev 11:1638–1644

Hemminki K, Li X (2002a) Cancer risks in Nordic immigrants and their offspring in Sweden. Eur J Cancer 38:2428–2434

Hemminki K, Li X (2002b) Cancer risks in twins: results from the Swedish family-cancer database. Int J Cancer 99:873–878

Hemminki K, Li X (2004) Familial risk in testicular cancer as a clue to a heritable and environmental aetiology. Br J Cancer 90:1765–1770

Henderson BE, Benton B, Jing J, Yu MC, Pike MC (1979) Risk factors for cancer of the testis in young men. Int J Cancer 23:598–602

Henderson BE, Bernstein L, Ross RK, Depue RH, Judd HL (1988a) The early in utero oestrogen and testosterone environment of blacks and whites: potential effects on male offspring. Br J Cancer 57:216–218

Henderson BE, Ross R, Bernstein L (1988b) Estrogens as a cause of human cancer: the Richard and Hinda Rosenthal Foundation award lecture. Cancer Res 48:246–253

Herbst H, Sauter M, Kuhler-Obbarius C, Loning T, Mueller-Lantzsch N (1998) Human endogenous retrovirus (HERV)-K transcripts in germ cell and trophoblastic tumours. APMIS 106:216–220

Holm M, Hoei-Hansen CE, Rajpert-De Meyts E, Skakkebaek NE (2003) Increased risk of carcinoma in situ in patients with testicular germ cell cancer with ultrasonic microlithiasis in the contralateral testicle. J Urol 170:1163–1167

Hopper JL, Carlin JB (1992) Familial aggregation of a disease consequent upon correlation between relatives in a risk factor measured on a continuous scale. Am J Epidemiol 136:1138–1147

Hosie S, Loff S, Witt K, Niessen K, Waag KL (2000) Is there a correlation between organochlorine compounds and undescended testes? Eur J Pediatr Surg 10:304–309

Husson G, Herrinton LJ (2003) Regarding "a case-control study of sexually transmitted disease and risk of testicular cancer". Ann Epidemiol 13:541–542

Huyghe E, Matsuda T, Thonneau P (2003) Increasing incidence of testicular cancer worldwide: a review. J Urol 170:5–11

International Agency for Research on Cancer (1999) Re-evaluation of some organic chemicals, hydrazine and hydrogen peroxide. Proceedings of the IARC Working Group on the Evaluation of Carcinogenic Risks to Humans. Lyon, France, 17-24 February 1998. IARC monographs on the evaluation of carcinogenic risks to humans / World Health Organization, International Agency for Research on Cancer, 71 Pt 1:1–315

Ikinger U, Wurster K, Terwey B, Mohring K (1982) Microcalcifications in testicular malignancy: diagnostic tool in occult tumor? Urology 19:525–528

Jacobsen R, Bostofte E, Engholm G, Hansen J, Olsen JH, Skakkebaek NE, Moller H (2000) Risk of testicular cancer in men with abnormal semen characteristics: cohort study. BMJ 321:789–792

Karagas MR, Weiss NS, Strader CH, Daling JR (1989) Elevated intrascrotal temperature and the incidence of testicular cancer in noncryptorchid men. Am J Epidemiol 129:1104–1109

Kavlock RJ, Daston GP, Derosa C, Fenner-Crisp P, Gray LE, Kaattari S, Lucier G, Luster M, Mac MJ, Maczka C, Miller R, Moore J, Rolland R, Scott G, Sheehan DM, Sinks T, Tilson HA (1996) Research needs for the risk assessment of health and environmental effects of endocrine disruptors: a report of the U.S. EPA-sponsored workshop. Environ Health Perspect 104(Suppl 4):715–740

Kelce WR, Stone CR, Laws SC, Gray LE, Kemppainen JA, Wilson EM (1995) Persistent DDT metabolite p, p'-DDE is a potent androgen receptor antagonist. Nature 375:581–585

Key TJ, Bull D, Ansell P, Brett AR, Clark GM, Moore JW, Chilvers CE, Pike MC (1996) A case-control study of cryptorchidism and maternal hormone concentrations in early pregnancy. Br J Cancer 73:698–701

Khoury MJ, Beaty TH, Liang KY (1988) Can familial aggregation of disease be explained by familial aggregation of environmental risk factors? Am J Epidemiol 127:674–683

Klebanoff MA (2007) Gestational age: not always what it seems. Obstet Gynecol 109:798–799

Knight JA, Marrett LD, Weir HK (1996) Occupation and risk of germ cell testicular cancer by histologic type in Ontario. J Occup Environ Med 38:884–890

Knutsson A, Damber L, Jarvholm B (2000) Cancers in concrete workers: results of a cohort study of 33,668 workers. Occup Environ Med 57:264–267

Kroman N, Frisch M, Olsen JH, Westergaard T, Melbye M (1996) Oestrogen-related cancer risk in mothers of testicular-cancer patients. Int J Cancer 66:438–440

Lam DL, Gerscovich EO, Kuo MC, McGahan JP (2007) Testicular microlithiasis: our experience of 10 years. J Ultrasound Med 26:867–873

Lambalk CB, Boomsma DI (1998) Genetic risk factors in tumours of the testis: lessons from twin studies. Twin Res 1:154–155

Lass A, Akagbosu F, Abusheikha N, Hassouneh M, Blayney M, Avery S, Brinsden P (1998) A programme of semen cryopreservation for patients with malignant disease in a tertiary infertility centre: lessons from 8 years' experience. Hum Reprod 13:3256–3261

Lee PA, Bellinger MF, Coughlin MT (1998) Correlations among hormone levels, sperm parameters and paternity in formerly unilaterally cryptorchid men. J Urol 160:1155–1157 discussion 1178

Leib-Mosch C, Brack-Werner R, Werner T, Bachmann M, Faff O, Erfle V, Hehlmann R (1990) Endogenous retroviral elements in human DNA. Cancer Res 50:5636S–5642S

Lenz S, Skakkebaek NE, Hertel NT (1996) Abnormal ultrasonic pattern in contralateral testes in patients with unilateral testicular cancer. World J Urol 14(Suppl 1):S55–S58

Lerchl A, Nieschlag E (1996) Decreasing sperm counts? A critical (re)view. Exp Clin Endocrinol Diabetes 104:301–307

Levin SM, Baker DB, Landrigan PJ, Monaghan SV, Frumin E, Braithwaite M, Towne W (1987) Testicular cancer in leather tanners exposed to dimethylformamide. Lancet 2:1153

Lipworth L, Dayan AD (1969) Rural preponderance of seminoma of the testis. Cancer 23:1119–1121

Logothetis CJ, Newell GR, Samuels ML (1985) Testicular cancer in homosexual men with cellular immune deficiency: report of 2 cases. J Urol 133:484–486

Longnecker MP, Klebanoff MA, Brock JW, Zhou H, Gray KA, Needham LL, Wilcox AJ (2002) Maternal serum level of 1, 1-dichloro-2, 2-bis(p-chlorophenyl)ethylene and risk of cryptorchidism, hypospadias, and polythelia among male offspring. Am J Epidemiol 155:313–322

Loughlin JE, Robboy SJ, Morrison AS (1980) Risk factors for cancer of the testis. N Engl J Med 303:112–113

Lower R, Boller K, Hasenmaier B, Korbmacher C, Muller-Lantzsch N, Lower J, Kurth R (1993) Identification of human endogenous retroviruses with complex mRNA expression and particle formation. Proc Natl Acad Sci USA 90:4480–4484

Lower R, Lower J, Kurth R (1996) The viruses in all of us: characteristics and biological significance of human endogenous retrovirus sequences. Proc Natl Acad Sci USA 93:5177–5184

Lyter DW, Bryant J, Thackeray R, Rinaldo CR, Kingsley LA (1995) Incidence of human immunodeficiency virus-related and nonrelated malignancies in a large cohort of homosexual men. J Clin Oncol 13:2540–2546

Marshall EG, Melius JM, London MA, Nasca PC, Burnett WS (1990) Investigation of a testicular cancer cluster using a case-control approach. Int J Epidemiol 19:269–273

McCredie M, Coates M, Grulich A (1994) Cancer incidence in migrants to New South Wales (Australia) from the Middle East, 1972–91. Cancer Causes Control 5:414–421

McGlynn KA, Devesa SS, Sigurdson AJ, Brown LM, Tsao L, Tarone RE (2003) Trends in the incidence of testicular germ cell tumors in the United States. Cancer 97:63–70

McGlynn KA, Devesa SS, Graubard BI, Castle PE (2005a) Increasing incidence of testicular germ cell tumors among black men in the United States. J Clin Oncol 23:5757–5761

McGlynn KA, Graubard BI, Nam JM, Stanczyk FZ, Longnecker MP, Klebanoff MA (2005b) Maternal hormone levels and risk of cryptorchism among populations at high and low risk of testicular germ cell tumors. Cancer Epidemiol Biomarkers Prev 14:1732–1737

McGlynn KA, Zhang Y, Sakoda LC, Rubertone MV, Erickson RL, Graubard BI (2006) Maternal smoking and testicular germ cell tumors. Cancer Epidemiol Biomarkers Prev 15: 1820–1824

McGlynn KA, Sakoda LC, Rubertone MV, Sesterhenn IA, Lyu C, Graubard BI, Erickson RL (2007) Body size, dairy consumption, puberty, and risk of testicular germ cell tumors. Am J Epidemiol 165:355–363

McMaster ML, Feuer EJ, Tucker MA (2006) New malignancies following cancer of the male genital tract. In: Curtis RE, Freedman DM, Ron E, Ries LAG, Hacker DG, Edwards BK, Tucker MA, Fraumeni JF Jr (eds) New malignancies among cancer survivors: SEER cancer registries, 1973–2000. National Cancer Institute, Bethesda, MD

Moller H (1989) Decreased testicular cancer risk in men born in wartime. J Natl Cancer Inst 81:1668–1669

Moller H (1993) Clues to the aetiology of testicular germ cell tumours from descriptive epidemiology. Eur Urol 23:8–13 discussion 14–15

Moller MB (1996) Association of testicular non-Hodgkin's lymphomas with elevated serum levels of human chorionic gonadotropin-like material. Oncology 53:94–98

Moller H (1997) Work in agriculture, childhood residence, nitrate exposure, and testicular cancer risk: a case-control study in Denmark. Cancer Epidemiol Biomarkers Prev 6:141–144

Moller H, Skakkebaek NE (1996) Risks of testicular cancer and cryptorchidism in relation to socio-economic status and related factors: case-control studies in Denmark. Int J Cancer 66:287–293

Moller H, Skakkebaek NE (1997) Testicular cancer and cryptorchidism in relation to prenatal factors: case-control studies in Denmark. Cancer Causes Control 8:904–912

Moller H, Skakkebaek NE (1999) Risk of testicular cancer in subfertile men: case-control study. BMJ 318:559–562

Moller H, Prener A, Skakkebaek NE (1996) Testicular cancer, cryptorchidism, inguinal hernia, testicular atrophy, and genital malformations: case-control studies in Denmark. Cancer Causes Control 7:264–274

Moller H, Cortes D, Engholm G, Thorup J (1998) Risk of testicular cancer with cryptorchidism and with testicular biopsy: cohort study. BMJ 317:729

Morris JD, Eddleston AL, Crook T (1995) Viral infection and cancer. Lancet 346:754–758

Morrison AS (1976a) Cryptorchidism, hernia, and cancer of the testis. J Natl Cancer Inst 56:731–733

Morrison AS (1976b) Some social and medical characteristics of Army men with testicular cancer. Am J Epidemiol 104:511–516

Moss AR, Osmond D, Bacchetti P, Torti FM, Gurgin V (1986) Hormonal risk factors in testicular cancer. A case-control study. Am J Epidemiol 124:39–52

Mueller N, Hinkula J, Wahren B (1988) Elevated antibody titers against cytomegalovirus among patients with testicular cancer. Int J Cancer 41:399–403

Muganda P, Mendoza O, Hernandez J, Qian Q (1994) Human cytomegalovirus elevates levels of the cellular protein p53 in infected fibroblasts. J Virol 68:8028–8034

New Zealand Health Information Service (2006) Cancer: new registrations and deaths 2002. Ministry of Health, New Zealand, Wellington

Newbold RR, Bullock BC, McLachlan JA (1985) Lesions of the rete testis in mice exposed prenatally to diethylstilbestrol. Cancer Res 45:5145–5150

Newell GR, Mills PK, Johnson DE (1984) Epidemiologic comparison of cancer of the testis and Hodgkin's disease among young males. Cancer 54:1117–1123

Nicholson PW, Harland SJ (1995) Inheritance and testicular cancer. Br J Cancer 71:421–426

Nistal M, Gonzalez-Peramato P, Regadera J, Serrano A, Tarin V, De Miguel MP (2006) Primary testicular lesions are associated with testicular germ cell tumors of adult men. Am J Surg Pathol 30:1260–1268

Noller KL, Fish CR (1974) Diethylstilbestrol usage: its interesting past, important present, and questionable future. Med Clin North Am 58:793–810

Office of Population Censuses and Surveys (Opcs) (1993) Cancer statistics – registrations, 1987, England and Wales. HMSO, London

Oliver RT (1990) Atrophy, hormones, genes and viruses in aetiology germ cell tumours. Cancer Surv 9:263–286

Olsen GW, Bodner KM, Ramlow JM, Ross CE, Lipshultz LI (1995) Have sperm counts been reduced 50 percent in 50 years? A statistical model revisited. Fertil Steril 63:887–893

Ono M, Kawakami M, Ushikubo H (1987) Stimulation of expression of the human endogenous retrovirus genome by female steroid hormones in human breast cancer cell line T47D. J Virol 61:2059–2062

Oosterhuis JW, Looijenga LH (2005) Testicular germ-cell tumours in a broader perspective. Nat Rev Cancer 5:210–222

Osterlind A (1986) Diverging trends in incidence and mortality of testicular cancer in Denmark, 1943–1982. Br J Cancer 53:501–505

Osterlind A, Berthelsen JG, Abildgaard N, Hansen SO, Hjalgrim H, Johansen B, Munck-Hansen J, Rasmussen LH (1991) Risk of bilateral testicular germ cell cancer in Denmark: 1960–1984. J Natl Cancer Inst 83:1391–1395

Otite U, Webb JA, Oliver RT, Badenoch DF, Nargund VH (2001) Testicular microlithiasis: is it a benign condition with malignant potential? Eur Urol 40:538–542

Paffenbarger RS Jr, Hyde RT, Wing AL (1987) Physical activity and incidence of cancer in diverse populations: a preliminary report. Am J Clin Nutr 45:312–317

Parker L (1997) Causes of testicular cancer. Lancet 350:827–828

Parkin DM, Iscovich J (1997) Risk of cancer in migrants and their descendants in Israel: II. Carcinomas and germ-cell tumours. Int J Cancer 70:654–660

Patja K, Pukkala E, Sund R, Iivanainen M, Kaski M (2006) Cancer incidence of persons with Down syndrome in Finland: a population-based study. Int J Cancer 118:1769–1772

Peckham MJ, McElwain TJ, Barrett A, Hendry WF (1979) Combined management of malignant teratoma of the testis. Lancet 2:267–270

Petersen PM, Skakkebaek NE, Vistisen K, Rorth M, Giwercman A (1999) Semen quality and reproductive hormones before orchiectomy in men with testicular cancer. J Clin Oncol 17:941–947

Peterson AC, Bauman JM, Light DE, McMann LP, Costabile RA (2001) The prevalence of testicular microlithiasis in an asymptomatic population of men 18 to 35 years old. J Urol 166:2061–2064

Petridou E, Roukas KI, Dessypris N, Aravantinos G, Bafaloukos D, Efraimidis A, Papacharalambous A, Pektasidis D, Rigatos G, Trichopoulos D (1997) Baldness and other correlates of sex hormones in relation to testicular cancer. Int J Cancer 71:982–985

Pettersson A, Kaijser M, Richiardi L, Askling J, Ekbom A, Akre O (2004) Women smoking and testicular cancer: one epidemic causing another? Int J Cancer 109:941–944

Pettersson A, Akre O, Richiardi L, Ekbom A, Kaijser M (2007a) Maternal smoking and the epidemic of testicular cancer – a nested case-control study. Int J Cancer 120:2044–2046

Pettersson A, Richiardi L, Nordenskjold A, Kaijser M, Akre O (2007b) Age at surgery for undescended testis and risk of testicular cancer. N Engl J Med 356:1835–1841

Pflieger-Bruss S, Schuppe HC, Schill WB (2004) The male reproductive system and its susceptibility to endocrine disrupting chemicals. Andrologia 36:337–345

Pharris-Ciurej ND, Cook LS, Weiss NS (1999) Incidence of testicular cancer in the United States: has the epidemic begun to abate? Am J Epidemiol 150:45–46

Pierik FH, Klebanoff MA, Brock JW, Longnecker MP (2007) Maternal pregnancy serum level of heptachlor epoxide, hexachlorobenzene, and beta-hexachlorocyclohexane and risk of cryptorchidism in offspring. Environ Res 105:364–369

Pike MC, Chilvers CE, Bobrow LG (1987) Classification of testicular cancer in incidence and mortality statistics. Br J Cancer 56:83–85

Pollan M, Gustavsson P, Cano MI (2001) Incidence of testicular cancer and occupation among Swedish men gainfully employed in 1970. Ann Epidemiol 11:554–562

Pourbagher MA, Kilinc F, Guvel S, Pourbagher A, Egilmez T, Ozkardes H (2005) Follow-up of testicular microlithiasis for subsequent testicular cancer development. Urol Int 74:108–112 discussion 113

Power DA, Brown RS, Brock CS, Payne HA, Majeed A, Babb P (2001) Trends in testicular carcinoma in England and Wales, 1971–99. BJU Int 87:361–365

Prener A, Hsieh CC, Engholm G, Trichopoulos D, Jensen OM (1992) Birth order and risk of testicular cancer. Cancer Causes Control 3:265–272

Prener A, Engholm G, Jensen OM (1996) Genital anomalies and risk for testicular cancer in Danish men. Epidemiology 7:14–19

Pukkala E, Weiderpass E (2002) Socio-economic differences in incidence rates of cancers of the male genital organs in Finland, 1971–95. Int J Cancer 102:643–648

Rajpert-De Meyts E, Jorgensen N, Brondum-Nielsen K, Muller J, Skakkebaek NE (1998) Developmental arrest of germ cells in the pathogenesis of germ cell neoplasia. APMIS 106:198–204 discussion 204–196

Raman JD, Nobert CF, Goldstein M (2005) Increased incidence of testicular cancer in men presenting with infertility and abnormal semen analysis. J Urol 174:1819–1822 discussion 1822

Rasmussen F, Gunnell D, Ekbom A, Hallqvist J, Tynelius P (2003) Birth weight, adult height, and testicular cancer: cohort study of 337,249 Swedish young men. Cancer Causes Control 14:595–598

Renshaw AA (1998) Testicular calcifications: incidence, histology and proposed pathological criteria for testicular microlithiasis. J Urol 160:1625–1628

Rhomberg W, Schmoll HJ, Schneider B (1995) High frequency of metalworkers among patients with seminomatous tumors of the testis: a case-control study. Am J Ind Med 28:79–87

Richiardi L, Akre O, Bellocco R, Ekbom A (2002) Perinatal determinants of germ-cell testicular cancer in relation to histological subtypes. Br J Cancer 87:545–550

Richiardi L, Askling J, Granath F, Akre O (2003) Body size at birth and adulthood and the risk for germ-cell testicular cancer. Cancer Epidemiol Biomarkers Prev 12:669–673

Richiardi L, Akre O, Lambe M, Granath F, Montgomery SM, Ekbom A (2004) Birth order, sibship size, and risk for germ-cell testicular cancer. Epidemiology 15:323–329

Richiardi L, Scelo G, Boffetta P, Hemminki K, Pukkala E, Olsen JH, Weiderpass E, Tracey E, Brewster DH, McBride ML, Kliewer EV, Tonita JM, Pompe-Kirn V, Kee-Seng C, Jonasson JG, Martos C, Brennan P (2006) Second malignancies among survivors of germ-cell testicular cancer: a pooled analysis between 13 cancer registries. Int J Cancer 120:623–631

Richiardi L, Pettersson A, Akre O (2007) Genetic and environmental risk factors for testicular cancer. Int J Androl 30:230–240

Ross RK, McCurtis JW, Henderson BE, Menck HR, Mack TM, Martin SP (1979) Descriptive epidemiology of testicular and prostatic cancer in Los Angeles. Br J Cancer 39:284–292

Ryder SJ, Crawford PI, Pethybridge RJ (1997) Is testicular cancer an occupational disease? A case-control study of Royal Naval personnel. J R Nav Med Serv 83:130–146

Sabroe S, Olsen J (1998) Perinatal correlates of specific histological types of testicular cancer in patients below 35 years of age: a case-cohort study based on midwives' records in Denmark. Int J Cancer 78:140–143

Safe SH (2000) Endocrine disruptors and human health – is there a problem? An update. Environ Health Perspect 108:487–493

Satge D, Sasco AJ, Cure H, Leduc B, Sommelet D, Vekemans MJ (1997) An excess of testicular germ cell tumors in Down's syndrome: three case reports and a review of the literature. Cancer 80:929–935

Sauter M, Schommer S, Kremmer E, Remberger K, Dolken G, Lemm I, Buck M, Best B, Neumann-Haefelin D, Mueller-Lantzsch N (1995) Human endogenous retrovirus K10: expression of Gag protein and detection of antibodies in patients with seminomas. J Virol 69:414–421

Schottenfeld D, Warshauer ME, Sherlock S, Zauber AG, Leder M, Payne R (1980) The epidemiology of testicular cancer in young adults. Am J Epidemiol 112:232–246

Serter S, Gumus B, Unlu M, Tuncyurek O, Tarhan S, Ayyildiz V, Pabuscu Y (2006) Prevalence of testicular microlithiasis in an asymptomatic population. Scand J Urol Nephrol 40: 212–214

Shah MN, Devesa SS, Zhu K, McGlynn KA (2007) Trends in testicular germ cell tumors in the United States. Int J Androl 30(4):206–213

Sharpe RM (2003) The 'oestrogen hypothesis' – where do we stand now? Int J Androl 26:2–15

Sharpe RM, Skakkebaek NE (1993) Are oestrogens involved in falling sperm counts and disorders of the male reproductive tract? Lancet 341:1392–1395

Sigurdson AJ, Chang S, Annegers JF, Duphorne CM, Pillow PC, Amato RJ, Hutchinson LP, Sweeney AM, Strom SS (1999) A case-control study of diet and testicular carcinoma. Nutr Cancer 34:20–26

Skakkebaek NE (1972) Possible carcinoma-in-situ of the testis. Lancet 2:516–517

Skakkebaek NE, Rajpert-De Meyts E, Main KM (2001) Testicular dysgenesis syndrome: an increasingly common developmental disorder with environmental aspects. Hum Reprod 16:972–978

Sonneveld DJ, Schaapveld M, Sleijfer DT, Meerman GJ, Van Der Graaf WT, Sijmons RH, Koops HS, Hoekstra HJ (1999) Geographic clustering of testicular cancer incidence in the northern part of The Netherlands. Br J Cancer 81:1262–1267

Sont WN, Zielinski JM, Ashmore JP, Jiang H, Krewski D, Fair ME, Band PR, Letourneau EG (2001) First analysis of cancer incidence and occupational radiation exposure based on the National Dose Registry of Canada. Am J Epidemiol 153:309–318

Srivastava A, Kreiger N (2000) Relation of physical activity to risk of testicular cancer. Am J Epidemiol 151:78–87

Stang A, Jockel KH, Baumgardt-Elms C, Ahrens W (2003) Firefighting and risk of testicular cancer: results from a German population-based case-control study. Am J Ind Med 43:291–294

Stone JM, Cruickshank DG, Sandeman TF, Matthews JP (1991) Laterality, maldescent, trauma and other clinical factors in the epidemiology of testis cancer in Victoria, Australia. Br J Cancer 64:132–138

Stoop H, Van Gurp R, De Krijger R, Geurts Van Kessel A, Koberle B, Oosterhuis W, Looijenga L (2001) Reactivity of germ cell maturation stage-specific markers in spermatocytic seminoma: diagnostic and etiological implications. Lab Invest 81:919–928

Storgaard L, Bonde JP, Olsen J (2006) Male reproductive disorders in humans and prenatal indicators of estrogen exposure. A review of published epidemiological studies. Reprod Toxicol 21:4–15

Strohsnitter WC, Noller KL, Hoover RN, Robboy SJ, Palmer JR, Titus-Ernstoff L, Kaufman RH, Adam E, Herbst AL, Hatch EE (2001) Cancer risk in men exposed in utero to diethylstilbestrol. J Natl Cancer Inst 93:545–551

Surveillance, Epidemiology and End Results (SEER) Program, (www.seer.cancer.gov) SEER*Stat Database: Incidence – SEER 9 Regs Limited-Use, Nov 2006 Sub (1973–2004) – Linked To County Attributes – Total U.S., 1969–2004 Counties, National Cancer Institute, DCCPS, Surveillance Research Program, Cancer Statistics Branch, released April 2007, based on the November 2006 submission

Swan SH, Elkin EP, Fenster L (1997) Have sperm densities declined? A reanalysis of global trend data. Environ Health Perspect 105:1228–1232

Swerdlow AJ, Stiller CA, Wilson LM (1982) Prenatal factors in the aetiology of testicular cancer: an epidemiological study of childhood testicular cancer deaths in Great Britain, 1953–73. J Epidemiol Community Health 36:96–101

Swerdlow AJ, Huttly SR, Smith PG (1987a) Prenatal and familial associations of testicular cancer. Br J Cancer 55:571–577

Swerdlow AJ, Huttly SR, Smith PG (1987b) Testicular cancer and antecedent diseases. Br J Cancer 55:97–103

Swerdlow AJ, Huttly SR, Smith PG (1989) Testis cancer: post-natal hormonal factors, sexual behaviour and fertility. Int J Cancer 43:549–553

Swerdlow AJ, Marmot MG, Grulich AE, Head J (1995) Cancer mortality in Indian and British ethnic immigrants from the Indian subcontinent to England and Wales. Br J Cancer 72:1312–1319

Swerdlow AJ, De Stavola BL, Swanwick MA, Maconochie NE (1997a) Risks of breast and testicular cancers in young adult twins in England and Wales: evidence on prenatal and genetic aetiology. Lancet 350:1723–1728

Swerdlow AJ, Higgins CD, Pike MC (1997b) Risk of testicular cancer in cohort of boys with cryptorchidism. BMJ 314:1507–1511

Talerman A, Kaalen JG, Fokkens W (1974) Rural preponderance of testicular neoplasms. Br J Cancer 29:176–178

Thune I, Lund E (1994) Physical activity and the risk of prostate and testicular cancer: a cohort study of 53,000 Norwegian men. Cancer Causes Control 5:549–556

Toledano MB, Jarup L, Best N, Wakefield J, Elliott P (2001) Spatial variation and temporal trends of testicular cancer in Great Britain. Br J Cancer 84:1482–1487

Toppari J, Larsen JC, Christiansen P, Giwercman A, Grandjean P, Guillette LJ Jr, Jegou B, Jensen TK, Jouannet P, Keiding N, Leffers H, McLachlan JA, Meyer O, Muller J, Rajpert-De Meyts E, Scheike T, Sharpe R, Sumpter J, Skakkebaek NE (1996) Male reproductive health and environmental xenoestrogens. Environ Health Perspect 104(Suppl 4):741–803

Travis LB, Fossa SD, Schonfeld SJ, McMaster ML, Lynch CF, Storm H, Hall P, Holowaty E, Andersen A, Pukkala E, Andersson M, Kaijser M, Gospodarowicz M, Joensuu T, Cohen RJ, Boice JD Jr, Dores GM, Gilbert ES (2005) Second cancers among 40,576 testicular cancer patients: focus on long-term survivors. J Natl Cancer Inst 97:1354–1365

United Kingdom Testicular Cancer Study Group (1994a) Aetiology of testicular cancer: association with congenital abnormalities, age at puberty, infertility, and exercise. BMJ 308:1393–1399

United Kingdom Testicular Cancer Study Group (1994b) Social, behavioural and medical factors in the aetiology of testicular cancer: results from the UK study. Br J Cancer 70:513–520

Van Den Eeden SK, Weiss NS, Strader CH, Daling JR (1991) Occupation and the occurrence of testicular cancer. Am J Ind Med 19:327–337

Van Montfrans JM, Dorland M, Oosterhuis GJ, Van Vugt JM, Rekers-Mombarg LT, Lambalk CB (1999) Increased concentrations of follicle-stimulating hormone in mothers of children with Down's syndrome. Lancet 353:1853–1854

Von Eckardstein S, Tsakmakidis G, Kamischke A, Rolf C, Nieschlag E (2001) Sonographic testicular microlithiasis as an indicator of premalignant conditions in normal and infertile men. J Androl 22:818–824

Walcott FL, Hauptmann M, Duphorne CM, Pillow PC, Strom SS, Sigurdson AJ (2002) A case-control study of dietary phytoestrogens and testicular cancer risk. Nutr Cancer 44:44–51

Waliszewski SM, Infanzon RM, Arroyo SG, Pietrini RV, Carvajal O, Trujillo P, Hayward-Jones PM (2005) Persistent organochlorine pesticides levels in blood serum lipids in women bearing babies with undescended testis. Bull Environ Contam Toxicol 75:952–959

Wanderas EH, Tretli S, Fossa SD (1995) Trends in incidence of testicular cancer in Norway 1955–1992. Eur J Cancer 31A:2044–2048

Wanderas EH, Fossa SD, Tretli S (1997) Risk of a second germ cell cancer after treatment of a primary germ cell cancer in 2201 Norwegian male patients. Eur J Cancer 33:244–252

Wanderas EH, Grotmol T, Fossa SD, Tretli S (1998) Maternal health and pre- and perinatal characteristics in the etiology of testicular cancer: a prospective population- and register-based study on Norwegian males born between 1967 and 1995. Cancer Causes Control 9:475–486

Weir HK, Kreiger N, Marrett LD (1998) Age at puberty and risk of testicular germ cell cancer (Ontario, Canada). Cancer Causes Control 9:253–258

Weir HK, Marrett LD, Moravan V (1999) Trends in the incidence of testicular germ cell cancer in Ontario by histologic subgroup, 1964–1996. CMAJ 160:201–205

Weir HK, Marrett LD, Kreiger N, Darlington GA, Sugar L (2000) Pre-natal and peri-natal exposures and risk of testicular germ-cell cancer. Int J Cancer 87:438–443

Westberg HB, Hardell LO, Malmqvist N, Ohlson CG, Axelson O (2005) On the use of different measures of exposure-experiences from a case-control study on testicular cancer and PVC exposure. J Occup Environ Hyg 2:351–356

Westergaard T, Olsen JH, Frisch M, Kroman N, Nielsen JW, Melbye M (1996) Cancer risk in fathers and brothers of testicular cancer patients in Denmark. A population-based study. Int J Cancer 66:627–631

Westergaard T, Andersen PK, Pedersen JB, Frisch M, Olsen JH, Melbye M (1998) Testicular cancer risk and maternal parity: a population-based cohort study. Br J Cancer 77:1180–1185

Whittemore AS, Paffenbarger RS Jr, Anderson K, Lee JE (1984) Early precursors of urogenital cancers in former college men. J Urol 132:1256–1261

Yang C, Chen S (1999) Two organochlorine pesticides, toxaphene and chlordane, are antagonists for estrogen-related receptor alpha-1 orphan receptor. Cancer Res 59:4519–4524

Zavos C, Andreadis C, Diamantopoulos N, Mouratidou D (2004) A hypothesis on the role of insulin-like growth factor I in testicular germ cell tumours. Med Hypotheses 63:511–514

Zhang ZF, Vena JE, Zielezny M, Graham S, Haughey BP, Brasure J, Marshall JR (1995) Occupational exposure to extreme temperature and risk of testicular cancer. Arch Environ Health 50:13–18

Zheng T, Holford TR, Ma Z, Ward BA, Flannery J, Boyle P (1996) Continuing increase in incidence of germ-cell testis cancer in young adults: experience from Connecticut, USA, 1935–1992. Int J Cancer 65:723–729

Part B
Pathology

Chapter 3
Prostate Cancer: A Pathological Perspective

Louis R. Bégin and Tarek A. Bismar

3.1 Introduction

This chapter provides a contemporary pathobiological perspective on various aspects of prostate cancer relating to diagnosis, phenotypical characterization, and prognostication. The emphasis is on conventional adenocarcinoma whose incidence has increased dramatically in the last two decades as a result of serum PSA screening. Following a brief histological overview of the normal prostate, the gross, microscopic, and immunophenotypical features of adenocarcinoma are described, including tumoral variants that can mimic benign conditions on biopsy assessment. In-depth discussion of the Gleason grading system is provided as it has a major impact on prognostic determination and treatment options. Taking into account recent modifications resulting from the 2005 ISUP Consensus Conference, the spectrum of histopathological patterns (grades) and methodology applied to biopsy or surgical specimens to obtain a Gleason score are described. Issues such as tumor quantification, extraprostatic extension (EPE), seminal vesicle invasion, surgical margin (SM) status and pelvic lymph node involvement are covered in terms of stringent definition and prognostic relevance. Cancer-related iatrogenic changes resulting from radiation therapy and androgen-deprivation therapy are outlined. Their recognition having an impact on patient management, entities such as high-grade prostatic intraepithelial neoplasia (HGPIN) (an accepted precursor lesion of many adenocarcinomas) and the descriptive designation of atypical small acinar proliferation (ASAP) are discussed. Accounting for no more than 5–10% of prostate cancer, we briefly describe the special subtypes of tumor, such as ductal adenocarcinoma, urothelial carcinoma, and small cell carcinoma, among others. Emerging biomarkers of potential prognostic interest are selectively and briefly outlined.

L.R. Bégin (✉)
Department of Pathology, McGill University and Hôpital du Sacré-Coeur de Montréal, 5400 Gouin Boulevard, Montreal, QC, H4J 1C5, Canada
e-mail: mdlrb@yahoo.ca

W.D. Foulkes and K.A. Cooney (eds.), *Male Reproductive Cancers:*
Epidemiology, Pathology and Genetics, Cancer Genetics,
DOI 10.1007/978-1-4419-0449-2_3, © Springer Science+Business Media, LLC 2010

3.2   Microanatomy and Histology As Related to Neoplasia

The prostate is characterized by three major distinctive glandular regions referred to as the *peripheral zone* (PZ), *central zone* (CZ), and *transition zone* (TZ). In addition, there is the anterior fibromuscular stroma which is a nonglandular area blending imperceptibly into the bladder neck and apical region (McNeal 1988). The PZ comprises about 70% of the prostate and is the site of origin of the majority (70–75%) of carcinomas, including most of those detected by transrectal ultrasound (TRUS)-guided needle biopsy. It is also the region most susceptible to inflammation which often results in glandular atrophy (McNeal et al. 1988; Young et al. 2000). Furthermore, the PZ is the preferential location for HGPIN (Qian and Bostwick 1995). In the current era of serum PSA screening, the biopsy approach is a systematic mapping of the PZ using an 18-gauge needle biopsy and the "obtainment" of 10 to 13 site-specific cores. For example, the commonly used 10-core biopsy template would map both sides from apex to base including extra cores from the lateral wings of the PZ (Amin et al. 2005). If there is a high clinical index of suspicion for malignancy, additional cores may be obtained from the TZ or from a hypoechoic and/or palpable nodule. The CZ, which is cone-shaped and surrounds the ejaculatory ducts, represents about 25% of the prostate and is generally resistant to HGPIN, carcinoma, and inflammation. Probably no more than 5–10% of carcinomas are native to the CZ (McNeal et al. 1988; Young et al. 2000). The TZ, mostly surrounding the proximal prostatic urethra, accounts for 5% of the normal adult prostate, yet it is almost the exclusive site for nodular hyperplasia which often results in significant enlargement of the prostate in late adulthood. About 15–20% of carcinomas are native to the TZ, and these are generally the tumors incidentally retrieved in transurethral resection of the prostate (TURP) or enucleation surgical specimens (Young et al. 2000). Nearly all well-differentiated (Gleason score 2–4) tumors are native to and often confined to the TZ. Incidentally, a diagnosis of Gleason score 2–4 adenocarcinoma is virtually never rendered on biopsy material obtained from the PZ (Epstein 2000). Interestingly, the TZ outer boundary seems to act as a barrier to intraprostatic spread of non-TZ carcinomas, although large non-TZ tumors may transgress this barrier and involve the TZ as well (McNeal et al. 1988).

Except for the main ducts near the urethra (periurethral ducts), the entire prostatic duct-acinar system is composed of a double-layered epithelium including an inner layer of columnar secretory cells and an outer layer of basal cells which are markedly flattened parallel to the basement membrane. Basal cells are typically inconspicuous on hematoxylin and eosin (H&E) staining. Secretory cells are immunoreactive for prostatic acid phosphatase (PAP), prostate-specific antigen (PSA) which is a serine protease, proPSA (precursor form of PSA) (Chan et al. 2003), prostate-specific membrane antigen (PSMA) which is a membrane glycoprotein having partial homology with the transferrin receptor (Bostwick et al. 2006), P501S (prostein) which is a novel prostate-specific protein (Kalos et al. 2004), and NKX3.1which is a prostate-specific nuclear protein related to the androgen-regulated homeobox gene (Gelmann et al. 2003). These markers are highly specific for benign and malignant prostatic epithelial cells and are not expressed in the seminal vesicles, ejaculatory ducts, or urothelium. These are relevant diagnostic markers for confirming the prostatic phenotype in the setting of metastasis and/or a poorly differentiated tumor (Chuang et al. 2007). Basal cells likely represent the epithelial proliferative (stem cell) compartment (Bonkhoff et al. 1994; De Marzo et al. 1998), are specifically immunoreactive for high molecular weight cytokeratin 34bE12 (cytokeratins 5, 10, 11) and p63 (a nuclear protein) but negative for PSA/PSMA/PAP, and do not display myoepithelial differentiation (Srigley et al. 1990). The presence of basal cells around prostatic glands is indicative of a benign or premalignant process, whereas malignant glands do not express basal cell markers. In the normal prostate there are scattered neuroendocrine (endocrine-paracrine) cells resting on the basal cell layer between secretory cells, mostly immunoreactive for chromogranin, synaptophysin, and serotonin, whereas other neuroendocrine markers are less consistently expressed (Bostwick et al. 2006).

The prostate does not have a true capsule but is rather outlined by a discontinuous fibrous or fibromuscular boundary which is poorly defined anteriorly and apically, and absent at the posterolateral angles near the base where the neurovascular bundles are inserted (Ayala et al. 1989). Anteriorly, the smooth muscle of the prostate merges with the extraprostatic smooth muscle, whereas the apical edge is poorly defined including some benign glands admixed with the skeletal muscle of the urogenital diaphragm. This information is relevant when defining and recognizing EPE which relates to appropriate pathological staging. The designation of capsular invasion or penetration is inappropriate and obsolete.

3.3   Gross Features

Most carcinomas native to the PZ, particularly those detected on the basis of serum PSA screening, involve the posterior or posterolateral aspect of the gland adjacent to the fibromuscular boundary outline. Therefore, they are occasionally palpable on digital rectal examination. On cut surface, in radical prostatectomy or enucleation specimens, tumor identification is often not feasible, particularly in unfixed specimens, small-sized tumors, and tumors of anterior or apical location with often admixed nodular hyperplasia (Epstein et al. 2004). Otherwise, the tumor appears more solid, firmer, smoother, and gray-white to yellow-orange as compared to the uninvolved tan spongy tissue (Fig. 3.1). The tumor contour is often ill-defined, and gross inspection is likely to underestimate the tumor size. The largest tumor diameter is often near and parallel to the outer fibromuscular boundary. Necrosis or hemorrhage is rarely seen. Tumors native to the TZ, usually discovered on TURP specimens, may appear as tissue chips with yellow-orange foci and/or a firmer consistency on palpation. Multifocality is observed in 50–85% of tumors and has been best documented on the basis of whole-mount prostate microscopic analysis. However, it is grossly apparent in no more than 10–20% of cases (Fig. 3.1a) as most

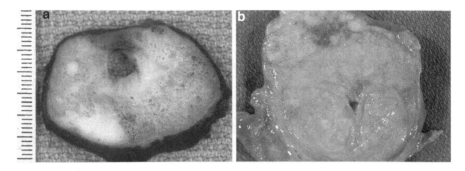

Fig. 3.1 (**a**) Organ-confined PZ cancer localized posteriorly with its largest diameter parallel to the inked prostatic outline (*lower left*). Note rounded, small additional tumor focus reflecting multicentricity (*upper left*); (**b**) Locally advanced PZ cancer with a major tumor component invading the periprostatic soft tissue posteriorly (*upper third*). The TZ shows nodular hyperplasia and is uninvolved by tumor (*lower half*)

tumor foci are of minute size, often contiguous to HGPIN in the background (Young et al. 2000; McNeal et al. 1991).

3.4 Microscopic and Diagnostic Features

The vast majority (about 95%) of prostate carcinomas are adenocarcinomas, i.e., proliferating and infiltrative gland patterns with various architectural features ranging from well-differentiated gland-forming tumors difficult to distinguish from benign glands to poorly differentiated tumors difficult to identify as of prostatic glandular origin. Such adenocarcinomas are often referred to as of the *usual, acinar*, or *conventional type*. On the other hand, the designation of adenocarcinoma without further qualification in clinical practice refers to this particular form of tumor. About 5% of carcinomas are of special type (Table 3.1) and are further discussed in the text (Randolph et al. 1997). The diagnosis of an adenocarcinoma of prostate at large, including minimal/minute tumor biopsy sampling (Grignon 1998; Epstein 2004), is based on a constellation of cytoarchitectural features which may be present in varying degrees and extent (Young et al. 2000; Epstein and Netto 2008; Humphrey 2003; Epstein et al. 2004). On the other hand, biopsy interpretation can be quite challenging, as many benign conditions can mimic adenocarcinoma, namely postatrophic microacinar hyperplasia, atypical adenomatous hyperplasia (AAH)/adenosis, sclerosing adenosis, verumontanum mucosal gland hyperplasia, and hyperplasia of mesonephric remnants (Eble 1998; Srigley 2004).

Architectural abnormalities include major features clearly indicative of invasion such as glands with a haphazard distribution between benign/native glands, confluent glands, cords, single cells, perineural invasion (PNI), and dissection of muscle fibers. There are also features such as small, closely packed glands, relatively monotonous-looking glands, glands clearly distinctive from nearby benign glands,

Table 3.1 Classification of primary carcinomas of the prostate[a]

Adenocarcinoma of the usual type (acinar, conventional) (90–95%)
Special types (5–10%)
Ductal adenocarcinoma
Mucinous adenocarcinoma
Signet ring cell carcinoma
Urothelial carcinoma
Squamous cell and adenosquamous carcinoma
Basal cell carcinoma
Small cell carcinoma
Large cell neuroendocrine carcinoma
Sarcomatoid carcinoma

[a]Modified from Young et al. (2000) AFIP Fascicle

glomerulations, and periglandular retraction from the surrounding stroma. Cytological abnormalities include: a single cell type without a basal cell constituent/phenotype, a sine qua non requirement; a tinctorial cytoplasmic alteration as compared to nearby benign glands, including a darker (amphophilic) or paler cytoplasm; a sharp, truncated luminal border; and nuclear changes including nucleomegaly, hyperchromasia, and distinctive to large nucleoli (nucleolomegaly). Generally, there is little variability in nuclear shape or size within one tumor, whereas in some cases nuclei are virtually indistinguishable from benign nuclei. Other features that can be seen in malignant glands are related to the intraluminal contents, namely wispy blue-tinged mucin (high specificity), flocculent granular vs. acellular dense pink secretions (limited specificity), and crystalloids (limited specificity). Corpora amylacea are very rarely seen in malignant glands.

Furthermore, three additional features virtually pathognomonic of adenocarcinoma can be seen and are particularly useful in the diagnosis of carcinoma on minimal tumor biopsy sampling (Baisden et al. 1999): PNI defined as wrapping of the nerve, seen in up to 10–20% of positive biopsies, which should be distinguished from perineural indentation by benign prostate glands; mucinous fibroplasia, also referred to as collagenous micronodules, characterized by delicate fibrous tissue with an ingrowth of fibroblasts, of intra- or extraluminal topography; and glomerulations characterized by glands with a cribriform proliferation that is not transluminal. Tumor necrosis, stromal myxoid or desmoplastic alteration within the prostate confinement, and inflammation are usually not seen. Mitoses are very uncommon. Angiolymphatic invasion is most unusual and its prevalence has been probably overestimated in the literature.

Three uncommon morphological variants are recognized within the microscopic spectrum of conventional adenocarcinoma and may occur as a dominant or minor tumor component. Their significance is mostly from a diagnostic perspective as they can mimic benign glandular conditions. These variants are potential diagnostic pitfalls particularly in biopsies with minimal tumor sampling. The variant with *atrophic-like features*, so-called atrophic carcinoma, is characterized by glands with scant cytoplasm that can mimic benign atrophic glands (Cina and Epstein 1997;

Egan et al. 1997). Clues for the diagnosis of malignancy include an infiltrative topography between larger benign glands, at least focal nuclear atypia (nucleomegaly and nucleolomegaly), and the coexistence with a nonatrophic carcinomatous component. The *pseudohyperplastic variant* is characterized by larger malignant glands with branching and papillary infolding mimicking normal glands or nodular hyperplasia (Humphrey et al. 1998; Levi and Epstein 2000). Some glands may have a straight even luminal border with abundant cytoplasm. Clues for an appropriate diagnosis include high density and close packing of these glands, and significant nuclear atypia. Despite its overall bland appearance, the pseudohyperplastic variant is usually encountered in the moderate or moderate to poorly differentiated spectrum (Gleason score 6–7) of adenocarcinoma and may show aggressive behavior such as EPE. The *foamy gland variant*, so-called foamy gland carcinoma, consists of glands with abundant foamy cytoplasm of nonlipidic, empty vacuolar nature, a very low nuclear to cytoplasmic ratio, and a bland-looking nuclear morphology (round, small, and hyperchromatic nuclei) (Nelson and Epstein 1996; Tran et al. 2001). Diagnostic clues include an infiltrative and/or packed morphology, often the presence of intraluminal pink dense secretions, and the coexistence of a nonfoamy carcinomatous component. Despite its bland cytology, this variant is considered a potentially aggressive subset often with an associated Gleason pattern 4 carcinomatous component and evidence of EPE in radical prostatectomy specimens (Tran et al. 2001). In all three of these tumor variants, the universal absence of basal cell immunoreactivity for cytokeratin 34bE12 and p63 is of key value in confirming their malignant nature.

3.5 Immunophenotype

Nearly all adenocarcinomas show cytoplasmic immunoreactivity for PSA and PAP although with more staining variability and less intensity in higher-grade/less-differentiated tumors (Goldstein 2002; Bostwick et al. 2006). Regarding the expression of PSMA, which is up-regulated in carcinoma, the most extensive and intense degree of staining is observed in poorly differentiated tumors, i.e., Gleason patterns 4 and 5 (Marchal et al. 2004). Since a small number of high-grade tumors may be reactive for only one of these markers, combined immunostaining may be useful in confirming the prostatic origin when PSA staining alone is negative. Furthermore, novel markers such as P501S (prostein), NKX3.1, and proPSA are expressed in the vast majority of adenocarcinomas (>90%), including poorly differentiated/high-grade tumors (Gelmann et al. 2003; Kalos et al. 2004; Parwani et al. 2006; Chuang et al. 2007), and therefore are of potential diagnostic utility in problematic cases.

Alpha-methylacyl-CoA racemase (AMACR, racemase, P504S protein) is an enzyme involved in beta-oxidation of branched-chain fatty acids and has been found to be overexpressed in the cytoplasm of a great majority of prostatic adenocarcinomas (Jiang et al. 2001). It is overexpressed in more than 85% of carcinomas detected by biopsies (Jiang et al. 2002; Magi-Galluzzi et al. 2003). AMACR is a very useful marker for the diagnosis of minimal adenocarcinoma, namely in the setting of an ASAP of uncertain nature, as it can increase the level of diagnostic confidence for malignancy in conjunction with negative basal cell immunoreactivity, since not all benign glands label uniformly with basal cell markers (Jiang et al. 2002; Magi-Galluzzi et al. 2003; Zhou et al. 2004). However, tumor variants such as atrophic-like, pseudohyperplastic, and foamy gland adenocarcinoma are immunoreactive for AMACR in only 60–70% of cases (Zhou et al. 2003; Epstein 2004). Triple (cocktail) immunostaining for basal cell markers (34bE12/p63) and AMACR is emerging as a favored technical approach as it can be applied on a single glass slide (Browne et al. 2004).

Carcinomatous cells are universally immunoreactive for cytokeratin AE1/AE3 (low and high molecular weight cytokeratin spectrum/cocktail). Cytoplasmic expression of cytokeratins 7 (CK7) and 20 (CK20) is observed in no more than half of adenocarcinomas and is relatively more common (prevalence and % of cells) in higher Gleason scores (Goldstein 2002). From a diagnostic perspective, CK7 and CK20 are markers of low specificity and of no ancillary value. Androgen receptor (AR) is a nuclear localized, androgen-binding protein complex present in secretory, basal, and stromal cells of the prostate. Nuclear staining, which does not distinguish active from inactive forms, has been observed in more than 85% of untreated adenocarcinomas with increased heterogeneity in higher-grade tumors (Magi-Galluzzi et al. 1997). Currently, AR immunostaining has no diagnostic or prognostic utility.

3.6   Gleason Histological Grading System

Originally designed in 1966 by Donald T. Gleason (Bailar et al. 1966; Gleason 1966) and subsequently refined in the following decades, the Gleason grading system has been endorsed by the World Health Organization (WHO) and the Armed Forces Institute of Pathology (AFIP), is now accepted throughout the world, and is widely used in clinical trials (Young et al. 2000; Epstein et al. 2004). Along with pathological staging, it is the most powerful prognostic determinant in terms of natural history in untreated patients and tumor progression (including PSA biochemical recurrence) following radical prostatectomy or radiation therapy (Albertsen et al. 1995; Egevad et al. 2002; Gleason and Mellinger 2002). Furthermore, in biopsy assessment, Gleason grading (score) has a major impact on therapeutic strategy as a patient with a high Gleason score (8–10) is unlikely to be a candidate for active surveillance (watchful waiting) or curative surgery. This grading system is strictly based on microscopic assessment of tumor architecture (at low to intermediate magnification) without consideration for the nuclear morphology. It recognizes five basic patterns (grades) with decreasing differentiation, including some morphological subsets within patterns 3, 4, and 5. Following the 2005 International Society of Urological Pathology (ISUP) Consensus Conference, a modified Gleason grading was adopted, providing some subtle yet stringent modifications in the recognition of some tumor patterns (namely patterns 3 and 4) and in the scoring methodology, particularly when applied to biopsy specimens (Epstein et al. 2005a). These modifications aimed at better standardization in daily pathological practice and were also influenced by the current mode of diagnosis of prostate cancer in the current era of PSA screening as well as the application of nomograms (e.g., Partin tables) in clinical management (Partin et al. 2001).

Gleason pattern 1 is a circumscribed nodule of closely packed but separate, uniform, rounded to oval, medium-sized glands. There is no infiltration between adjacent benign glands. This pattern is exceedingly rare, mostly confined to the TZ, and virtually never diagnosed on needle biopsies (Epstein 2000). *Gleason pattern 2* is a fairly circumscribed nodule of more loosely arranged medium-sized glands not quite as uniform as pattern 1 (Fig. 3.2a). Minimal infiltration between adjacent benign glands can be seen. This pattern is usually encountered in the TZ, but occasionally found in the PZ. *Gleason pattern 3* is mostly characterized by variably sized individual glands, most often small-sized (smaller than seen in patterns 1 or 2), infiltrating in and among benign glands (Fig. 3.2b). The presence of smoothly circumscribed rounded small cribriform nodules of the same size of normal glands is also a morphological subset of relatively uncommon occurrence. Carcinomatous histological variants such as atrophic-like, pseudohyperplastic, and often foamy gland, represent a Gleason pattern 3. *Gleason pattern 4* is basically characterized by ill-defined glands with poorly formed glandular lumina and often fused microacinar glands (Fig. 3.2c). Morphological subsets include large cribriform glands not fulfilling the caliber of pattern 3 (Fig. 3.2d) or cribriform glands with an irregular border, and the rare hypernephromatoid pattern of fused glands with clear or very pale-staining cytoplasm (Fig. 3.2e). In *Gleason pattern 5*, there is essentially no glandular differentiation, i.e., an almost complete loss of lumina, the tumor being composed of solid sheets, cords, or single tumor cells invading the stroma (Fig. 3.2f). Comedocarcinoma with central necrosis surrounded by papillary, cribriform, or solid masses (without any basal cell constituent immunoreactive for cytokeratin 34BE12/p63 at their periphery) is also defined as a pattern 5.

Taking into account the marked degree of intratumoral architectural/pattern heterogeneity in prostate cancer (Aihara et al. 1994), the Gleason grading methodology for obtaining a score (sum) is based on recognition of a primary pattern defined as the most prevalent in surface area, a secondary pattern defined as the second most prevalent in surface area, and occasionally a tertiary pattern (the least prevalent of the three). If the tumor is composed of only one pattern, the Gleason score is obtained by doubling the numerical value of this pattern, e.g., pattern 3 + 3 for a score of 6. If the tumor includes two patterns, the score is obtained by the sum of the primary and secondary patterns, e.g., 3 + 4 for a score of 7. If three patterns are encountered, a Gleason score is obtained differently depending on the nature of tissue material. For *biopsy/*TUPR/*enucleation specimens*, the primary pattern is added to the worse (numerically the higher) pattern of the remaining two, e.g., primary pattern 3 (50%), secondary pattern 4 (40%), and tertiary pattern 5 (10%) would result in a score of 8 (3 + 5). In other words, the higher pattern of the remaining two is incorporated as the secondary pattern. *For radical prostatectomy specimens*, the score is obtained by the sum of the primary and secondary patterns, and

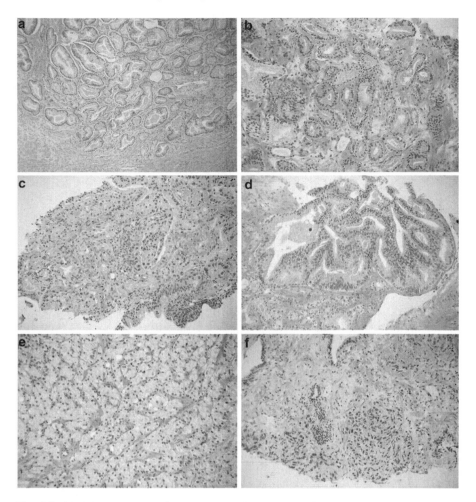

Fig. 3.2 (**a**) Adenocarcinoma Gleason pattern 2, characterized by a circumscribed nodule of medium- to large-sized, individualized glands with some irregular spacing; (**b**) Gleason pattern 3 with small glands anarchically infiltrating between benign native glands (*extreme left*); (**c**) Gleason pattern 4 with confluent pattern of more or less poorly formed glands; (**d**) Gleason pattern 4 with large rounded cribriform tumor component; (**e**) Gleason pattern 4 of confluent nests/cords of tumor cells with clear cytoplasm, so-called hypernephromatoid; (**f**) Gleason pattern 5 with solid tumor without glandular differentiation (*lower half*)

recording of a tertiary pattern with its relative percentage if worse (numerically higher) than the remaining two. Recognition and recording of a tertiary Gleason pattern 5 in a prostatectomy specimen has prognostic significance, namely in predicting PSA biochemical recurrence and tumor progression (Mosse et al. 2004; Hattab et al. 2006).

The following practical considerations are relevant to the contemporary use of the Gleason grading system and its clinical interpretation. On needle biopsy assessment, each core (sample) of the mapping is generally assigned an individual Gleason score rather than a composite score on the overall positive tissue sampling. This approach seems to be a better predictor of pathological stage at radical prostatectomy (Kunz and Epstein 2003), whereby the highest score will be the one clinically selected for therapeutic strategy (Rubin et al. 2004). In other words, the biopsy site sample with the highest Gleason score is the one mostly considered when using nomograms and making clinical decisions, independent of the overall percentage involvement. In general, whatever the type of tissue specimen, if a secondary pattern is less than 5% of the tumor and of lower grade than the primary pattern, it is ignored and not accounted for in the score (Epstein et al. 2005a). A score 2 is never assigned on biopsy, is of very rare occurrence, and is strictly given on a radical prostatectomy or TURP specimen (Epstein 2000). Similarly, a score 3–4 should rarely, if ever be made on biopsy (Epstein 2000). In radical prostatectomy specimens, as cancer multifocality is highly prevalent, each separate "dominant" (at least >5 mm) tumor nodule should be individually assigned a score as well as any-sized focus with a high-grade morphology, i.e., Gleason patterns 4 and 5.

Regarding the interobserver reproducibility of Gleason grading, the level of agreement has generally been moderate among general pathologists (Allsbrook et al. 2001a) and substantially better among uropathologists (Allsbrook et al. 2001b). The major issue is undergrading, namely pattern 3 being misinterpreted as patterns 1 or 2 (Steinberg et al. 1997). However, educational efforts and the use of Web-based tutorials significantly improve the level of reproducibility in Gleason grading (Kronz et al. 2000).

The concordance of Gleason score between biopsy and radical prostatectomy specimens is within one score in more than 90% of cases, and therefore relatively good (Bostwick 1994; Spires et al. 1994; Steinberg et al. 1997). However, biopsy undergrading is a reality and occurs in about one-third of cases, largely resulting from sampling issues. The concordance tends to be decreased in low-grade tumors or if a minimal volume of tumor is sampled on biopsy.

The frequency and rate of Gleason score (grade) progression in prostate cancer is unknown, but it is generally agreed that high-grade disease correlates with a larger volume of tumor (McNeal et al. 1990; Aihara et al. 1994; Epstein et al. 2004). However, some high-grade tumors may be of relatively small size de novo, suggesting that dedifferentiation does not necessarily always result from time progression and large tumor volume (Epstein et al. 1994).

In clinical practice, *Gleason score grouping* is often used for prognostic categorization with regard to treatment and prognosis, the following scheme being currently used and differing slightly from the TNM 2002 scheme (Epstein et al. 2005b): *well differentiated* for Gleason scores 2–4, most patients being cured following therapy; *moderately differentiated* for Gleason scores 5–6; *moderately to poorly differentiated* for Gleason score 7, the prognosis being significantly worse than for scores 5–6; and *poorly differentiated* for Gleason scores 8–10, encountered in less than 10% of carcinomas at radical prostatectomy, and a highly aggressive disease often presenting at high stage. Over 90% of carcinomas encountered in radical prostatectomy specimens are moderately or moderately to poorly differentiated tumors, i.e., within a Gleason score 5–7 range. Regarding Gleason score 7, there is some evidence that a tumor with a primary pattern 4 has a more aggressive outcome than one with a primary pattern 3, although there are some conflicting results (Chan et al. 2000; Sakr et al. 2000; Lau et al. 2001; Epstein et al. 2005b). In Partin nomograms, patients with a score 7 (4+3), i.e., with primary pattern 4, are considered differently from patients with a score 7 (3+4).

3.7   Pathological Prognostic Determinants other than Grading

In addition to grading, features of key importance in reporting prostate cancer include tumor quantification, EPE, invasion of seminal vesicles, and SM status. These parameters are validated prognostic determinants, some of which are incorporated in the current pathological staging system (TNM) and are useful in clinical management (Epstein et al. 2005b; Srigley 2006).

On biopsy, *tumor quantification* is provided as the number of positive cores (samples), the relative percentage of tumor in each core vs. a global percentage, and/or the tumor length involvement (mm) of each core vs. a global tumor length. This information is relevant as it may help to predict pathological stage and SM status, extensive biopsy involvement being generally indicative of an adverse outcome (Bismar et al. 2003). However, minimal tumor involvement is not necessarily predictive of a favorable outcome due to sampling limitations. It is generally agreed that tumor volume is an important prognostic determinant which correlates with Gleason score, pathological stage, SM status, and tumor progression following prostatectomy (McNeal 1992; Epstein et al. 2004). On the other hand, although there is conflicting information, tumor volume in prostatectomy specimens has not been convincingly shown to be an independent prognostic determinant when controlling for other pathological parameters (Kikuchi et al. 2004; Epstein et al. 2005b). As tumor volume assessment is not easy in daily practice, recording the maximum tumor diameter is a simple and reproducible quantitative methodology that correlates reasonably well with total tumor volume (Renshaw et al. 1999), and has been shown to be a significant predictor of biochemical recurrence in one study (Eichelberger et al. 2005). The ratio of tumor positive tissue blocks to the total number of blocks submitted (positive-block ratio) is also a valid method of quantification which was shown to be an independent predictor of PSA recurrence in a recent study (Marks et al. 2007).

EPE is defined as tumor invasion into the adjacent periprostatic soft tissue (Fig. 3.3a). As the prostate is lacking a true capsule (Ayala et al. 1989), definitional microscopic criteria when EPE is not grossly evident must be stringent, yet they are often subtle. EPE occurs predominantly posteriorly and posterolaterally via PNI in PZ cancer, whereas it occurs anteriorly by direct stromal invasion in TZ cancer. Posterolaterally, EPE implies the presence of tumor in the loose extraprostatic fibrous tissue and/or fat, or significant extension beyond the fibromuscular boundary/

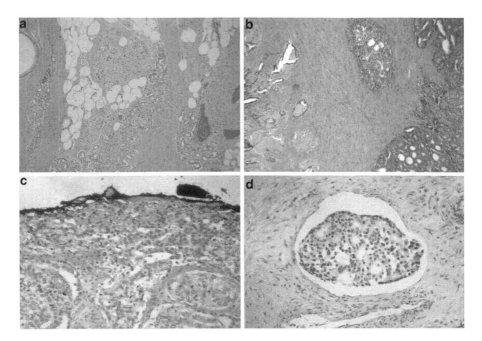

Fig. 3.3 (**a**) Extraprostatic extension (EPE) of adenocarcinoma with small-sized malignant glands at the level of fat and large nerves in the periprostatic soft tissue; (**b**) Seminal vesicle invasion (SVI) with adenocarcinoma within the muscularis propria (*right half*). Note the glandular constituent of the seminal vesicle in the left third; (**c**) Positive surgical marginal status with carcinoma in contact with the ink at the level of transection; (**d**) Intraluminal carcinomatous embolus characteristic of angiolymphatic invasion, usually observed in large volume and advanced tumor

outline of the prostate. A dense desmoplastic response to tumor may occur in periprostatic adipose tissue resulting in an irregular bulge in the surface contour (Epstein et al. 2005b). Furthermore, one of the most common modes of EPE in this region is involvement of a neurovascular bundle exiting the posterolateral angle of the body near the base. Anteriorly and apically, EPE is defined as the presence of tumor beyond the adjacent benign glandular outline of the prostate although determination of EPE in this location may be difficult. Some pathologists believe that assessment of EPE at the apex is not feasible (Epstein et al. 2005b). EPE is often subjectively qualified as *focal* vs. *nonfocal* or *extensive*, a distinction not accounted for in the current pT3a staging. The extent of EPE can also be quantitatively assessed, namely by measuring with an ocular micrometer the distance that the tumor protrudes perpendicularly beyond the outer margin of the prostate. In a recent study, this so-called *radial distance* of EPE was found to be an independent predictor of PSA recurrence and therefore of potential value for substaging pT3a tumors (Sung et al. 2007). In the last two decades, the incidence of EPE in radical prostatectomies has significantly decreased as a result of early diagnosis on the basis of PSA screening (Epstein et al. 2005b). EPE is occasionally confirmed on biopsy when malignant glands are seen within fat at the tip of the core. On the other hand, the presence of tumor among skeletal muscle or ganglion cells is not equivalent of EPE, as these elements are commonly found within the prostate per se.

Seminal vesicle invasion (SVI) is defined as the presence of tumor within the muscularis propria of the seminal vesicle at the extraprostatic level, i.e., the free part, and not at the level of ejaculatory ducts (Fig. 3.3b). SVI is a significant prognostic determinant most often associated with concomitant EPE. Evidence of SVI at large in radical prostatectomy specimens has an adverse prognostic impact with a 5-year biochemical PSA progression-free mean rate of about 35% in men with otherwise negative pelvic lymph nodes (Epstein et al. 2005b). On the other hand, SVI is not necessarily indicative of a uniformly poor prognosis when patients are substratified taking into account other pathological parameters (Debras et al. 1998; Tefilli et al. 1998; Epstein et al. 2000). Three pathways of invasion may result in SVI, namely extension via the ejaculatory duct complex, spreading through the base of the prostate or via the periprostatic/periseminal vesicle soft tissue, or as a discontinuous localized tumor deposit presumably of metastatic nature (Ohori et al. 1993). As their glandular epithelium looks alike, the distinction between the ejaculatory duct and the seminal vesicle is not always easy on a biopsy specimen, and therefore stringent criteria of recognition must be used. One should rely on the presence of a muscularis propria which is an intrinsic constituent of the seminal vesicle but not the ejaculatory duct, and correlation with appropriate topographic information as provided by the biopsy operator.

Regarding the SM status, a positive margin is defined as carcinomatous cells in apposition with the inked (India ink) margin of the prostatectomy specimen, having excluded false cuts and artifactual tissue crevices (Fig. 3.3c). A positive SM may result from two possible scenarios. First, it may result from transection of an "intraprostatic" tumor and therefore be compatible with organ-confined disease as the presence or absence of EPE cannot be determined at that level. This phenomenon is most often seen posterolaterally at the neurovascular bundles or apically. It is often referred to as an iatrogenic positive margin (stage pT2+), implying that one cannot exclude EPE at that level. Second, it may result from an inability to widely excise the EPE component of a tumor, the preferential site being the posterolateral aspect in the region of neurovascular bundles. In TZ cancer, the positive margin is usually anterior concomitantly with EPE at that level. A positive SM is usually further qualified as *focal* or *extensive*. The SM status is an important prognostic determinant following surgery, as patients with a positive SM have an increased risk of progression as compared to those with a negative SM, multifocal and extensive involvement being associated with a higher risk of progression (Epstein et al. 2005b). Importantly, a *microscopically* positive margin at the bladder neck is not considered as pT4 disease in terms of pathological stage.

Angiolymphatic invasion is an extremely rare observation in biopsy specimens (Fig. 3.3d). In prostatectomy specimens, although there is a wide range of prevalence reported (Epstein et al. 2005b), it is a relatively uncommon finding nowadays as it is more likely to be encountered in volumetrically large and advanced disease. Furthermore, some overestimation may potentially result from the presence of retraction space artifact around tumor. There is some evidence that this finding could be an independent predictor of progression, yet it is not definitely conclusive (Herman et al. 2000; Epstein et al. 2005b).

PNI is defined as tumor juxtaposed intimately along, around, or within a nerve, and is observed in about 10–20% of needle biopsy specimens (Epstein and Netto 2008; Bismar et al. 2003). There is substantial evidence that its presence in biopsies correlates with EPE in radical prostatectomy specimens (Amin et al. 2005) (although there is conflicting information in this regard), and that its value as an independent prognostic determinant is questionable (Bismar et al. 2003). PNI is usually reported in biopsies as this information may be clinically required for treatment purposes, e.g., planning nerve-sparing surgery. On the other hand, PNI is a ubiquitous (>75%) finding in prostatectomy specimens and has not been shown to be an independent prognostic determinant (Epstein et al. 2005b).

3.8 Mode of Tumor Spreading

As already discussed, local tumor spread usually occurs within periprostatic soft tissue (stage pT3a) and/or as seminal vesicle involvement (stage pT3b). Whereas EPE is a relatively common microscopic finding in radical prostatectomy specimens following a clinical assumption of organ-confined disease, clinically detectable/grossly visible disease (Fig. 3.1b) is encountered less often today than in the past. In some cases, clinical/gross invasion of the bladder neck region (stage pT4) can occur particularly in large tumors and be associated with obstructive uropathy. Spreading to the rectal wall (stage pT4) is of rare occurrence as the interposed Denonvillier's fascia provides a natural barrier of resistance.

Distant disease occurs as lymphatic or hematogenous spread via the angiolymphatic route of invasion. Regarding *lymphatic spread*, the natural route of lymphatic drainage for the prostate is the pelvic lymph nodes. The first ones usually involved are the obturator and hypogastric, followed by external iliac, common iliac, presacral, and presciatic. The prevalence of periprostatic/periseminal vesicle lymph nodes being rare (<5%) in radical prostatectomy specimens, their involvement alone with metastasis conveys the same prognostic significance as with pelvic lymph nodes (Kothari et al. 2001). Very rarely, supraclavicular or axillary lymph nodes (often left-sided) may be involved. The overall incidence of pelvic lymph node metastases at the time of radical prostatectomy has markedly decreased over the last decades, estimated at less than 2%, as a result of earlier diagnosis and more selective surgery (Catalona and Smith 1998). The extent of pelvic lymphadenectomy during radical prostatectomy is a subject of controversy. If a lymphadenectomy specimen is provided, it is safe to submit all the adipose tissue for histological examination as lymph nodes can be difficult to visualize grossly. The presence of pelvic lymph node metastases is of poor prognostic significance. Indeed, without further treatment, distant hematogenous metastases appear within 5 years in more than 85% of such patients (Epstein et al. 2004). However, it is unclear if the number of positive lymph nodes and/or evidence of perinodal soft tissue involvement has significance in prognostic substratification (Epstein et al. 2005b). The concept of "isolated tumor cells" (single cells or clusters of cells ≤0.2 mm) and micrometastasis (tumor cell aggregate ≤0.2 cm), as applied in breast cancer staging, is not currently incorporated in the 2002 TNM pathological staging system for prostate cancer.

Bone is the preferential site of distant *hematogenous dissemination*, namely pelvic bones followed by dorsal and lumbar vertebrae, ribs, cervical vertebrae, femur, skull, sacrum, and humerus (Epstein et al. 2004). Tumor embolization through the paravertebral vascular plexus is probably the pathway involved in vertebral metastases. Intraosseous/bone marrow metastatic involvement is usually associated with osteoblastic changes, i.e., a production of a large amount of reactive woven bone. Lung and liver metastases usually occur in terminal disease and are not necessarily clinically apparent. In a setting of distant metastases, the mortality rate is about 15% at 3 years, 80% at 5 years, and 90% at 10 years (Epstein et al. 2004).

3.9 Iatrogenic Histological Changes Resulting from Therapy

3.9.1 Radiation Therapy Effect

As it allows for a relatively precise delivery of ionizing radiation, brachytherapy (interstitial seed implants) and/or three-dimensional external beam radiation therapy are currently used in the treatment of clinically localized prostate cancer. Needle biopsy sampling may be done to monitor treatment response. It is also useful in the setting of biochemical PSA failure to confirm and characterize tumor recurrence and potentially select patients in which salvage prostatectomy might be considered. Biopsy findings have prognostic relevance as positive biopsies without evidence of treatment effect are associated with a worse outcome than negative biopsies, whereas carcinoma with treatment effect has an intermediate prognosis (Epstein et al. 2004). In order to provide a meaningful biopsy interpretation following radiation therapy, a minimal interval from treatment completion to biopsy of 18 months is desirable. Practically speaking, microscopic assessment is looking at the following scenarios: no detectable tumor; the presence of altered carcinoma, i.e., with significant radiation effect; the presence of unaltered carcinoma; or a combination of the latter two. In positive biopsies, the histological appearance of carcinoma is variable ranging from cases with profound treatment effect to others showing no apparent therapy effect (Gaudin 1998). Significant treatment effect is observed in about 40–50% of patients (Cheng et al. 1999; Gaudin et al. 1999).

Adenocarcinoma with radiation effect is characterized by a decreased number of glands which are often poorly formed or of markedly attenuated caliber, with a haphazard topographic distribution, and which may result in clustered or individual cells. Artifactual retraction from the surrounding stroma is frequently observed among malignant glands and cell clusters. Unlike irradiated benign glands, carcinomatous cells usually have a large amount of clear or vacuolated cytoplasm, whereas nuclei lack the striking degree of atypia usually seen in benign glands. Nuclear enlargement may or may not be apparent, and there is often a loss of nucleolomegaly. In fact, architectural evidence of invasion and the absence of a basal cell constituent (negativity for cytokeratin 34bE12 and p63) are major diagnostic determinants of malignancy in a postradiation setting as benign glands show varying degrees of atrophy and nuclear atypia that can mimic malignancy. The expression of cytokeratin AE1/AE3, PSA, and PAP persists within tumor cells. Gleason grading is not applied to carcinoma with radiation effect as there is a phenomenon of iatrogenic (artifactual) grade inflation.

3.9.2   Androgen-Deprivation Therapy Effect

Of common use in metastatic disease, androgen-deprivation (total androgen blockade) therapy has also been studied in combination with radiation therapy or radical prostatectomy to treat clinically localized disease. The available data on androgen-deprivation-related changes in the prostate are mostly based on the study of prostatectomy specimens (Têtu et al. 1991; Vaillancourt et al. 1996; Reuter 1997; Bullock et al. 2002). Following many months of androgen deprivation, a significant decrease in tumor volume and major cytoarchitectural alterations occur in most adenocarcinomas (Gaudin 1998). The residual adenocarcinoma is characterized by marked alteration and loss of glandular architecture, attenuation of the glandular caliber, including poorly formed glands, and loss of stromal-epithelial cohesion. Tumor cells show prominent cytoplasmic clearing with an ill-defined outline, loss of tinctorial affinity, decreased nuclear size, and loss of nucleolar prominence. Glands with a discontinuous, flattened epithelial lining, variable degrees of luminal dilatation, or even rupture and extravasated, blue-tinged mucin can be observed. Microcystic mucin-containing spaces without residual lining epithelium are occasionally seen. Tumor identification may be difficult in the presence of minute cell clusters or isolated tumor cells only. In such instances, immunohistochemical staining is required to confirm the presence of residual carcinoma whose cells will be immunoreactive for cytokeratin AE1/AE/PSA but negative for cytokeratin 34bE12. Because of iatrogenic artifactual grade inflation, no tumor grade is provided following androgen-deprivation therapy.

3.10   Putative Precursor Lesions of Prostatic Adenocarcinoma

3.10.1   Prostatic Intraepithelial Neoplasia (PIN)

Prostatic intraepithelial neoplasia (PIN) is defined as a neoplastic transformation of the secretory epithelium of native glands/acini, showing an intraepithelial spectrum of cytological changes culminating in those similar to carcinoma (Young et al. 2000,

Sakr 2004). PIN is currently stratified as low-grade PIN and high-grade PIN (HGPIN), the latter showing much more significant cytological alteration, namely, distinctive nucleoli. In practice, low-grade PIN is not reported as it lacks diagnostic reproducibility and its high prevalence does not convey significant information as a risk factor for carcinoma (Epstein and Netto 2008). HGPIN is histologically characterized by cellular/nuclear stratification, cytoplasmic amphophilia, nuclear enlargement and hyperchromasia, and distinctive to prominent nucleoli (Fig. 3.4). These changes usually result in glands with a darker tinctorial quality that stand out on lower magnification. HGPIN may depict the following architectural patterns: a tufting pattern including undulating mounds and humps; a micropapillary pattern with finger-like projections; a cribriform pattern; and a flat pattern composed of one or two cell layers, of uncommon occurrence. Variants of HGPIN resembling histological subsets of prostatic adenocarcinoma, e.g., foamy cell type, signet ring cell type, have also been described (Reyes et al. 1997).

Based on autopsy studies, HGPIN seems to appear about a decade earlier than prostatic adenocarcinoma (Sakr et al. 1994). The overall incidence of HGPIN is reasonably estimated at 5–8% in biopsy material and about 2% in TURP specimens (Epstein and Herawi 2006; Akhavan et al. 2007), although variation in reporting is affected by the number of biopsy cores obtained, the type of population studied, and the reproducibility issue. HGPIN is present in more than 85% of prostatectomy specimens.

There is strong evidence for a relationship between HGPIN and adenocarcinoma of the prostate, particularly for tumors native to the PZ. The incidence and extent of HGPIN increases with age and both lesions show a similar topographic distribution, have common cytological alterations, and share molecular features and biomarker expression including p27, p53, C-MYC, AMACR, and the newly described TMPRSS2-ERG gene fusion associated with prostate cancer, among several other features (Sakr et al. 1996; Sakr and Partin 2001; Humphrey 2003). Interestingly, Perner et al. have recently detected the latter fusion gene in 19% of HGPIN lesions

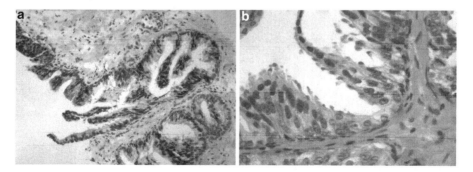

Fig. 3.4 (**a**) Native glands with a tufting and micropapillary pattern of prostatic intraepithelial neoplasia (PIN); (**b**) The presence of nucleomegaly and nucleolar prominence at the basal pole defines high-grade PIN

contiguous to adenocarcinoma but not in isolated HGPIN lesions, suggesting that only a subset of HGPIN lesions shares a strong association with prostate cancer (Perner et al. 2007).

Patients with a diagnosis of HGPIN alone on biopsy have a 30–35% risk of cancer detection in subsequent follow-up biopsies, based on an assessment of the largest studies (Sakr 2004, Epstein and Netto 2008). On the other hand, a cancer is unlikely to be found if it was not detected on the first two follow-up biopsies (Epstein and Netto 2008). Data appear inconsistent when it comes to the association between certain types (e.g., architectural patterns) or the extent of HGPIN and the subsequent risk of cancer detection, depending on the study design and whether other parameters such as serum PSA are compounded in the analysis (Bishara et al. 2004; Herawi et al. 2006; Netto and Epstein 2006; Brimo et al. 2007).

3.10.2 Atypical Adenomatous Hyperplasia (AAH)

AAH, also called adenosis, is a well-circumscribed, lobular proliferation of small glands with nuclear/cytoplasmic similarity to nearby normal or hyperplastic glands. A basal cell constituent is present usually with a discontinuous pattern of immuno-reactivity for cytokeratin 34bE12/p63. AAH is usually retrieved as an incidental finding in TURP material from the TZ, but it may be uncommonly encountered in biopsy specimens. Although it has been suggested that AAH could be a precursor to low-grade TZ adenocarcinoma on the basis of circumstantial evidence, there is no proof of a relationship between AAH and prostate cancer (Young et al. 2000; Epstein and Netto 2008; Humphrey 2003; Meyer et al. 2006).

3.10.3 Glandular Atrophy

Glandular atrophy is an extremely common observation in the prostate. It is already present in about two-thirds of men by the age of 30, the incidence and extent increasing with age. It is mostly localized in the PZ and retrieved in more than 90% of biopsy specimens (Humphrey 2003). Whereas varying patterns of glandular atrophy have been described (Srigley 2004), there has been a recent consensus effort to standardize the recognition and designation of various forms of glandular atrophy (De Marzo et al. 2006). Four distinct subtypes are currently recognized, namely, simple atrophy, simple atrophy with cyst formation, postatrophic hyperplasia, and partial atrophy (De Marzo et al. 2006). Acknowledging the ubiquitous nature of glandular atrophy, the main importance of appropriately diagnosing its various forms is the distinction from adenocarcinoma, as glandular atrophy is a mimicker of malignancy, particularly in biopsy material (Srigley 2004). The other reason for renewed interest in glandular atrophy is its potential involvement in the pathogenesis of prostate cancer and/or HGPIN (Humphrey 2003). Indeed, features such as increased proliferative activity as detected by Ki-67, increased expression of BCL-2, activation of glutathione S-transferase P1 (GSTP1), and morphological evidence of merging with HGPIN have been reported in simple atrophy/postatrophic hyperplasia (De Marzo et al. 1999; Putzi and De Marzo 2000; Nakayama et al. 2003). However, a recent study failed to show the presence of the TMPRSS2-ERG fusion gene in any atrophic lesion (Perner et al. 2007). Although the hypothesis of glandular atrophy being a precursor lesion of adenocarcinoma and/or HGPIN is appealing, further studies (possibly including animal models) are required before reaching any conclusion (De Marzo et al. 2007).

3.11 Atypical Small Acinar Proliferation (ASAP)

ASAP is a descriptive designation rather than a specific diagnostic entity. It is encountered mostly in biopsy specimens and defined as a focus of glandular proliferation/grouping of uncertain nature, often with cytoarchitectural features suspicious but below the diagnostic threshold of adenocarcinoma (Cheville et al. 1997). An interpretation of ASAP often results from the limited size of the atypical glandular focus on the H&E section, precluding further immunohistochemical staining for basal cell markers (cytokeratin 34bE12/p63) and AMACR in order to elucidate its nature. On the other hand, it is well established that many cases of ASAP represent an adenocarcinoma that has been minimally and marginally sampled, a retrospective review of cases initially diagnosed as ASAP having shown that up to 20% of ASAP lesions were reinterpreted as adenocarcinoma (Humphrey 2003). Therefore, the interpretation of ASAP is significantly subjective, as it is partly related to the level of experience and confidence of the observer.

In clinical practice, an interpretation of ASAP implies close follow-up/monitoring including repeat biopsies usually within 3 months, as an adenocarcinoma will be detected in 40–50% of such patients on repeat biopsies (Iczkowski et al. 1998; Brimo et al. 2007). The repeat biopsy sampling should target the whole prostate and not be confined to the area of previous ASAP, as the carcinoma subsequently diagnosed is often geographically detected at a significant distance from the original area of ASAP (Renshaw et al. 1998; Girasole et al. 2006).

3.12 Special Types of Prostatic Carcinoma

The following special types of carcinoma account for no more than 5–10% of prostate cancer at large (Table 3.1) (Randolph et al. 1997; Young et al. 2000). Some of them are assigned a Gleason pattern (grade) by default. Sarcomatoid carcinoma of the prostate (Shannon et al. 1992; Hansel and Epstein 2006) and large cell neuroendocrine carcinoma of the prostate (Evans et al. 2006), the latter being encountered in advanced disease, are extremely rare and highly aggressive types of tumor not further discussed.

3.12.1   Ductal Adenocarcinoma

Ductal (prostatic duct) adenocarcinoma, formerly qualified as endometrioid, originates centrally from the periprostatic ducts or peripherally from the acini. It is most often associated with an adenocarcinomatous component of the usual type. In its pure form, it accounts for less than 1% of prostatic carcinomas (Yang et al. 2004). It is characterized by a papillary and cribriform growth pattern with a pseudostratified, cuboidal to tall columnar cell constituent (Fig. 3.5a). Tumor cells express PSA, PAP, and AMACR. Rarely, a discontinuous basal cell constituent (immunoreactive for cytokeratin 34bE12/p63) may be seen when there is spreading within pre-existing ducts (Herawi and Epstein 2007). Ductal adenocarcinoma is considered a Gleason pattern 4 by default, unless it exhibits zonal (comedo) necrosis which conveys a Gleason pattern 5. The prognosis is generally considered to be worse than conventional adenocarcinoma, particularly when growing around large centrally located ducts (Guo and Epstein 2006), and hormonal therapy seems to be less effective (Yang et al. 2004; Eade et al. 2007).

3.12.2   Mucinous Adenocarcinoma

Mucinous (colloid) adenocarcinoma is characterized by lakes of extracellular mucin containing cribriform and anastomosing strands or nests of tumor cells, including occasional glandular formations (Fig. 3.5b). Tumors cells express PSA and PAP but not CEA, in contrast to mucinous tumors of rectal or bladder derivation. At least 25% of a resected tumor must have this appearance in order to be classified as a mucinous type, and as such accounts for less than 0.5% of prostatic carcinomas. Its mucinous nature appears grossly gelatinous and conveys an atypical signal intensity on MRI whose interpretation may be problematic (Young et al. 2000). Mucinous adenocarcinoma is reported to be more aggressive than the usual type, has a greater propensity to develop bone metastasis, and is assigned a Gleason pattern 4 by default.

3.12.3   Signet Ring Cell Carcinoma

Signet ring cell carcinoma is a rare tumor with at least a 25% component of widely infiltrative, clustered, or single tumor cells with an optically clear vacuole displacing the nucleus (Fig. 3.5c). Immunoreactivity for PSA and PAP is observed in most cases, whereas CEA is expressed in about 20% of these. Most tumors are negative for intracytoplasmic mucin in contrast to similar tumors in other organs. It is assigned a Gleason pattern 5. This is an aggressive tumor, often with advanced-stage disease at presentation, yet the proliferation index is relatively low (less than 10%) (Torbenson et al. 1998).

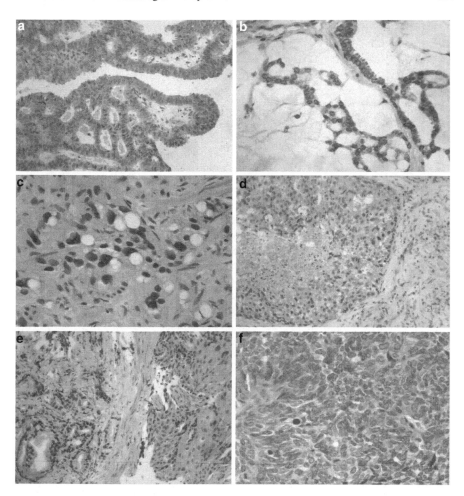

Fig. 3.5 (**a**) Ductal type adenocarcinoma with a cribriform/papillary architecture and a pseudostratified cuboidal to columnar epithelial constituent; (**b**) Mucinous adenocarcinoma with malignant glands and cell cords lying within copious extracellular mucin; (**c**) Signet ring cell carcinoma characterized by single tumor cells with a large cytoplasmic vacuole displacing the nucleus at the periphery; (**d**) Urothelial carcinoma with solid sheet of large cohesive tumor cells and zonal necrosis; (**e**) Adenosquamous carcinoma with a coexisting glandular (*left half*) and squamous (*right half*) differentiation; (**f**) Small cell carcinoma in which cells have a high nuclear to cytoplasmic ratio and a finely dispersed chromatin

3.12.4   Urothelial Carcinoma

Primary urothelial (transitional cell) carcinoma accounts for less than 1% of prostate cancer and is usually diagnosed in TURP material. The age distribution is similar to its urinary bladder counterpart (mean age in the 60s) and patients often present with urinary obstructive symptoms and/or hematuria. This tumor presumably arises from the urothelial lining of the proximal (periurethral) portion of prostatic ducts via a dysplasia/carcinoma-in situ sequence of progression similarly to bladder cancer (Grignon 2004). On the other hand, one should always consider the more common scenario of secondary spread from the bladder: most often via retrograde involvement of the duct-acinar system by a urothelial carcinoma in situ component with concomitant involvement of the prostatic urethra, usually without stromal invasion; less commonly via direct invasion by a deeply penetrating tumor often located around the trigone. Therefore, a cystoscopy and appropriate (random) biopsy sampling of the bladder should be performed before concluding to a primary urothelial carcinoma of the prostate. Histologically, most tumors are characterized by a high-grade morphology with significant nuclear pleomorphism, mitotic activity, apoptosis, and punctate necrosis, whereas the invasive component is often associated with a desmoplastic stromal response (Fig. 3.5d). Such features are helpful clues in the distinction from a poorly differentiated/Gleason pattern 5 adenocarcinoma, although the differential diagnosis can be problematic. In such a setting, immunoreactivity for cytokeratin 34bE12/p63/p53/S100P and negativity for PSA/PAP are strongly supportive of a urothelial phenotype (Grignon 2004; Chuang et al. 2007). Invasion of the prostatic stroma (stage pT2 for primary tumor vs. pT4 for secondary tumor), EPE and SVI are determinants of adverse outcome. In one study, all patients with urothelial carcinoma in situ were alive at 5 years in contrast to no survivors for those with evidence of SVI (Cheville et al. 1998). Distant spread occurs to regional lymph nodes and bone, bone metastases being characteristically osteolytic (Grignon 2004).

3.12.5 Squamous Cell Carcinoma/Adenosquamous Carcinoma

Primary tumors of the prostate with squamous differentiation are rare and secondary spread from a bladder or urethral cancer must be excluded (Young et al. 2000; van der Kwast 2004). The origin of squamous cell carcinoma is unclear, putatively from the basal cell showing a divergent differentiation pathway. More than half of adenosquamous carcinomas (Fig. 3.5e) develop many years after a diagnosis of conventional adenocarcinoma treated with hormonal or radiation therapy. Most patients present with urinary obstruction, hematuria, and bone pain resulting from osteolytic metastases (Kim et al. 1999). The squamous component per se is negative for the expression of PSA/PAP, and therefore most such tumors are not associated with an increased serum PSA even in a metastatic setting (Humphrey 2003). These tumors are highly aggressive, often with rapid bone dissemination, and do not respond to radiation or androgen-deprivation therapy, although a response to chemotherapy has been reported in a few cases (Little et al. 1993; Imamura et al. 2000).

3.12.6 Basal Cell Carcinoma

Basal cell carcinoma of the prostate, formerly designated basaloid and adenoid cystic carcinomas, is a poorly defined entity. It is usually diagnosed on TURP material in an elderly individual presenting with symptoms of urinary obstruction

(Tan and Billis 2004). This neoplasm is characterized by an insular and cord-like growth pattern of basaloid epithelial cells with peripheral palisading often reminiscent of adenoid cystic tumors of the salivary glands (Grignon et al. 1988). Features often seen in this tumor, such as desmoplastic stromal response, central (comedo) necrosis, or perineural invasion are clues allowing distinction from benign florid basal cell hyperplasia. Basal cell markers such as cytokeratin 34bE12/p63 are often (yet inconsistently) expressed, whereas varying degrees of S-100 protein immunoreactivity have been reported (Tan and Billis 2004). In contrast to basal cell hyperplasia, there is a strong bcl-2 expression and a high Ki-67 index (McKenney et al. 2004). Although the natural history is not well elucidated, most patients seem to have an indolent course. A subset of tumors showing large solid nests with often central necrosis, a high Ki-67 index, and less immunoreactivity for basal cell markers behave aggressively (Ali and Epstein 2007).

3.12.7   Small Cell Carcinoma

Small cell carcinoma is an extremely rare and aggressive type of prostate cancer. Most patients present with advanced-stage disease including visceral (lung, liver, brain) and occasionally osteolytic bone metastases, usually without significant serum PSA elevation (Losi et al. 1994). In more than one-third of patients there is a prior history of conventional adenocarcinoma with some form of treatment often including hormonal therapy. The latter observation may reflect the emergence of a selective bias, i.e., cancer progression via the development of a hormone-insensitive clone (Humphrey 2003). This tumor is mostly characterized by diffuse sheets of cells with very little cytoplasm, nuclear molding, a finely dispersed chromatin, and inconspicuous nucleoli (Fig. 3.5f). Tumor necrosis, apoptosis, and high mitotic activity are usually seen. Tumor cells are immunoreactive for cytokeratin AE1/AE3 (dot-like pattern) and TTF-1, but generally negative for PSA/PAP (Leibovici et al. 2007). Therefore, in the absence of an associated conventional adenocarcinomatous component, distinction from metastatic small cell carcinoma of lung can be difficult. Use of neuroendocrine markers (chromogranin, synaptophysin) alone is not sufficient to make a diagnosis of small cell carcinoma since these may be expressed focally in Gleason pattern 5 adenocarcinoma of the usual type (di Sant' Agnese 2000). Small cell carcinoma is resistant to androgen-deprivation therapy, but chemotherapy regimens used for its pulmonary counterpart have prolonged survival in many patients (Palmgren et al. 2007).

3.13   Emerging Biomarkers of Potential
Prognostic Significance

The incidence of prostate cancer is on the rise as a result of serum PSA screening and increased life expectancy. Currently, it is estimated that 1 in 7 males will develop an adenocarcinoma of the prostate, yet only 1 in 26 will die from it.

Such disparity between incidence and mortality implies that a large number of tumors which would otherwise be slowly growing and indolent are probably overtreated. Therefore, much of the investigative work on prostate focuses on searching for biomarkers that could be predictive of tumor progression, particularly at an early/low-volume stage of disease, most of which has a Gleason score 5–7 range. Using gene expression studies, comparative genomic hybridization (CGH), single nucleotide polymorphism (SNP), and proteomics platforms coupled with bioinformatics, several individual and multiplex panels have been described and validated using high throughput tissue microarray technology to help predict tumor progression (Rubin 2004). A brief discussion of a few promising biomarkers, although not necessarily applied to current clinical practice, follows.

DNA ploidy is routinely assessed in some laboratories for predicting tumor progression after radical prostatectomy, independent of the Gleason score and other pathological parameters. However, its value as an independent prognostic determinant has so far not been proven, as reported results are somewhat conflictual (Humphrey et al. 1991; Di Silverio et al. 1996).

Microvessel density (angiogenesis) refers to neovascularization around cancer cells. In some studies, the density of microvessels has been associated with cancer progression after prostatectomy (Strohmeyer et al. 2000). However, there is a subjectivity issue in many of the analyses, namely in selecting maximal neovascularization "hot spots" vs. doing a random sampling (Rubin et al. 1999).

p53 protein overexpression, as a reflection of p53 gene mutations, has been associated with tumor progression following prostatectomy, independent of Gleason score and other pathological parameters (Bauer et al. 1996). However, a p53 abnormality is only present in about 15% of clinically localized cancers as compared to 60% of hormone refractory metastatic tumors (Humphrey 2003). Its immunohistochemical assessment in clinical practice is not currently advocated (Epstein et al. 2005b).

The AR is a 910-amino acid nuclear protein that mediates androgen hormonal signals for the growth, differentiation, and survival of prostatic cells (Trapman and Brinkmann 1996). AR protein expression occurs in epithelial, stromal, and basal cells of the prostate. It is observed in a majority of prostate carcinomas and does not correlate with an androgen dependent vs. independent therapeutic status. There is increasing heterogeneity in AR expression in higher histological grades and pathological stages (Epstein 2004). Expression levels of AR as well as the increase in AR mRNA transcript have been shown to be key factors in disease recurrence following treatment. Higher levels of AR have been associated with aggressive clinicopathological features, advanced disease stage, and biochemical failure after radical prostatectomy (Chen et al. 2004; Li et al. 2004). In addition, AR amplification has been demonstrated in 15–30% of hormone refractory tumors (Ford et al. 2003; Lee and Tenniswood 2004). Germ line abnormalities in the AR, manifested by shorter CAG repeats in exon 1, have been associated with features such as increased susceptibility to prostate cancer, higher grade at diagnosis, metastasis, and even mortality (Giovannucci et al. 1997; Stanford et al. 1997), but its biological significance in prostate carcinogenesis has been questioned (Zeegers et al. 2004).

Somatic mosaicism of the CAG repeats has been detected in prostate cancer and adjacent benign tissue but not in the normal parenchyma, suggesting that AR CAG repeats may be an important genetic event in carcinogenesis at the level of precancerous tissue (Alvarado et al. 2005).

As previously discussed, AMACR expression is widely used as an adjunct diagnostic immunohistochemical marker in clinical practice. Recently, its expression was shown to be heterogeneous within an individual tumor, this heterogeneity correlating with a higher Gleason score (Murphy et al. 2007). It has also been reported that patients whose tumors express lower levels of AMACR have a 3.7 fold and 4.1 fold higher risk for PSA recurrence and cancer-related death, respectively, as compared to tumors expressing higher levels of AMACR, independent of other clinical parameters. Furthermore, among those tumors with both low AMACR expression and high Gleason score, the risk of dying from their cancer was 18 times higher (Rubin et al. 2005).

The recent discovery of the fusion gene between the androgen-regulated TMPRSS2 gene and one gene of the ETS family of transcription factors (the *TMPRSS2-ETS* family fusion gene) has gained significant interest regarding its potential clinical value as a diagnostic and prognostic marker in prostate cancer (Tomlins et al. 2005). It has been reported that the expression variants of this fusion gene (*ERG*, *ETV1*, and *ETV4*) could define new molecular subtypes of prostate cancer, in addition to pointing to aggressive phenotypes of tumor as correlations with biochemical PSA failure and cancer-related death were established (Tomlins et al. 2006; Wang et al. 2006; Demichelis et al. 2007; Mehra et al. 2007). Furthermore, recently, the presence of this fusion gene has been associated with various histopathological features of prostate cancer such as macronucleoli and signet ring cell or cribriform patterns (Mosquera et al. 2007). This new fusion gene is discussed in detail in the molecular genetics section.

3.14   Conclusions

Biopsy histological assessment remains the time-honored gold standard for diagnosing prostate cancer. The current use of biopsy guns providing thin core tissue samplings, in conjunction with TRUS imaging, allows targeting specific areas of clinical concern and systematic histological mapping of the prostate. Once cancer is detected, this biopsy approach provides further key information such as tumor phenotype, distribution, quantification, and grade, all of which have an established impact on prognostic assessment and patient management. Furthermore, this procedure is currently the ultimate tool in monitoring patients with a diagnosis of HGPIN and/or ASAP. Immunohistochemical staining for markers such as cytokeratin 34bE12, p63, and AMACR is of ancillary value in the diagnosis of minimal cancer, namely in the differential setting of ASAP. The Gleason scheme for grading prostate cancer, designed more than four decades ago, is now widely used in clinical practice throughout the world. Indeed, the Gleason score is a powerful independent prognostic determinant which is used in clinically valid nomograms and is a required parameter in clinical research, a Gleason score 8–10 range implying high-grade/aggressive disease. A major need and challenge in the management of prostate cancer, particularly in our current era of early detection in which most patients have low-volume/low-stage disease with a Gleason score 5–7 range, is to identify clinically useful biomarkers that could refine prognostication and allow patient substratification namely for conservative management vs. intervention. Ideally, such biomarkers should be applicable to formalin-fixed paraffin-embedded biopsy material, as it is the tissue available on first hand and at the primary step in decision making/therapeutic strategy. Bioinformatic analysis of microarray data, and techniques such as fluorescence in situ hybridization (FISH) and reverse transcription polymerase chain reaction (RT-PCR) analysis, investigating molecular phenotypes, are likely to play a major role in this regard. The recent discovery and current investigative work on the *TMPRSS2-ETS* family fusion gene in prostate cancer, correlating the fusion status with varying clinicopathological and outcome parameters, is an example of the current direction taken in the pathobiological and translational research on prostate cancer.

References

Aihara M, Wheeler TM, Ohori M, Scardino PT (1994) Heterogeneity of prostate cancer in radical prostatectomy specimens. Urology 43:60–66

Akhavan A, Keith JD, Bastacky SI, Cai C, Wang Y, Nelson JB (2007) The proportion of cores with high-grade prostatic intraepithelial neoplasia on extended-pattern needle biopsy is significantly associated with prostate cancer on site-directed repeat biopsy. BJU Int 99:765–769

Albertsen PC, Fryback DG, Storer BE, Kolon TF, Fine J (1995) Long-term survival among men with conservatively treated localized prostate cancer. JAMA 274:626–631

Ali TZ, Epstein JI (2007) Basal cell carcinoma of the prostate: a clinicopathologic study of 29 cases. Am J Surg Pathol 31:697–705

Allsbrook WC, Mangold KA, Johnson MH, Lane RB, Lane CG, Epstein JI (2001a) Interobserver reproducibility of Gleason grading of prostatic carcinoma: general pathologist. Hum Pathol 32:81–88

Allsbrook WC, Mangold KA, Johnson MH, Lane RB, Lane CG, Amin MB, Bostwick DG, Humphrey PA, Jones EC, Reuter VE, Sakr W, Sesterhenn IA, Troncoso P, Wheeler TM, Epstein JI (2001b) Interobserver reproducibility of Gleason grading of prostatic carcinoma: urologic pathologists. Hum Pathol 32:74–80

Alvarado C, Beitel LK, Sircar K, Aprikian A, Trifiro M, Gottlieb B (2005) Somatic mosaicism and cancer: a micro-genetic examination into the role of the androgen receptor gene in prostate cancer. Cancer Res 65:8514–8518

Amin M, Boccon-Gibod L, Egevad L, Epstein JI, Humphrey PA, Mikuz G, Newling D, Nilsson S, Sakr W, Srigley JR, Wheeler TM, Montironi R (2005) Prognostic and predictive factors and reporting of prostate carcinoma in prostate needle biopsy specimens. Scand J Urol Nephrol Suppl 216:20–33

Ayala AG, Ro JY, Babaian R, Troncoso P, Grignon DJ (1989) The prostatic capsule: does it exist? Its importance in the staging and treatment of prostatic carcinoma. Am J Surg Pathol 13:21–27

Bailar JC, Mellinger GT, Gleason DF (1966) Survival rates of patients with prostatic cancer, tumor stage, and differentiation – preliminary report. Cancer Chemother Rep 50:129–136

Baisden BL, Kahane H, Epstein JI (1999) Perineural invasion, mucinous fibroplasia, and glomerulations: diagnostic features of limited cancer on prostate needle biopsy. Am J Surg Pathol
23:918–924

Bauer JJ, Sesterhenn IA, Mostofi FK, McLeod DG, Srivastava S, Moul JW (1996) Elevated levels
of apoptosis regulator proteins p53 and bcl-2 are independent prognostic biomarkers in surgi-
cally treated clinically localized prostate cancer. J Urol 156:1511–1516

Bishara T, Ramnani DM, Epstein JI (2004) High-grade prostatic intraepithelial neoplasia on
needle biopsy: risk of cancer on repeat biopsy related to number of involved cores and morphologic pattern. Am J Surg Pathol 28:629–633

Bismar TA, Lewis JS, Vollmer RT, Humphrey PA (2003) Multiple measures of carcinoma extent
versus perineural invasion in prostate needle biopsy tissue in prediction of pathologic stage in
a screening population. Am J Surg Pathol 27:432–440

Bonkhoff H, Stein U, Remberger K (1994) Multidirectional differentiation in the normal, hyperplastic, and neoplastic human prostate: simultaneous demonstration of cell-specific epithelial
markers. Hum Pathol 25:42–46

Bostwick DG (1994) Gleason grading of prostatic needle biopsies. Correlation with grade in 316
matched prostatectomies. Am J Surg Pathol 18:796–803

Bostwick DG, Ma J, Qian J, Josefson D, Liu L (2006) Immunohistology of the prostate, bladder,
testis and kidney. In: Dabbs DJ (ed) Diagnostic immunohistochemistry. Churchill Livingstone,
Pittsburgh, pp 509–610

Brimo F, Vollmer RT, Corcos J, Humphrey PA, Bismar TA (2007) Outcome for repeated biopsy
of the prostate: roles of serum PSA, small atypical glands and prostatic intraepithelial neoplasia. Am J Clin Pathol 128:648–651

Browne TJ, Hirsch MS, Brodsky G, Welch WR, Loda MF, Rubin MA (2004) Prospective evaluation of AMACR (P504S) and basal cell markers in the assessment of routine prostate needle
biopsy specimens. Hum Pathol 35:1462–1468

Bullock MJ, Srigley JR, Klotz LH, Goldenberg SL (2002) Pathologic effects of neoadjuvant
cyproterone acetate on nonneoplastic prostate, prostatic intraepithelial neoplasia, and adenocarcinoma: a detailed analysis of radical prostatectomy specimens from a randomized trial.
Am J Surg Pathol 26:1400–1413

Catalona WJ, Smith DS (1998) Cancer recurrence and survival rates after anatomic radical retropubic prostatectomy for prostate cancer: intermediate-term results. J Urol 160:2428–2434

Chan TY, Partin AW, Walsh PC, Epstein JI (2000) Prognostic significance of Gleason score 3 + 4
versus Gleason score 4 + 3 tumor at radical prostatectomy. Urology 56:823–827

Chan TY, Mikolajczyk SD, Lecksell K, Shue MJ, Rittenhouse HG, Partin AW, Epstein JI (2003)
Immunohistochemical staining of prostate cancer with monoclonal antibodies to the precursor
of prostate-specific antigen. Urology 62:177–181

Chen CD, Welsbie DS, Tran C, Baek SH, Chen R, Vessella R, Rosenfeld MG, Sawyers CL (2004)
Molecular determinants of resistance to antiandrogen therapy. Nat Med 10:33–39

Cheng L, Cheville JC, Bostwick DG (1999) Diagnosis of prostate cancer in needle biopsies after
radiation therapy. Am J Surg Pathol 23:1173–1183

Cheville JC, Reznicek MJ, Bostwick DG (1997) The focus of "atypical glands, suspicious for
malignancy" in prostatic needle biopsy specimens: incidence, histologic features, and clinical
follow-up of cases diagnosed in a community practice. Am J Clin Pathol 108:633–640

Cheville JC, Dundore PA, Bostwick DG, Lieber MM, Batts KP, Sebo TJ, Farrow GM (1998) Transitional
cell carcinoma of the prostate: clinicopathologic study of 50 cases. Cancer 82:703–707

Chuang AY, DeMarzo AM, Veltri RW, Sharma RB, Bieberich CJ, Epstein JI (2007)
Immunohistochemical differentiation of high-grade prostate carcinoma from urothelial carcinoma. Am J Surg Pathol 31:1246–1255

Cina SJ, Epstein JI (1997) Adenocarcinoma of the prostate with atrophic features. Am J Surg
Pathol 21:289–295

De Marzo AM, Meeker AK, Epstein JI, Coffey DS (1998) Prostate stem cell compartments:
expression of the cell cycle inhibitor p27Kip1 in normal, hyperplastic, and neoplastic cells.
Am J Pathol 153:911–919

De Marzo AM, Marchi VL, Epstein JI, Nelson WG (1999) Proliferative inflammatory atrophy of the prostate: implications for prostatic carcinogenesis. Am J Pathol 155:1985–1992

De Marzo AM, Platz EA, Epstein JI, Ali T, Billis A, Chan TY, Cheng L, Datta M, Egevad L, Ertoy-Baydar D, Farre X, Fine SW, Iczkowski KA, Ittmann M, Knudsen BS, Loda M, Lopez-Beltran A, Magi-Galluzzi C, Mikuz G, Montironi R, Pikarsky E, Pizov G, Rubin MA, Samaratunga H, Sebo T, Sesterhenn IA, Shah RB, Signoretti S, Simko J, Thomas G, Troncoso P, Tsuzuki TT, van Leenders GJ, Yang XJ, Zhou M, Figg WD, Hoque A, Lucia MS (2006) A working group classification of focal prostate atrophy lesions. Am J Surg Pathol 30:1281–1291

De Marzo AM, Platz EA, Sutcliffe S, Xu J, Grönberg H, Drake CG, Nakai Y, Isaacs WB, Nelson WG (2007) Inflammation in prostate carcinogenesis. Nat Rev Cancer 7:256–269

Debras B, Guillonneau B, Bougaran J, Chambon E, Vallancien G (1998) Prognostic significance of seminal vesicle invasion on the radical prostatectomy specimen. Rationale for seminal vesicle biopsies. Eur Urol 33:271–277

Demichelis F, Fall K, Perner S, Andrén O, Schmidt F, Setlur SR, Hoshida Y, Mosquera JM, Pawitan Y, Lee C, Adami HO, Mucci LA, Kantoff PW, Andersson SO, Chinnaiyan AM, Johansonn JE, Rubin MA (2007) TMPRSS2:ERG gene fusion associated with lethal prostate cancer in a watchful waiting cohort. Oncogene 26:4596–4599

di Sant' Agnese PA (2000) Divergent neuroendocrine differentiation in prostatic carcinoma. Semin Diagn Pathol 17:149–161

Di Silverio F, D'Eramo G, Buscarini M, Sciarra A, Casale P, Di Nicola S, Loreto A, Seccareccia F, De Vita R (1996) DNA ploidy, Gleason score, pathological stage and serum PSA levels as predictors of disease-free survival in C-D1 prostatic cancer patients submitted to radical retropubic prostatectomy. Eur Urol 30:316–321

Eade TN, Al-Saleem T, Horwitz EM, Buyyounouski MK, Chen DY, Pollack A (2007) Role of radiotherapy in ductal (endometrioid) carcinoma of the prostate. Cancer 109:2011–2015

Eble JN (1998) Variants of prostatic hyperplasia that resemble carcinoma. J Urol Pathol 8:3–19

Egan AJ, Lopez-Beltran A, Bostwick DG (1997) Prostatic adenocarcinoma with atrophic features: malignancy mimicking a benign process. Am J Surg Pathol 21:931–935

Egevad L, Granfors T, Karlberg L, Bergh A, Stattin P (2002) Prognostic value of the Gleason score in prostate cancer. BJU Int 89:538–542

Eichelberger LE, Koch MO, Eble JN, Ulbright TM, Juliar BE, Cheng L (2005) Maximum tumor diameter is an independent predictor of prostate-specific antigen recurrence in prostate cancer. Mod Pathol 18:886–890

Epstein JI (2000) Gleason score 2–4 adenocarcinoma of the prostate on needle biopsy: a diagnosis that should not be made. Am J Surg Pathol 24:477–478

Epstein JI (2004) Diagnosis and reporting of limited adenocarcinoma of the prostate on needle biopsy. Mod Pathol 17:307–315

Epstein JI, Herawi M (2006) Prostate needle biopsies containing prostatic intraepithelial neoplasia or atypical foci suspicious for carcinoma: implications for patient care. J Urol 175:820–834

Epstein JI, Netto GJ (2008) Biopsy interpretation of the prostate. Lippincott Williams & Wilkins, Philadelphia

Epstein JI, Carmichael MJ, Partin AW, Walsh PC (1994) Small high grade adenocarcinoma of the prostate in radical prostatectomy specimens performed for nonpalpable disease: pathogenetic and clinical implications. J Urol 151:1587–1592

Epstein JI, Partin AW, Potter SR, Walsh PC (2000) Adenocarcinoma of the prostate invading the seminal vesicle: prognostic stratification based on pathologic parameters. Urology 56:283–288

Epstein JI, Algaba F, Allsbrook WC, Bastacky S, Boccon-Gibod L, De Marzo AM, Egevad L, Furusato M, Hamper UM, Helap B, Humphrey PA, Iczkowski KA, Lopez-Beltran A, Montironi R, Rubin MA, Sakr WA, Samaratunga H, Parkin DM (2004) Acinar adenocarcinoma. In: Eble JN, Sauter G, Epstein JI, Sesterhenn IA (eds) World Health Organization classification of tumours: pathology and genetics of tumours of the urinary system and male genital organs. International Agency for Research on Cancer, Lyon, pp 162–192

Epstein JI, Allsbrook WC, Amin MB, Egevad LL, ISUP Grading Committee (2005a) The 2005 International Society of Urological Pathology (ISUP) Consensus Conference on Gleason Grading of Prostatic Carcinoma. Am J Surg Pathol 29:1228–1242

Epstein JI, Amin M, Boccon-Gibod L, Egevad L, Humphrey PA, Mikuz G, Newling D, Nilsson S, Sakr W, Srigley JR, Wheeler TM, Montironi R (2005b) Prognostic factors and reporting of prostate carcinoma in radical prostatectomy and pelvic lymphadenectomy specimens. Scand J Urol Nephrol Suppl 216:34–63

Evans AJ, Humphrey PA, Belani J, van der Kwast TH, Srigley JR (2006) Large cell neuroendocrine carcinoma of prostate. A clinicopathologic summary of 7 cases of a rare manifestation of advanced prostate cancer. Am J Surg Pathol 30:684–693

Ford OH, Gregory CW, Kim D, Smitherman AB, Mohler JL (2003) Androgen receptor gene amplification and protein expression in recurrent prostate cancer. J Urol 170:1817–1821

Gaudin PB (1998) Histopathologic effects of radiation and hormonal therapies on benign and malignant prostate tissues. J Urol Pathol 8:55–67

Gaudin PB, Zelefsky MJ, Leibel SA, Fuks Z, Reuter VE (1999) Histopathologic effects of three-dimensional conformal external beam radiation therapy on benign and malignant prostate tissues. Am J Surg Pathol 23:1021–1031

Gelmann EP, Bowen C, Bubendorf L (2003) Expresion of NKX3.1 in normal and malignant tissues. Prostate 55:111–117

Giovannucci E, Stampfer MJ, Krithivas K, Brown M, Dahl D, Brufsky A, Talcott J, Hennekens CH, Kantoff PW (1997) The CAG repeat within the androgen receptor gene and its relationship to prostate cancer. Proc Natl Acad Sci USA 94:3320–3323

Girasole CR, Cookson MS, Putzi MJ, Chang SS, Smith JA, Wells N, Oppenheimer JR, Shappell SB (2006) Significance of atypical and suspicious small acinar proliferations, and high grade prostatic intraepithelial neoplasia on prostate biopsy: implications for cancer detection and biopsy strategy. J Urol 175:929–933

Gleason DF (1966) Classification of prostatic carcinomas. Cancer Chemother Rep 50:125–128

Gleason DF, Mellinger GT (2002) Prediction of prognosis for prostatic adenocarcinoma by combined histological grading and clinical staging 1974. J Urol 167:953–958

Goldstein NS (2002) Immunophenotypic characterization of 225 prostate adenocarcinomas with intermediate or high Gleason scores. Am J Clin Pathol 117:471–477

Grignon DJ (1998) Minimal diagnostic criteria for adenocarcinoma of the prostate. J Urol Pathol 8:31–43

Grignon DJ (2004) Urothelial carcinoma. In: Eble JN, Sauter G, Epstein JI, Sesterhenn IA (eds) World Health Organization classification of tumours: pathology and genetics of tumours of the urinary system and male genital organs. International Agency for Research on Cancer, Lyon, pp 202–204

Grignon DJ, Ro JY, Ordonez NG, Ayala AG, Cleary KR (1988) Basal cell hyperplasia, adenoid basal cell tumor, and adenoid cystic carcinoma of the prostate gland: an immunohistochemical study. Hum Pathol 19:1425–1433

Guo CC, Epstein JI (2006) Intraductal carcinoma of the prostate on needle biopsy: histologic features and clinical significance. Mod Pathol 19:1528–1535

Hansel DE, Epstein JI (2006) Sarcomatoid carcinoma of the prostate: a study of 42 cases. Am J Surg Pathol 30:1316–1321

Hattab EM, Kock MO, Eble JN, Lin H, Cheng L (2006) Tertiary Gleason pattern 5 is a powerful predictor of biochemical relapse in patients with Gleason score 7 prostatic adenocarcinoma. J Urol 175:1695–1699

Herawi M, Epstein JI (2007) Immunohistochemical antibody cocktail staining (p63/HMWCK/AMACR) of ductal adenocarcinoma and Gleason pattern 4 cribriform and noncribriform acinar adenocarcinomas of the prostate. Am J Surg Pathol 31:889–894

Herawi M, Kahane H, Cavallo C, Epstein JI (2006) Risk of prostate cancer on first re-biopsy within 1 year following a diagnosis of high grade prostatic intraepithelial neoplasia is related to the number of cores sampled. J Urol 175:121–124

Herman CM, Wilcox GE, Kattan MW, Scardino PT, Wheeler TM (2000) Lymphovascular invasion as a predictor of disease progression in prostate cancer. Am J Surg Pathol 24:859–863

Humphrey PA (2003) Prostate pathology. American Society of Clinical Pathologists, Chicago

Humphrey PA, Walther PJ, Currin SM, Vollmer RT (1991) Histologic grade, DNA ploidy, and intraglandular tumor extent as indicators of tumor progression of clinical stage B prostatic carcinoma. A direct comparison. Am J Surg Pathol 15:1165–1170

Humphrey PA, Kaleem Z, Swanson PE, Vollmer RT (1998) Pseudohyperplastic prostatic adeno-carcinoma. Am J Surg Pathol 22:1239–1246

Iczkowski KA, Bassler TJ, Schwob VS, Bassler IC, Kunnel BS, Orozco RE, Bostwick DG (1998) Diagnosis of "suspicious for malignancy" in prostate biopsies: predictive value for cancer. Urology 51:749–757

Imamura M, Nishiyama H, Ohmori K, Nishimura K (2000) Squamous cell carcinoma of the prostate without evidence of recurrence 5 years after operation. Urol Int 65:122–124

Jiang Z, Woda BA, Rock KL, Xu Y, Savas L, Khan A, Pihan G, Cai F, Babcook JS, Rathanaswami P, Reed SG, Xu J, Fanger GR (2001) P504S: a new molecular marker for the detection of prostate carcinoma. Am J Surg Pathol 25:1397–1404

Jiang Z, Wu CL, Woda BA, Dresser K, Xu J, Fanger GR, Yang XJ (2002) P504S/alpha-methylacyl-CoA racemase: a useful marker for diagnosis of small foci of prostatic carcinoma on needle biopsy. Am J Surg Pathol 26:1169–1174

Kalos M, Askaa J, Hylander BL, Repasky EA, Cai F, Vedvick T, Reed SG, Wright GL, Fanger GR (2004) Prostein expression is highly restricted to normal and malignant prostate tissues. Prostate 60:246–256

Kikuchi E, Scardino PT, Wheeler TM, Slawin KM, Ohori M (2004) Is tumor volume an indepen-dent prognostic factor in clinically localized prostate cancer? J Urol 172:508–511

Kim YW, Park YK, Park JH, Lee J, Lee SJ, Kim JI, Yang MH (1999) Adenosquamous carcinoma of the prostate. Yonsei Med J 40:396–399

Kothari PS, Scardino PT, Ohorin M, Kattan MW, Wheeler TM (2001) Incidence, location, and significance of periprostatic and periseminal vesicle lymph nodes in prostate cancer. Am J Surg Pathol 25:1429–1432

Kronz JD, Silberman MA, Allsbrook WC, Epstein JI (2000) A web-based tutorial improves prac-ticing pathologists' Gleason grading of images of prostate carcinoma specimens obtained by needle biopsy: validation of a new medical education paradigm. Cancer 89:1818–1823

Kunz GM, Epstein JI (2003) Should each core with prostate cancer be assigned a separate Gleason score? Hum Pathol 34:911–914

Lau WK, Blute ML, Bostwick DG, Weaver AL, Sebo TJ, Zincke H (2001) Prognostic factors for survival of patients with pathological Gleason score 7 prostate cancer: differences in outcome between primary Gleason grades 3 and 4. J Urol 166:1692–1697

Lee EC, Tenniswood MP (2004) Emergence of metastatic hormone-refractory disease in prostate cancer after anti-androgen therapy. J Cell Biochem 91:662–670

Leibovici D, Spiess PE, Agarwal PK, Tu SM, Pettaway CA, Hitzhusen K, Millikan RE, Pisters LL (2007) Prostate cancer progression in the presence of undetectable or low serum prostate-specific antigen level. Cancer 109:198–204

Levi AW, Epstein JI (2000) Pseudohyperplastic prostatic adenocarcinoma on needle biopsy and simple prostatectomy. Am J Surg Pathol 24:1039–1046

Li R, Wheeler T, Dai H, Frolov A, Thompson T, Ayala G (2004) High level of androgen receptor is associ-ated with aggressive clinicopathologic features and decreased biochemical recurrence-free survival in prostate: cancer patients treated with radical prostatectomy. Am J Surg Pathol 28:928–934

Little NA, Wiener JS, Walther PJ, Paulson DF, Anderson EE (1993) Squamous cell carcinoma of the prostate: 2 cases of a rare malignancy and review of the literature. J Urol 149:137–139

Losi L, Brausi M, Di GC (1994) Rare prostatic carcinomas: histogenesis and morphologic pattern. Pathologica 86:366–370

Magi-Galluzzi C, Xu X, Hlatky L, Hahnfeldt P, Kaplan I, Hsiao P, Chang C, Loda M (1997) Heterogeneity of androgen receptor content in advanced prostate cancer. Mod Pathol 10:839–845

Magi-Galluzzi C, Luo J, Isaacs WB, Hicks JL, De Marzo AM, Epstein JI (2003) Alpha-methylacyl-CoA racemase: a variably sensitive immunohistochemical marker for the diagnosis of small prostate cancer foci on needle biopsy. Am J Surg Pathol 27:1128–1133

Marchal C, Redondo M, Padilla M, Caballero J, Rodrigo I, Garcia J, Quian J, Boswick DG (2004) Expression of prostate specific membrane antigen (PSMA) in prostatic adenocarcinoma and prostatic intraepithelial neoplasia. Histol Histopathol 19:715–718

Marks RA, Lin H, Koch MO, Cheng L (2007) Positive-block ratio in radical prostatectomy specimens is an independent predictor of prostate-specific antigen recurrence. Am J Surg Pathol 31:877–881

McKenney JK, Amin MB, Srigley JR, Jimenez RE, Ro JY, Grignon DJ, Young RH (2004) Basal cell proliferations of the prostate other than usual basal cell hyperplasia: a clinicopathologic study of 23 cases, including four carcinomas, with a proposed classification. Am J Surg Pathol 28:1289–1298

McNeal JE (1988) Normal histology of the prostate. Am J Surg Pathol 12:619–633

McNeal JE (1992) Cancer volume and site of origin of adenocarcinoma in the prostate: relationship to local and distant spread. Hum Pathol 23:258–266

McNeal JE, Redwine EA, Freiha FS, Stamey TA (1988) Zonal distribution of prostatic adenocarcinoma. Correlation with histologic pattern and direction of spread. Am J Surg Pathol 12:897–906

McNeal JE, Villers AA, Redwine EA, Freiha FS, Stamey TA (1990) Histologic differentiation, cancer volume, and pelvic lymph node metastasis in adenocarcinoma of the prostate. Cancer 66:1225–1233

McNeal JE, Villers A, Redwine EA, Freiha FS, Stamey TA (1991) Microcarcinoma in the prostate: its association with duct-acinar dysplasia. Hum Pathol 22:644–652

Mehra R, Tomlins SA, Shen R, Nadeem O, Wang L, Wei JT, Pienta KJ, Ghosh D, Rubin MA, Chinnaiyan AM, Shah RB (2007) Comprehensive assessment of TMPRSS2 and ETS family gene aberrations in clinically localized prostate cancer. Mod Pathol 20:538–544

Meyer F, Têtu B, Bairati I, Lacombe L, Fradet Y (2006) Prostatic intraepithelial neoplasia in TURP specimens and subsequent prostate cancer. Can J Urol 13:3255–3260

Mosquera JM, Perner S, Demichelis F, Kim R, Hofer MD, Mertz KD, Paris PL, Simko J, Collins C, Bismar TA, Chinnaiyan AM, Rubin MA (2007) Morphological features of TMPRSS2-ERG gene fusion prostate cancer. J Pathol 212:91–101

Mosse CA, Magi-Galluzzi C, Tsuzuki T, Epstein JI (2004) The prognostic significance of tertiary Gleason pattern 5 in radical prostatectomy specimens. Am J Surg Pathol 28:394–398

Murphy AJ, Hughes CA, Lannigan G, Sheils O, O'Leary J, Loftus B (2007) Heterogeneous expression of alpha-methylacyl-CoA racemase in prostatic cancer correlates with Gleason score. Histopathol 50:243–251

Nakayama M, Bennett CJ, Hicks JL, Epstein JI, Platz EA, Nelson WG, De Marzo AM (2003) Hypermethylation of the human glutathione S-transferase-pi gene (GSTP1) CpG island is present in a subset of proliferative inflammatory atrophy lesions but not in normal or hyperplastic epithelium of the prostate: a detailed study using laser-capture microdissection. Am J Pathol 163:923–933

Nelson RS, Epstein JI (1996) Prostatic carcinoma with abundant xanthomatous cytoplasm. Foamy gland carcinoma. Am J Surg Pathol 20:419–426

Netto GJ, Epstein JI (2006) Widespread high-grade prostatic intraepithelial neoplasia on prostatic needle biopsy: a significant likelihood of subsequently diagnosed adenocarcinoma. Am J Surg Pathol 30:1184–1188

Ohori M, Scardino PT, Lapin SL, Seale-Hawkins C, Link J, Wheeler TM (1993) The mechanisms and prognostic significance of seminal vesicle involvement by prostate cancer. Am J Surg Pathol 17:1252–1261

Palmgren JS, Karavadia SS, Wakefield MR (2007) Unusual and underappreciated: small cell carcinoma of the prostate. Semin Oncol 34:22–29

Partin AW, Mangold LA, Lamm DM, Walsh PC, Epstein JI, Pearson JD (2001) Contemporary update of prostate cancer staging nomograms (Partin Tables) for the new millennium. Urology 58:843–848

Parwani AV, Marlow C, Demarzo AM, Mikolajczyk SD, Rittenhouse HG, Veltri RW, Chan TY (2006) Immunohistochemical staining of precursor forms of prostate-specific antigen (proPSA) in metastatic prostate cancer. Am J Surg Pathol 30:1231–1236

Perner S, Mosquera JM, Demichelis F, Hofer MD, Paris PL, Simko J, Collins C, Bismar TA, Chinnaiyan AM, De Marzo AM, Rubin MA (2007) TMPRSS2-ERG fusion prostate cancer: an early molecular event associated with invasion. Am J Surg Pathol 31:882–888

Putzi MJ, De Marzo AM (2000) Morphologic transitions between proliferative inflammatory atrophy and high-grade prostatic intraepithelial neoplasia. Urology 56:828–832

Qian J, Bostwick DG (1995) The extent and zonal location of prostatic intraepithelial neoplasia and atypical adenomatous hyperplasia: relationship with carcinoma in radical prostatectomy specimens. Pathol Res Pract 191:860–867

Randolph TL, Amin MB, Ro JY, Ayala AG (1997) Histologic variants of adenocarcinoma and other carcinomas of prostate: pathologic criteria and clinical significance. Mod Pathol 10:612–629

Renshaw AA, Santis WF, Richie JP (1998) Clinicopathological characteristics of prostatic adeno-carcinoma in men with atypical prostate needle biopsies. J Urol 159:2018–2021

Renshaw AA, Richie JP, Loughlin KR, Jiroutek M, Chung A, D'Amico AV (1999) Maximum diameter of prostatic carcinoma is a simple, inexpensive, and independent predictor of pros-tate-specific antigen failure in radical prostatectomy specimens. Validation in a cohort of 434 patients. Am J Clin Pathol 111:641–644

Reuter VE (1997) Pathological changes in benign and malignant prostatic tissue following andro-gen deprivation therapy. Urology 49:16–22

Reyes AO, Swanson PE, Carbone JM, Humphrey PA (1997) Unusual histologic types of high-grade prostatic intraepithelial neoplasia. Am J Surg Pathol 21:1215–1222

Rubin MA (2004) Using molecular markers to predict outcome. J Urol 172:S18–S21

Rubin MA, Buyyounouski M, Bagiella E, Sharir S, Neugut A, Benson M, de la Taille A, Katz AE, Olsson CA, Ennis RD (1999) Microvessel density in prostate cancer: lack of correlation with tumor grade, pathologic stage, and clinical outcome. Urology 53:542–547

Rubin MA, Bismar TA, Curtis S, Montie JE (2004) Prostate needle biopsy reporting: how are the surgical members of the Society of Urologic Oncology using pathology reports to guide treat-ment of prostate cancer patients? Am J Surg Pathol 28:946–952

Rubin MA, Bismar TA, Andrén O, Mucci L, Kim R, Shen R, Ghosh D, Wei JT, Chinnaiyan AM, Adami HO, Kantoff PW, Johansson JE (2005) Decreased alpha-methylacyl CoA racemase expression in localized prostate cancer is associated with an increased rate of biochemical recurrence and cancer-specific death. Cancer Epidemiol Biomarkers Prev 14:1424–1432

Sakr WA (2004) Prostatic intraepithelial neoplasia. In: Eble JN, Sauter G, Epstein JI, Sesterhenn IA (eds) World Health Organization classification of tumours: pathology and genetics of tumours of the urinary system and male genital organs. International Agency for Research on Cancer, Lyon, pp 193–198

Sakr WA, Partin AW (2001) Histological markers of risk and the role of high-grade prostatic intraepithelial neoplasia. Urology 57:115–120

Sakr WA, Grignon DJ, Crissman JD, Heilbrun LK, Casin BJ, Pontes JJ, Haas GP (1994) High grade prostatic intraepithelial neoplasia (HGPIN) and prostatic adenocarcinoma between the ages of 20–69: an autopsy study of 249 cases. In Vivo 8:439–443

Sakr WA, Grignon DJ, Haas GP, Heilbrun LK, Pontes JE, Crissman JD (1996) Age and racial distribution of prostatic intraepithelial neoplasia. Eur Urol 30:138–144

Sakr WA, Tefilli MV, Grignon DJ, Banerjee M, Dey J, Gheiler EL, Tiguert R, Powell IJ, Wood DP (2000) Gleason score 7 prostate cancer: a heterogeneous entity? Correlation with pathologic parameters and disease-free survival. Urology 56:730–734

Shannon RL, Ro JY, Grignon DJ, Ordonez NG, Johnson DE, Mackay B, Têtu B, Ayala AG (1992) Sarcomatoid carcinoma of the prostate. A clinicopathologic study of 12 patients. Cancer 69:2676–2682

Spires SE, Cibull ML, Wood DP, Miller S, Spires SM, Banks ER (1994) Gleason histologic grad-ing in prostatic carcinoma. Correlation of 18-gauge core biopsy with prostatectomy. Arch Pathol Lab Med 118:705–708

Srigley JR (2004) Benign mimickers of prostatic adenocarcinoma. Mod Pathol 17:328–348

Srigley JR (2006) Key issues in handling and reporting radical prostatectomy specimens. Arch Pathol Lab Med 130:303–317

Srigley JR, Dardick I, Hartwick RW, Klotz L (1990) Basal epithelial cells of human prostate gland are not myoepithelial cells. A comparative immunohistochemical and ultrastructural study with the human salivary gland. Am J Pathol 136:957–966

Stanford JL, Just JJ, Gibbs M, Wicklund KG, Neal CL, Blumenstein BA, Ostrander EA (1997) Polymorphic repeats in the androgen receptor gene: molecular markers of prostate cancer risk. Cancer Res 57:1194–1198

Steinberg DM, Sauvageot J, Piantadosi S, Epstein JI (1997) Correlation of prostate needle biopsy and radical prostatectomy Gleason grade in academic and community settings. Am J Surg Pathol 21:566–576

Strohmeyer D, Rössing C, Strauss F, Bauerfeind A, Kaufmann O, Loening S (2000) Tumor angiogenesis is associated with progression after radical prostatectomy in pT2/pT3 prostate cancer. Prostate 42:26–33

Sung MT, Lin H, Koch MO, Davidson DD, Cheng L (2007) Radial distance of extraprostatic extension measured by ocular micrometer is an independent predictor of prostate-specific antigen recurrence. A new proposal for the substaging of pT3a prostate cancer. Am J Surg Pathol 31:311–318

Tan PH, Billis A (2004) Basal cell carcinoma. In: Eble JN, Sauter G, Epstein JI, Sesterhenn IA (eds) World Health Organization classification of tumours: pathology and genetics of tumours of the urinary system and male genital organs. International Agency for Research on Cancer, Lyon, p 206

Tefilli MV, Gheiler EL, Tiguert R, Banerjee M, Sakr W, Grignon DJ, Pontes JE, Wood DP (1998) Prognostic indicators in patients with seminal vesicle involvement following radical prostatectomy for clinically localized prostate cancer. J Urol 160:802–806

Têtu B, Srigley JR, Boivin JC, Dupont A, Monfette G, Pinault S, Labrie F (1991) Effect of combination endocrine therapy (LHRH agonist and flutamide) on normal prostate and prostatic adenocarcinoma. A histopathologic and immunohistochemical study. Am J Surg Pathol 15:111–120

Tomlins SA, Rhodes DR, Perner S, Dhanasekaran SM, Mehra R, Sun XW, Varambally S, Cao X, Tchinda J, Kuefer R, Lee C, Montie JE, Shah RB, Pienta KJ, Rubin MA, Chinnaiyan AM (2005) Recurrent fusion of TMPRSS2 and ETS transcription factor genes in prostate cancer. Science 310:644–648

Tomlins SA, Mehra R, Rhodes DR, Smith LR, Roulston D, Helgeson BE, Cao X, Wei JT, Rubin MA, Shah RB, Chinnaiyan AM (2006) TMPRSS2:ETV4 gene fusions define a third molecular subtype of prostate cancer. Cancer Res 66:3396–3400

Torbenson M, Dhir R, Nangia A, Becich MJ, Kapadia SB (1998) Prostatic carcinoma with signet ring cells: a clinicopathologic and immunohistochemical analysis of 12 cases, with review of the literature. Mod Pathol 11:552–559

Tran TT, Sengupta E, Yang XJ (2001) Prostatic foamy gland carcinoma with aggressive behavior: clinicopathologic, immunohistochemical, and ultrastructural analysis. Am J Surg Pathol 25:618–623

Trapman J, Brinkmann AO (1996) The androgen receptor in prostate cancer. Pathol Res Pract 192:752–760

Vaillancourt L, Têtu B, Fradet Y, Dupont A, Gomez J, Cusan L, Suburu ER, Diamond P, Candas B, Labrie F (1996) Effect of neoadjuvant endocrine therapy (combined androgen blockade) on normal prostate and prostatic carcinoma. A randomized study. Am J Surg Pathol 20:86–93

van der Kwast TH (2004) Squamous neoplasms. In: Eble JN, Sauter G, Epstein JI, Sesterhenn IA (eds) World Health Organization classification of tumours: pathology and genetics of tumours of the urinary system and male genital organs. International Agency for Research on Cancer, Lyon, p 205

Wang J, Cai Y, Ren C, Ittmann M (2006) Expression of variant TMPRSS2/ERG fusion messenger RNAs is associated with aggressive prostate cancer. Cancer Res 66:8347–8351

Yang XJ, Cheng L, Helpap B, Samaratunga H (2004) Ductal adenocarcinoma. In: Eble JN, Sauter
    G, Epstein JI, Sesterhenn IA (eds) World Health Organization classification of tumours:
    pathology and genetics of tumours of the urinary system and male genital organs. International
    Agency for Research on Cancer, Lyon, pp 199–201
Young RH, Srigley JR, Amin MB, Ulbright TM, Cubilla AL (2000) Tumors of the prostate gland,
    seminal vesicles, male urethra, and penis. In: Atlas of tumor pathology, ed. Armed Forces
    Institute of Pathology, Washington, DC
Zeegers MP, Kiemeney LA, Nieder AM, Ostrer H (2004) How strong is the association between
    CAG and GGN repeat length polymorphisms in the androgen receptor gene and prostate can-
    cer risk? Cancer Epidemiol Biomarkers Prev 13:1765–1771
Zhou M, Jiang Z, Epstein JI (2003) Expression and diagnostic utility of alpha-methylacyl-CoA-
    racemase (P504S) in foamy gland and pseudohyperplastic prostate cancer. Am J Surg Pathol
    27:772–778
Zhou M, Aydin H, Kanane H, Epstein JI (2004) How often does alpha-methylacyl-CoA-racemase
    contribute to resolving an atypical diagnosis on prostate needle biopsy beyond that provided
    by basal cell markers? Am J Surg Pathol 28:239–243

Chapter 4
Testicular Tumor Pathology

Kirk J. Wojno and Louis R. Bégin

4.1 Introduction

Most neoplasms of the testis are of germ cell origin. More than half of germ cell tumors contain more than one histologic type and are referred to as malignant mixed germ cell tumors. The American Cancer Society estimates that 8,400 new cases of testicular germ cell tumors will be diagnosed in 2009 in the United States (American Cancer Society. http://www.cancer.org). The incidence varies by country and socio-economic status and ranges from one to ten per 100,000 (Eble et al. 2004) with the highest incidence in developed European countries such as Germany, Denmark, Norway, and Switzerland (Ferlay et al. 2001). The incidence of testicular germ cell tumors, specifically, seminoma has been increasing in populations of European descent (Coleman et al. 1993). There is speculation that the increased incidence in developed countries is related to a high-fat western diet and lack of physical activity associated with higher socioeconomic status. Due to advances in treatment, the overall 5-year survival rate for testicular germ cell tumors is 96% and is even greater for localized disease (American Cancer Society. http://www.cancer.org). This chapter deals exclusively with adult germ cell tumors; however, excellent reviews of pediatric germ cell tumors are available elsewhere (Wojno and Bloom 1997).

4.2 Pathogenesis

The cause of testicular germ cell tumors is unknown. It has been theorized that the development of testicular germ cell tumors starts in fetal life with abnormal differentiation of primordial germ cells. There are strong associations with congenital abnormalities of the male genitalia such as cryptorchidism, intersex syndromes,

L.R. Bégin (✉)
Department of Pathology, McGill University and Hôpital du Sacré-Coeur de Montréal, 5400 Gouin Boulevard West, Montreal, QC, H4J 1C5, Canada
e-mail: mdlrb@yahoo.ca

W.D. Foulkes and K.A. Cooney (eds.), *Male Reproductive Cancers:*
Epidemiology, Pathology and Genetics, Cancer Genetics,
DOI 10.1007/978-1-4419-0449-2_4, © Springer Science+Business Media, LLC 2010

hypospadias, inguinal hernia, and atrophy. The association is strongest with cryptorchidism with a three- to fivefold increased risk of germ cell tumor (Richiardi et al. 2007). The association of germ cell tumors with intrauterine growth retardation with low birth weight suggests prenatal risk factors may be important. Please see chapters by McGlynn (pp. 51–83) and Rapley (pp. 317–335) for a detailed discussion of risk factors for testicular cancer.

4.3   Intratubular Germ Cell Neoplasia

Intratubular germ cell neoplasia (IGCN) is the presence of malignant appearing germ cells in abnormal seminiferous tubules, i.e., typically reduced diameter, decreased spermatogenesis, and thickened tubular walls. The malignant appearing germ cells are large (15–25 microns) and have abundant clear-to-vacuolated cytoplasm and a distinct cytoplasmic membrane (Fig. 4.1). They also have significant nuclear enlargement (~10 microns), hyperchromasia, and coarse chromatin with prominent nucleoli. The overall cell size and nuclear size is significantly larger than residual Sertoli cells (Young 2008; Bahrami et al. 2007). IGCN is almost uniformly found adjacent to malignant germ cell tumors if enough residual seminiferous tubules are available for microscopic examination. The natural history of untreated IGCN discovered in a testis without a germ cell tumor is that 90% progress to malignant germ cell tumors within 7 years (Zhou and Magi-Galluzzi 2007).

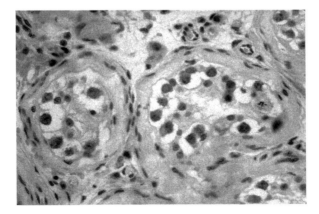

Fig 4.1 Intratubular germ cell neoplasia (IGCN) involving two seminiferous tubules with decreased caliber and thickened peritubular basement membrane. Note the presence of enlarged germ cells with clear cytoplasm and enlarged hyperchromatic round nuclei. These cells are aligned along the basal pole of the tubule with displacement of Sertoli cells toward the lumen.

4.4 Histologically Pure Germ Cell Tumors

The tumor most commonly encountered in the pure form is the classic seminoma. Only rare nonseminomatous germ cell tumors are histologically pure. All germ cell tumors including seminoma need to be adequately sampled to rule out other germ cell components. The extent of sampling can in part be dictated by other laboratory data. Elevated serum markers for hCG and AFP in a seminoma should prompt an aggressive search for mixed germ cell components.

4.4.1 Seminoma

Seminoma accounts for more than one third of malignant germ cell tumors. It typically affects men in their early 40s (Biermann et al. 2007) and Meticulous gross examination is essential for proper staging. Tumors are usually large at time of detection and have often replaced the entire testicle (Fig. 4.2a). The thick fibrous capsule of the tunica albuginea is typically taut from the pressure of the expansile tumor. This confining capsule should be carefully inspected for defects and alterations at gross

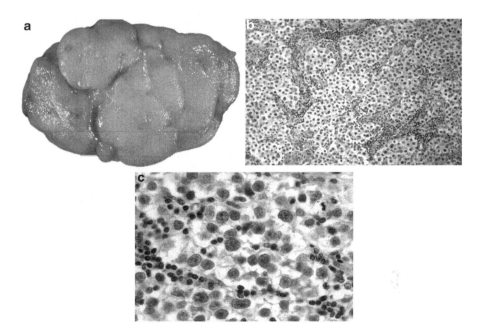

Fig 4.2 Seminoma: (**a**) hemisection of testis showing extensive replacement by a lobulated, soft, and bulging tumor with a homogeneous pale tan and glistening appearance; (**b**) solid sheets of tumor cells with evenly spaced nuclei and the presence of an intervening delicate fibrovascular framework including lymphocytes; (**c**) Seminoma cells with distinct cytoplasmic outline, a clear to granular cytoplasm, and round nuclei with a prominent nucleolus

examination in order to obtain an appropriate tissue sampling for histological examination. Such sampling of areas suspicious for capsular encroachment by tumor is an important step for appropriate assignment of pathologic stage. Seminoma is notoriously discohesive and care must be taken to minimize artifactual displacement of tumor cells into vascular channels. This form of artifactual false-positive angiolymphatic invasion is a common source of incorrect stage assignment, and appropriate examination of the rete testis and submission of appropriate sections can yield additional prognostic information (Hoskin et al. 1986).

Seminoma is composed of malignant germ cells without specific terminal differentiation. The cells are much larger than normal spermatogonia. They are relatively nondescript cells with a distinct cellular outline, abundant clear or vacuolated cytoplasm, and a large central hyperchromatic sometimes vesicular nucleus with prominent nucleoli. The tumor cells are typically arranged in sheets or lobules (Fig. 4.2b, c). An intense inflammatory infiltrate (mostly lymphocytes) is typically present and may include plasma cells, eosinophils, histiocytes, and granulomatous features. The malignant germ cells may be the major component or difficult to find within an intense inflammatory infiltrate. Syncytiotrophoblastic giant cells may be present singly or in small clusters, but not as an expansile hemorrhagic mass. The latter is indicative of a choriocarcinoma component which would imply a malignant mixed germ cell tumor.

The immunophenotype of the seminoma cell is characterized by membranous positivity for placental alkaline phosphatase (PLAP) and cytoplasmic expression of CD117 (c-kit). Focal positivity in rare tumor cells can be observed for cytokeratin or CD30. More extensive cytokeratin or CD30 positivity would be indicative of an embryonal carcinoma component in a malignant mixed germ cell tumor. Alpha fetoprotein (AFP) expression indicates a yolk sac tumor component. Inhibin positivity can be seen in a variant of Leydig cell tumor that mimic seminoma but not in seminoma per se. OCT3/4 is usually expressed in IGCN, seminoma, and embryonal carcinoma (de Jong et al. 2005; Zhou and Magi-Galluzzi 2007). D2-40 is a germ cell marker more specific for seminoma than OCT3/4 and does not stain embryonal carcinoma (Iczkowski et al. 2008) (Table 4.1).

From a diagnostic perspective, molecular and genetic profiling is rarely needed in primary testicular tumors; however, it may be useful in determining the nature of a poorly

Table 4.1 Antibodies used for iimmunohistochemical staining

Abbreviation	Antibody name
CK20	Cytokeratin 20
Cytokeratin AE1/3	Cocktail of low and high molecular weight cytokeratins
CAM5.2	Cytokeratins 8, 18, and 19
CK7	Cytokeratin 7
Cytokeratin 34bE12	High molecular weight cytokeratins 5, 10, and 11
EMA	Epithelial membrane antigen
PLAP	Placental alkaline phosphatase
OCT3/4	Octamer 3/4 (embryonic stem cell transcription factor)
CD30	Cluster designation 30
AFP	Alpha fetoprotein

differentiated neoplasm in a midline or metastatic location. If a germ cell tumor is sus-pected clinically or morphologically then isochromosome 12p can be used to document the germ cell origin. This chromosomal aberration is encountered in 98% of germ cell tumors and is not seen in other tumor types (Wehle et al. 2008). Therefore it has high sensitivity and specificity for germ cell tumors, but it does not distinguish between vari-ous types of germ cell tumors.

4.5   Histologically Mixed Germ Cell Tumors

The vast majority of nonseminomatous germ cell tumors in adults are composed of mixtures of morphologically distinct germ cell neoplasms showing various patterns of differentiation often recapitulating various stages of embryonic development. The finding of a pure nonseminomatous germ cell tumor in an adult should prompt a vigorous search for other components. If not found, other components may have regressed or become necrotic. The rare pure nonseminomatous tumors seen in adults are typically small and have not had the opportunity to develop other patterns of differentiation. For the most part, the specific combination of the components does not have prognostic significance, except for tumors with high percentages of embryonal carcinoma or choriocarcinoma which have a more aggressive course (Bahrami et al. 2007; Pizzocaro et al. 2003; Moul et al. 1994). Therefore the rela-tive proportion of tumor made of these various components should be reported and taken into consideration both prognostically and therapeutically. Due to the mor-phologic complexity and heterogeneity within each component of mixed germ cell tumors they will be described separately. The common coexistence of certain patterns such as the fact that embryonal carcinoma and yolk sac tumor are almost always found together in the typical adult mixed germ cell tumor will be high-lighted (Ulbright et al. 1999; Emerson and Ulbright 2007).

Embryonal carcinoma is a very frequent component of mixed germ cell tumors (~87%). It is only rarely seen in pure form and as such mostly observed in children. It is encountered in a younger adult population than for seminoma (Ulbright et al. 1999). The percentage of embryonal carcinoma affects the prognosis and therefore should be reported. Determination of this percentage needs to take into account fea-tures and representative proportional sampling. Biased sampling based on oversam-pling of unusual gross or certain gross patterns for histological examination can lead to over- or under-reporting of the percentage of embryonal carcinoma. Careful atten-tion to this fact at the time of grossing can minimize this type of error. The gross appearance of embryonal carcinoma is typically a firm variegated white mass that may have hemorrhagic and/or necrotic foci (Fig. 4.3a). The gross appearance may appear softer and of gray discoloration when mixed with yolk sac tumor. The main histologic feature is that of malignant epithelium that can have various patterns including glandular, solid, tubulopapillary, and the so-called embryoid body pattern (Ulbright et al. 1999). The malignant epithelial constituent is characterized by cohesive aggre-gates of neoplastic cells of polygonal, cuboidal, or columnar shape (Fig. 4.3b).

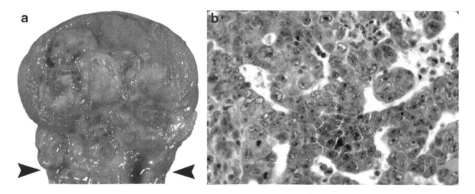

Fig 4.3 Embryonal carcinoma (EC): (**a**) a large intratesticular bulging tumor involving the root of the spermatic cord (between arrowheads). The cut surface is variegated with predominantly soft and gray white areas, zones of yellow granular necrosis and hemorrhagic foci; (**b**) glandular papillary pattern including a syncytial arrangement of cells with dense abundant cytoplasm. Nuclei are large with an irregular thickened membrane and varying number of markedly enlarged nucleoli, lacking an evenly spaced pattern

The malignant epithelium of embryonal carcinoma should have limited terminal differentiation reminiscent of embryonic development. Although glandular and tubulopapillary patterns are allowed, the finding of any terminal differentiation such as squamous, or intestinal epithelium would be considered teratomatous or carcinoma arising in a teratoma rather that embryonal carcinoma.

Immunoperoxidase staining for cytokeratins shows positivity in embryonal carcinoma and help distinguish it from other neoplasms such as seminoma or yolk sac tumor which are typically cytokeratin negative. Embryonal carcinoma is positive for cytokeratin AE1/3, CAM5.2, and CK7, but negative or weakly positive for CK20, and cytokeratin 34bE12. Other useful markers positive in embryonal carcinoma include PLAP, OCT3/4, and CD30. Positive staining for AFP usually indicates a yolk sac tumor component which may be otherwise difficult to identify morphologically (Biermann et al. 2006; Emerson and Ulbright 2005).

Due to the relatively cohesive nature of embryonal carcinoma, artifactual angiolymphatic invasion due to cutting artifact is less common. Since the documentation of angiolymphatic invasion affects stage and prognosis, care must be taken to avoid false positive interpretations.

Yolk sac tumor is a very frequent component of mixed germ cell tumors as it is often associated with embryonal carcinoma in mixed germ cell tumors (Ulbright et al. 1999). It is only very rarely seen in pure form in adults. In its pure form it is encountered mostly in infants and very young children.

The gross features in a pure form are a soft consistency and a yellow color (Fig. 4.4a). When associated with embryonal carcinoma it is firmer in consistency and more gray-white in color. As with embryonal carcinoma the yolk sac tumor can have numerous morphologic patterns that are often mixed together. The reticular/microcystic pattern is most common (Ulbright et al. 1999). It is characterized by loose connective tissue

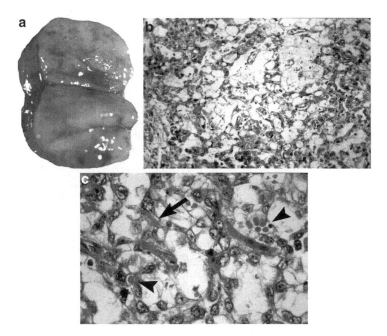

Fig 4.4   Yolk sac tumor (YST): (**a**) hemisection of testis with a pure form of YST showing a solid and homogeneous yellow glistening cut surface; (**b**) typical reticular/microcystic pattern of loosely textured tumor cells creating a meshwork of spaces; (**c**) anastomosing network of frequently vacuolated YST tumor cells with relatively uniform nuclei including distinct nucleoli. Note the presence of hyaline globules (*arrowheads*) and basement membrane deposits (*arrow*) which are hallmarks of YST

stroma punctuated by small cysts lined by flattened cells with little cytoplasm (Fig. 4.4b, c). Even though these cells may resemble flattened endothelial cells they do not stain with endothelial markers. Other patterns include macrocystic, papillary, endodermal sinus, solid, glandular-alveolar, polyvesicular vitelline, hepatoid, and parietal pattern.

Immunoperoxidase stain for AFP is usually positive at least focally. Staining for cytokeratin AE1/3 is positive but of weaker intensity than embryonal carcinoma. Low molecular weight cytokeratins are usually more expressed. Staining for EMA, inhibin, and CD30 is negative. These stains can help for the differential diagnosis with seminoma (AFP negativity), embryonal carcinoma (CD30 positivity), and granulosa cell tumor (inhibin positivity) (Emerson and Ulbright 2005). If serum AFP is elevated in a seminoma, than then intensive search for a yolk sac tumor component, or immunoperoxidase staining to rule out yolk sac tumor morphologically mimicking a seminoma should be undertaken. Since yolk sac tumor often coexists with embryonal carcinoma and some patterns of both neoplasms can be difficult to distinguish from each other, immunoperoxidase stains are often required not so much for diagnosis, but to determine the accurate percentage of embryonal carcinoma as it is prognostically significant (Bahrami et al. 2007; Pizzocaro et al. 2003; Moul et al. 1994).

Teratoma in its pure form is uncommon in adults, but when it does occur it must be considered a malignant germ cell tumor due to the significant risk of metastasis (Wojno and Bloom 1997). Teratoma in a pure form in prepubertal children is a benign neoplasm. By definition a teratoma is a neoplasm composed of all three embryonic layers (ectoderm, mesoderm, endoderm). The tissue from each layer may be either mature or embryonic in nature.

The gross morphology of teratoma is tremendously heterogeneous and can include all forms of recognizable mature tissue such as teeth, hair, bone, cartilage, etc. Immature tissue can have a varied gross morphology. Both cystic and solid components can be present (Fig. 4.5a). The full histologic spectrum of tissue types can be seen in teratoma, in both mature (Fig. 4.5b) and immature (Fig. 4.5c) forms. For example a teratoma could include skin (ectoderm), muscle (mesoderm), and intestinal epithelium (endoderm). Fetal tissue (immature component) can also be focally present, not to be misinterpreted as malignant transformation within a mature component. An example of true malignant transformation would be an invasive moderately differentiated squamous cell carcinoma with expansile growth and overgrowth of the surrounding teratoma of the germ cell tumor. If malignant transformation is limited to the testis there is no apparent change in prognosis

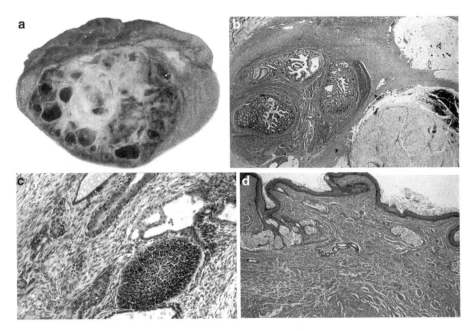

Fig 4.5 Teratoma: (**a**) hemisection of testis showing a well circumscribed, ovoid and firm, partly solid and multicystic tumor with an intracystic fluid content; (**b**) mature component including glands with intestinal-type epithelial lining (*left half*) and lobules of fat (*right half*); (**c**) immature component with stromal hypercellularity and primitive epithelial elements forming a solid nest and tubules; (**d**) outline of a dermoid cyst (teratoma variant) showing a cutaneous lining (*top*) with pilocebaceous/adnexal structures within dermis

(Ulbright 2005). It is difficult to know for sure if such malignancy has metastasized and there is always the possibility of undetected metastasis. If it is detected in a metastatic location, the prognosis is poor.

Dermoid and epidermoid cysts are also considered teratomas. The dermoid cyst is less common and contains skin appendages (Fig. 4.5d) and is typically benign as long as it is not associated with other teratomatous elements or associated with IGCN (Ulbright 2008). The epidermoid cyst is lined by squamous epithelium lacking skin appendages and contains keratinous debris. As long as it is not associated with other teratomatous elements or IGCN, it is considered benign. Therefore, in general, with both types of cysts it is important to rule out concomitant IGCN. The potential pitfall is when adjacent scar tissue is seen, raising the possibility of an adjacent burnt out germ cell neoplasm. The latter scenario is quite challenging and may require close follow-up to rule out a malignant evolution (Ulbright 2008).

A malignant small round blue cell component of teratoma with neural differentiation is considered to be a primitive neuroectodermal tumor (PNET), the latter being considered part of the spectrum of teratomatous differentiation. Although pure PNET of the testis does occur, it is most often seen as a focal component of a malignant mixed germ cell tumor (Michael et al. 1997). PNET in a prepubertal teratoma indicates a malignant germ cell tumor. In the adult, its finding does not appear to alter the overall prognosis of a malignant mixed germ cell tumor. Only PNET in a metastasis is considered to have a worse prognosis.

Carcinoid tumor which is considered a teratoma may be pure or part of an otherwise conventional teratoma. Morphologically it resembles a carcinoid in other locations. These tumors are typically not associated with a carcinoid syndrome. In a pure form, the possibility of a metastasis should be considered, especially if a carcinoid syndrome is present. Immunostains can be helpful in excluding other tumor types such as prostate cancer (PSA positivity), or Sertoli cell tumor (inhibin positivity) (Stroosma and Delaere 2008).

Due to the diversity of tissues in teratoma there is no specific immunoperoxidase stain to aid in the diagnosis. AFP can be seen in intestinal and hepatic type tissue and PLAP can be seen in glandular type tissue. In the setting of dermoid and epidermoid cysts, immunostaining for PLAP and CD117 is useful to rule out a concomitant IGCN component. Immunostaining for CD99 and vimentin is useful in diagnosing PNET whereas neuroendocrine markers (chromogranin and synaptophysin) will be expressed in a carcinoid tumor (Ulbright 2005).

Choriocarcinoma is a highly malignant carcinoma composed of an intimate admixture of syncytiotrophoblasts and cytotrophoblasts. Choriocarcinoma is less common that the other types of germ cell tumor previously discussed, but like them it is rare in a pure form and usually occurs as part of a malignant mixed germ cell tumor. Choriocarcinoma is seen in about 15% of malignant mixed germ cell tumors (Ulbright 2008). The greater the percentage of choriocarcinoma in a malignant mixed germ cell tumor, the worse the prognosis, and therefore the specimen should be sampled in such a way that an accurate percentage can be reported. Choriocarcinoma is a hemorrhagic neoplasm and therefore hemorrhagic areas should be sampled but not over-represented in the tumor sampling. Germ cell tumors with extensive component of choriocarcinoma are often metastatic at the time of diagnosis with the lungs being a common site of metastasis. Consequently, a vigorous metastatic workup is warranted in such cases (Sesterhenn and Davis 2004).

Grossly the tumor is often composed of gray white fleshy tissue peripherally located around a red hemorrhagic mass. Sometimes the hemorrhagic mass predominates. Trophoblastic differentiation occurs with a spectrum of morphology from the small cytotrophoblastic cell to the large multinucleated syncytiotrophoblastic giant cell (Fig. 4.6). Cytotrophoblasts are round-to-ovoid cells with pale cytoplasm, distinct cell borders, and irregular nuclei with vesicular chromatin and visible nucleoli. These cells tend to grow in sheets often surrounded by syncytiotrophoblasts. Intermediate trophoblasts are larger and more irregularly shaped mononucleated cells with more abundant cytoplasm, but with similar nuclear features. This cell constituent tends to have an infiltrative growth pattern. Syncytiotrophoblasts are very large multinucleated cells with an irregular cell border and amphophilic cytoplasm. Syncytiotrophoblasts often caps a cluster of cyto- or intermediate trophoblasts similarly to umbrella cells capping underlying urothelial cells in the bladder. This resemblance is only coincidental but it provides a useful mental image. Hemorrhage and irregular vascular channels as well as an expansile growth pattern are also characteristic.

The immunophenotype of each trophoblastic cell type is different. All cell types express cytokeratin and PLAP, but the staining is heterogeneous and not all cells will stain. The syncytiotrophoblast stains positively for hCG, human placental lactogen (hPL), EMA, and inhibin. The cytotrophoblast is negative for hPL and hCG, while the intermediate trophoblast is positive for hPL and inhibin (Ulbright et al. 1997).

Problems in the differential diagnosis often occur if there are only small foci of such tumor, especially within a background of seminoma or solid embryonal carcinoma as both of these tumors may include a few scattered syncytiotrophoblastic cells (not to be misinterpreted as a choriocarcinoma component). The distinguishing features between

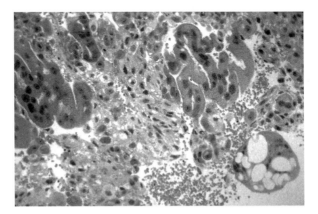

Fig 4.6 Choriocarcinoma characterized by an intimate admixture of sheets of cohesive mononucleated cytotrophoblastic cells and large multinucleated syncytiotrophoblastic cells with abundant amphophilic cytoplasm including vacuoles

scattered syncytiotrophoblasts and a small focus of genuine choriocarcinoma rest on finding at least two cell types (i.e., a biphasic cellular proliferation, most often cytotrophoblasts and syncytiotrophoblasts) and an expansile growth pattern.

Choriocarcinoma produces hCG which is a useful tumor marker that can be measured in the serum. It is useful for staging and monitoring for disease recurrence.

Pure choriocarcinoma is treated as a stage III malignant germ cell tumor due to its aggressive behavior.

Seminoma, while often pure in its classic form, can be part of a malignant mixed germ cell tumor. There is debate in the literature as to whether it represents a phenomenon of dedifferentiation or it is a metachronous neoplasia (Young 2008).

4.6   Tumor Markers

Serum tumor marker evaluation including AFP, hCG, and LDH is an important part of the preoperative work of a testicular mass. Serum AFP levels are elevated in tumors with a yolk sac tumor component, whereas serum hCG levels are elevated in tumors with a choriocarcinoma component. LDH is not tumor specific and is elevated in approximately 50% of germ cell tumors. Its level typically correlates with tumor burden. Comparison of pre- and postoperative tumor marker levels gives tremendous information regarding tumor removal as well as specifying which markers are useful for clinical monitoring and follow up (Kinkade 1999).

4.7   Staging

Pathologic documentation of invasion through the tunica albuginea into the tunica vaginalis is a challenging task that requires meticulous gross dissection. The tunica vaginalis is a thin serous lining covering the tunica albuginea. Documentation of invasion of tumor through the tunica albuginea with involvement of the tunica vaginalis on a histologic slide is a demanding task. It requires careful correlation between the gross and histologic findings.

Pathologic staging of testicular tumors is relatively straightforward. The TNM system is most widely employed (Greene et al. 2002) (Table 4.2). The primary tumor stage is pT1 when limited to the testis, pT2 when tumor invades through the tunica albuginea and involves the tunica vaginalis or if there is angiolymphatic invasion, pT3 when tumor invades the spermatic cord, and pT4 when tumor invades the scrotum. The latter stage is usually obvious at the time of surgery, while pT3 requires careful gross dissection and appropriate tissue sampling for histology to document focal extension of tumor into the spermatic cord. Angiolymphatic invasion can be problematic in that many germ cell tumor types are discohesive and tumor cells are artifactually introduced into lymphatic channels or vascular spaces. Careful attention to microscopic details usually allows the pathologist to differentiate

Table 4.2 AJCC TNM pathological stage (adapted from Greene et al. (2002)

pTX: Primary tumor cannot be assessed

pT0: No evidence of primary tumor (e.g., histologic scar in testis)

pTis: Intratubular germ cell neoplasia

pT1: Tumor limited to the testis and epididymis without vascular/lymphatic invasion; tumor may invade into the tunica albuginea but not the tunica vaginalis

pT2: Tumor limited to the testis and epididymis with vascular/lymphatic invasion, or tumor extending through the tunica albuginea with involvement of the tunica vaginalis

pT3: Tumor invades the spermatic cord with or without vascular/lymphatic invasion

pT4: Tumor invades the scrotum with or without vascular/lymphatic invasion

NX: Regional lymph nodes cannot be assessed

N0: No regional lymph node metastasis

N1: Metastasis with a lymph node mass 2 cm or less in greatest dimension; or no more than 5 lymph nodes positive, no more than, 2 cm in greatest dimension

N2: Metastasis with a lymph node mass larger than 2 cm but no more than 5 cm in greatest dimension; or more than 5 lymph nodes positive, none more than 5 cm in greatest dimension

N3: Metastasis with a lymph node mass more than 5 cm in greatest dimension

MX: Presence of distant metastasis cannot be assessed

M0: No distant metastasis

M1: Distant metastasis

M1a: Nonregional nodal or pulmonary metastasis

M1b: Distant metastasis other than to nonregional lymph nodes and lungs

SX: Marker studies not available or not performed

S0: Marker study levels within normal limits

S1: Lactate dehydrogenase (LDH) less than $1.5 \times N$, and

Human chorionic gonadotropin (hCG) less than 5,000 (mIU/mL), and

Alpha-fetoprotein (AFP) less than 1,000 (ng/mL)

S2: LDH $1.5-10 \times N$ or

hCG 5,000–50,000 (mIU/mL), or

AFP 1,000–10,000 (ng/mL)

S3: LDH more than $10 \times N$, or

hCG more than 50,000 (mIU/mL), or AFP more than 10,000 (ng/mL)

true angiolymphatic invasion from cutting artifact contamination. pTis is reserved for IGCN, and pT0 for scars indicative of regressed tumors. As with all TNM classifications the "x" is reserved for acknowledging that the information is not available, i.e., pTx.

Lymph node staging is based on number and size of lymph node metastasis. The lymph node stage is: pN1 when no more than 5 positive lymph nodes are identified with none greater than 2 cm, or a single whole mass of multiple positive nodes not exceeding 2 cm, pT2 when more than 5 positive lymph nodes are identified with none greater than 5 cm or single whole lymph node mass measuring between 2 and 5 cm, and pT3 when a positive lymph node or lymph node mass is greater than 5 cm. pN0 or pNx are reserved for negative lymph nodes or those not assessed, respectively.

Distant metastasis staging is divided into two groups. Stage M1a is assigned for nonregional lymph node metastasis or pulmonary metastasis. Other distant metastases to locations other than lungs or lymph nodes are designated M1b. M0 or Mx are reserved for no distant metastasis or when they cannot be assessed.

Serum marker staging is based on measurement of LDH, hCG, and AFP prior to treatment. Serum marker stage is S1 for LDH less than 1.5 times normal and hCG less than 5,000 mIU/ml and AFP less than 1,000 ng/ml; stage S2 for LDH between 1.5 and 10 times normal, or hCG between 5,000 and 50,000 mIU/ml, or AFP between 1,000 and 10,000 ng/ml; and stage S3 for LDH greater than 10 times normal, or hCG greater than 50,000 mIU/ml, or AFP greater than 10,000 ng/ml. Testicular serum tumor markers have a unique place in cancer staging in that they are included as part of the staging of a testicular tumor.

The overall stage grouping of testicular tumors is based on combining various elements of the pTNM staging assignment. Stage 0 is reserved for intratubular lesions. Stage I is split into three groups with negative nodes or metastasis. It is further subdivided into two groups without, and one with, positive serum markers. Stage Ia is for pT1 with negative nodes, stage Ib for pT2-4, both with negative markers. Stage Is is for any pT with any positive S stage. Stage II is divided into three groups A, B, C based on lymph node stage (N1, N2, N3) and serum marker stage of S1 or less. Stage III is divided into three groups A, B, C based on regional or distant metastasis at various serum stage levels. Stage IIIA for distant metastasis for lymph nodes or lungs and normal or low level serum markers S1, stage IIIB for regional or distant lymph node metastasis with Moderately elevated serum markers S2, and stage IIIC is for any regional or distant metastasis to lung or lymph nodes with markedly elevated serum markers, or any distant metastasis other than lung or lymph nodes.

As can be seen pattern of metastasis is typical to regional retroperitoneal lymph nodes than more distant lymph node sites and lungs. More unusual sites of metastasis beyond that mentioned are typical of advanced stage (Greene et al. 2002).

4.8 Sex Cord Stromal Tumors

Sex cord stromal tumors are tumors of the nongerm cell components of the testis and include Leydig cell, Sertoli cell, granulosa cell, fibroma-thecoma, and undifferentiated sex cord stroma categories as well as mixtures of the aforementioned. These tumors are typically benign; however, 10% can behave in a malignant fashion without obvious histologic correlate (Cheville 1999). These aggressive tumors usually manifest their malignant behavior within a few years and often lead to mortality within a 5 years interval. Therefore, several years of follow-up are warranted to rule out a potentially aggressive neoplasm.

Leydig cell tumor is the most common of sex cord stromal tumors (Al-Agha 2007). The tumor may occur at any age, but only the adult form will be addressed here. It typically presents as a painless testicular mass. Functional tumors may be associated with impotence and gynecomastia. Elevated serum markers for androgens, estrogens, and progestins and decreased serum levels of gonadotropins may be detected.

Grossly the tumor is yellow-tan to mahogany-brown and varies in size from small to 10 cm, but is usually encountered in the 3 to 5 cm range. Tumor cells are polygonal in shape with distinct cell borders and abundant eosinophilic cytoplasm (Fig. 4.7a). Refractile eosinophilic Reinke crystals are seen in fewer than half of cases. Lipofuscin pigment is present in approximately 15% of cases and is responsible for the gross mahogany color when present in great abundance (Young 2008). The nucleus is round with a central nucleolus. Some nuclear anaplasia and atypia can be seen, but mitotic figures are rare. Positive immunoperoxidase staining for inhibin and vimentin can be helpful in confirming the diagnosis.

Sertoli cell tumors are a morphologically heterogeneous group of neoplasms with at least five distinctive variants reported in the literature (Young 2008; Emerson and Ulbright 2007; Ulbright 2008). The morphologic features of these specific variants are beyond the scope of this chapter and of little prognostic significance. The significance lies in the pathologist's ability to correctly identify Sertoli cell differentiation and distinguish it from a germ cell neoplasm. The classic type of Sertoli cell tumor is typically yellow-tan to white and is smaller and firmer than a Leydig cell tumor. Microscopically, the cells of Sertoli cell tumor are arranged in tubules, nests, cords, and sheets (Fig. 4.7b). The epithelial aggregates may be present within a fibrous stroma. The cells have a slightly amphophilic cytoplasm and oval nuclei with small nucleoli. Immunoperoxidase stains may be useful in confirming the diagnosis. Sertoli cell tumors characteristically express inhibin, vimentin, and cytokeratin. Otherwise, they are negative for markers specifically ascribed to germ cell tumors (PLAP, AFP, HCG, and CD30) and EMA (Young 2008).

Adult granulosa cell tumor is a rare testicular tumor. The tumor typically has a cystic gray tan gelatinous appearance. Microscopically these tumors resemble their ovarian counterpart. The cells have oval-to-spindled nuclei with indistinct cytoplasm.

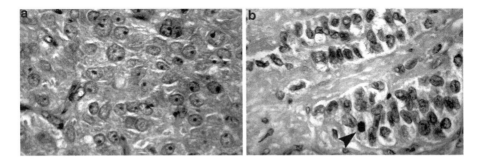

Fig 4.7 Sex cord stromal tumor: (**a**) Leydig cell type showing a solid pattern of large polygonal cells with abundant slightly granular cytoplasm. Nuclei are round with a single central nucleolus; (**b**) Sertoli cell type (of not otherwise specified category) showing thick cords of cells with an intervening fibrous stroma. Tumor cells have a pale cytoplasm and relatively bland nuclei. Note the presence of one mitosis (*arrowhead*)

A prominent nuclear groove is a key diagnostic feature. A microfollicular pattern with Call-Exner bodies is characteristic. These bodies are composed of eosinophilic material surrounded by palisading cells. Nuclear anaplasia and atypia is uncommon. Mitotic figures are rare. Tumor cells have an immunophenotype including positivity for vimentin and inhibin as do other sex cord stromal tumors. CD99 (MIC2), S-100 protein, actin, and desmin are also expressed which can help in the distinction from other sex cord stromal tumors (Young 2005).

Fibroma-thecoma is a very rare tumor of the testis. Grossly the tumor is firm and yellow to white and lacks any evidence of hemorrhage or necrosis. It is composed of compact spindle cells with varying amounts of collagenous stroma. There is no significant nuclear atypia. Tumors cells are positive with immunoperoxidase staining for vimentin and smooth muscle actin. Since this is a benign tumor, it is important to distinguish it from a sarcoma or an unclassified sex cord stromal tumor as the latter can have a malignant potential (Cheville 1999).

Mixed sex cord stromal tumors do occur and are characterized by many morphological types of sex cord stromal differentiation (Young 2008).

Mixed germ cell sex cord stromal tumors are composed of both sex cord stromal elements and neoplastic germ cells similar to seminoma cells. Gonadoblastoma is the prototypical lesion in this category. It is composed of a mixture of germ cells and sex cord stromal cells present in a nested organoid pattern. The nests contain hyaline structures of basement membrane material surrounded by the cellular elements. Calcifications are common. The so-called unclassified type of this neoplasm is of questionable existence as most such cases represent sex cord stromal tumors with entrapped non neoplastic germ cells rather than a true proliferation of germ cells (Ulbright et al. 2000). This whole subject is somewhat controversial and should be approached with caution. Several years of clinical follow-up is an appropriate management as it is the case with sex cord stromal tumors at large.

Unclassified sex cord stromal tumor is a wastebasket category for tumors that do not have enough morphological and/or immunophenotypic features to fit into a specific category. These tumors with an unusual morphology characteristically express vimentin and inhibin, are negative for germ cell tumor markers, and lack specific cytoarchitectural features. These rare tumors are difficult to prognosticate but tend to follow the general behavior of sex cord stromal tumors, i.e., 10% behaving in a malignant fashion (Magro et al. 2007).

4.9 Rete Testis Carcinoma

Rete testis carcinoma is an adenocarcinoma arising in the rete testis at the hilum of the testis. It typically has a gray-white color and firm consistency. Tubular, papillary, and solid architectural patterns can be seen. Finding an in situ component is a useful diagnostic feature. Metastasis from another site needs to be excluded clinically. Immunoperoxidase staining is not specific as the phenotype is similar to adenocarcinomas in other locations, namely tumor cells positive for cytokeratin,

EMA, CEA, vimentin, and negative for AFP, hCG, and PLAP. Negative cytogenetics for isochromosome 12p is useful in excluding a germ cell tumor. This neoplasm occurs at an older age than germ cell tumors and has quite aggressive behavior (Menon et al. 2002; Jones et al. 2000).

4.10 Epididymal Tumors

Carcinoma within the epididymis is metastatic until proven otherwise and often originates from the prostate. Primary neoplasm of the epididymis is often a papillary cystadenoma which can be a morphologic mimic of renal cell carcinoma. The benign papillary cystadenoma typically occurs in the head of the epididymis and can be sporadic or associated with von Hippel-Lindau disease. Immunoperoxidase stains for cytokeratins and EMA are positive. A benign papillary mesothelioma can also occur at this location. Immunohistochemistry can be useful in this differential diagnosis by proving mesothelial differentiation (calretinin positivity) (Amin 2005).

4.11 Mesothelial Neoplasms

Both benign and malignant mesothelial neoplasms may involve the testis. Adenomatoid tumor is a benign mesothelial tumor that is often paratesticular but can appear to involve the testis by external compression. Malignant mesothelioma also arises from the mesothelial lining on the surface of the testis (tunica vaginalis) and can involve a hydrocele sac. The tumor can be a solid mass or spread as a thickening along a mesothelial surface. Papillary, tubular, solid, and spindle cell morphologies are encountered. A useful immunoperoxidase stain that marks mesothelial cells is calretinin. Negative staining for LeuM1 and CEA which typically stain adenocarcinomas can also help with this differential diagnosis (Amin 2005).

4.12 Lymphoid Neoplasms

Primary lymphomas of the testis are not usually associated with systemic disease at the time of presentation, yet they are quite aggressive. They occur in older men (>50 years). They typically expand the interstitial compartment between the seminiferous tubules. They are mostly of diffuse large cell morphology with a B cell immunophenotype. Immunoperoxidase stains for lymphoid markers easily separate this neoplasm from spermatocytic seminoma which also occurs in this age group. Relapse often occurs in extranodal sites and survival is generally poor (Verma et al. 2008).

4.13 Metastatic Tumors

Prostate cancer is the tumor phenotype most commonly encountered as a metastasis to the testis or paratesticular region. It is frequently encountered in patients with hormone refractory metastatic adenocarcinoma of prostate. Metastasis from other tumor sites does occur but much less frequently, usually occurring in a setting of known widespread disease (Ulbright and Young 2008). Immunoperoxidase staining can be useful in confirming the primary site of origin but is often not necessary.

4.14 Conclusion

Testicular cancer is one of the few cancers other than hematological malignancies that is curable with standard chemotherapy even when widely metastatic. The potential curability, as well as the fact that this is a disease affecting primarily young men, emphasizes the need for accurate pathological interpretation. Many molecular genetic studies of testicular cancer report findings for all germ cell tumors and inferences for certain histological subtypes are limited due to the small number of cases examined. Future studies will likely focus on identifying the specific genetic expression patterns for seminoma and nonseminomatous germ cell tumors. Whereas some progress has been made toward this goal (see Chap. by Nathanson, Sect. 6.5), none of this work has yet been translated into clinical practice. Future research in this area will require close interaction between pathologists, molecular biologists, and clinicians, as well as access to a large number of clinical specimens, to more fully elucidate the molecular differences between the various types of testicular cancers. This work should improve our diagnostic abilities as well as define more accurate treatments for this relatively rare, but important, cancer.

References

Al-Agha OM, Axiotis CA (2007) An in-depth look at Leydig cell tumor of the testis. Arch Pathol Lab Med 131(2):311–317

American Cancer Society. http://www.cancer.org/docroot/CRI/content/CRI_2_4_1X_What_are_the_key_statistics_for_testicular_cancer_41.asp?sitearea=

Amin MB (2005) Selected other problematic testicular and paratesticular lesions: rete testis neoplasms and pseudotumors, mesothelial lesions and secondary tumors. Mod Pathol 18 (Suppl 2):S131–S145

Bahrami A, Ro JY, Ayala AG (2007) An overview of testicular germ cell tumors. Arch Pathol Lab Med 131(8):1267–1280

Biermann K, Heukamp LC, Steger K, Zhou H, Franke FE, Sonnack V, Brehm R, Berg J, Bastian PJ, Muller SC, Wang-Eckert L, Buettner R (2007) Genome-wide expression profiling reveals new insights into pathogenesis and progression of testicular germ cell tumors. Cancer Genomics Proteomics 4(5):359–367

Biermann K, Klingmüller D, Koch A, Pietsch T, Schorle H, Büttner R, Zhou H (2006) Diagnostic value of markers M2A, OCT3/4, AP-2gamma, PLAP and c-KIT in the detection of extragonadal seminomas. Histopathology 49(3):290–297

Cheville JC (1999) Classification and pathology of testicular germ cell and sex cord-stromal tumors. Urol Clin North Am 26(3):595–609

Coleman MP, Esteve J, Damiecki P, Arslan A, Renard H (1993) Trends in cancer incidence and mortality. IARC Sci Publ 121:1–806

de Jong J, Stoop H, Dohle GR, Bangma CH, Kliffen M, van Esser JW, van den Bent M, Kros JM, Oosterhuis JW, Looijenga LH (2005) Diagnostic value of OCT3/4 for pre-invasive and invasive testicular germ cell tumours. J Pathol 206((2):242–249

Emerson RE, Ulbright TM (2005) The use of immunohistochemistry in the differential diagnosis of tumors of the testis and paratestis. Semin Diagn Pathol 22(1):33–50

Emerson RE, Ulbright TM (2007) Morphological approach to tumours of the testis and paratestis. J Clin Pathol 60(8):866–880

Ferlay J, Bray F, Pissani P, Parkin DM (2001) GLOBOCAN 2000, Cancer incidence, mortality and prevalence worldwide. IARC Press, Lyon

Greene FL, Page DL, Fleming ID, Fritz A, Balch CM, Haller DG, Morrow M (2002) AJCC Cancer Staging Manual, 6th edn. Springer, New York

Hoskin P, Dilly S, Easton D, Horwich A, Hendry W, Peckham MJ (1986) Prognostic factors in stage I non-seminomatous germ-cell testicular tumors managed by orchiectomy and surveillance: implications for adjuvant chemotherapy. J Clin Oncol 4(7):1031–1036

Iczkowski KA, Butler SL, Shanks JH, Hossain D, Schall A, Meiers I, Zhou M, Torkko KC, Kim SJ, MacLennan GT (2008) Trials of new germ cell immunohistochemical stains in 93 extragonadal and metastatic germ cell tumors. Hum Pathol 39(2):275–281

Jones EC, Murray SK, Young RH (2000) Cysts and epithelial proliferations of the testicular collecting system (including rete testis). Semin Diagn Pathol 17(4):270–293

Kinkade S (1999) Testicular cancer. Am Fam Physician 59(9):2539–2544, 2549–2550

Levin HS (2007) Neoplasms of the testis. In: Zhou M, Magi-Galluzzi C (eds) Genitourinary Pathology. Churchill Livingstone/Elsevier, Philadelphia, pp 534–622

Magro G, Gurrera A, Gangemi P, Saita A, Greco P (2007) Incompletely differentiated (unclassified) sex cord/gonadal stromal tumor of the testis with a "pure" spindle cell component: report of a case with diagnostic and histogenetic considerations. P. Pathol Res Pract 203(10):759–762

Menon PK, Vasudevarao, Sabhiki A, Kudesia S, Joshi DP, Mathur UB (2002) A case of carcinoma rete testis: histomorphological, immunohistochemical and ultrastructural findings and review of literature. Indian J Cancer 39(3):106–111

Michael H, Hull MT, Ulbright TM, Foster RS, Miller KD (1997) Primitive neuroectodermal tumors arising in testicular germ cell neoplasms. Am J Surg Pathol 21(8):896–904

Moul JW, McCarthy WF, Fernandez EB, Sesterhenn IA (1994) Percentage of embryonal carcinoma and of vascular invasion predicts pathological stage in clinical stage I nonseminomatous testicular cancer. Cancer Res 54:362–364

Pizzocaro G, Nicolai N, Miceli R, Artusi R, Salvioni R, Piva L, Marubini E (2003) Prognostic value of vascular invasion and percent of embryonal carcinoma in non-seminomatous testis cancer in clinical stage I (CS1) patients submitted to retroperitoneal lymph-node dissection (RPLND) alone. Proc Am Soc Clin Oncol 22: abstract 1662

Richiardi L, Pettersson A, Akre O (2007) Genetic and environmental risk factors for testicular cancer. Int J Androl 30(4):230–240

Sesterhenn IA, Davis CJ Jr (2004) Pathology of germ cell tumors of the testis. Cancer Control 11(6):374–387

Stroosma OB, Delaere KP (2008) Carcinoid tumours of the testis. BJU Int 101(9):1101–1105

Ulbright TM (2005) Germ cell tumors of the gonads: a selective review emphasizing problems in differential diagnosis, newly appreciated, and controversial issues. Mod Pathol 18 (Suppl 2):S61–S79

Ulbright TM (2008) The most common, clinically significant misdiagnoses in testicular tumor pathology, and how to avoid them. Adv Anat Pathol 15(1):18–27

Ulbright TM, Amin MB, Young RH (1999) Tumors of the testis, adnexa, spermatic cord, and scrotum. In: Atlas of tumor pathology, ed. Armed Forces Institute of Pathology, Washington, DC

Ulbright TM, Srigley JR, Reuter VE, Wojno K, Roth LM, Young RH (2000) Sex cord-stromal tumors of the testis with entrapped germ cells: a lesion mimicking unclassified mixed germ cell sex cord-stromal tumors. Am J Surg Pathol 24(4):535–542

Ulbright TM, Young RH (2008) Metastatic carcinoma to the testis: a clinicopathologic analysis of 26 nonincidental cases with emphasis on deceptive features. Am J Surg Pathol 32(11):1683–1693

Ulbright TM, Young RH, Scully RE (1997) Trophoblastic tumors of the testis other than classic choriocarcinoma: "monophasic" choriocarcinoma and placental site trophoblastic tumor: a report of two cases. Am J Surg Pathol 21(3):282–288

Verma N, Lazarchick J, Gudena V, Turner J, Chaudhary UB (2008) Testicular lymphoma: an update for clinicians. Am J Med Sci 336(4):336–341

Wehle D, Yonescu R, Long PP, Gala N, Epstein J, Griffin CA (2008) Fluorescence in situ hybridization of 12p in germ cell tumors using a bacterial artificial chromosome clone 12p probe on paraffin-embedded tissue: clinical test validation. Cancer Genet Cytogenet 183(2):99–104

Wojno K, Bloom D (1997) Testicular tumors. In: Crawford ED, Das S (eds) Current Genitourinary Cancer Surgery. Williams & Wilkins, Baltimore, pp 582–594

Woodward PJ, Heidenreich A, Looijenga LHJ, Oosterhuis JW, McLeod DG, Moller H, Manivel JC, Mostofi FK, Hailemariam S, Parkinson MC, Grigor K, True L, Jacobsen GK, Oliver TD, Talerman A, Kaplan GW, Ulbright TM, Sesterhenn IA, Rushton HG, Michael H, Reuter VE (2004) Germ cell tumors. In: Eble JN, Sauter G, Epstein JI, Sesterhenn IA (eds) World Health Organization classification of tumours: pathology and genetics of tumors of the urinary system and male genital organs. International Agency for Research on Cancer, Lyon, pp 221–249

Young RH (2005) Sex cord-stromal tumors of the ovary and testis: their similarities and differences with consideration of selected problems. Mod Pathol 18 (Suppl 2):S81–S98

Young RH (2008) Testicular tumors – some new and a few perennial problems. Arch Pathol Lab Med 132(4):548–564

Part C
Molecular Genetics

Chapter 5
Somatic Molecular Genetics of Prostate Cancer

Laure Humbert and Mario Chevrette

5.1 Introduction

Despite progress in diagnosis and treatment, prostate cancer is still one of the most frequent lethal diseases in men in Western countries. Today, an increasing number of prostate cancers are detected through elevated serum prostate-specific antigen (PSA) levels. PSA detection is very sensitive. Determining free versus total PSA serum level has enabled the achievement of better specificity (Balk et al. 2003), however, this tool remains imperfect. Many patients undergo unnecessary diagnostic procedures, experiencing physiological and psychological stress. Similarly, current techniques such as imaging and biopsies are not optimal thus, hopes are high for the discovery of new molecular markers for prostate cancer. Studying prostate cancer progression may reveal new insights into the molecular mechanisms of cancer development to help improve prevention, provide better tools for diagnosis, as well as for prognosis and treatment.

There is no site-specific inherited prostate cancer susceptibility gene, but epidemiological studies have demonstrated familial clustering of prostate cancer suggesting an important role of hereditary factors in the development of the disease. Almost 25% of all prostate cancer occurs in family clusters and about 9% can be attributed to hereditary prostate cancer with an autosomal dominant transmission (Carter et al. 1993; Gronberg et al. 1997; Schaid et al. 1998; Langeberg et al. 2007). Men having an affected first-degree relative have two- to threefold higher risk of developing prostate cancer compared with men with no family history (Johns and Houlston 2003). Studies of twins showed higher frequency for prostate cancer in monozygotic as compared to dizygotic twins (Lichtenstein et al. 2000). Several chromosomes may harbor high-penetrance prostate cancer susceptibility genes. Molecular studies have identified three candidate susceptibility genes: the *HPC2/ELAC2*

M. Chevrette (✉)
Division of Urology, Department of Surgery, The Research Institute of the McGill University Health Center, McGill University, Montreal, QC, Canada
e-mail: mario.chevrette@mcgill.ca

W.D. Foulkes and K.A. Cooney (eds.), *Male Reproductive Cancers:*
Epidemiology, Pathology and Genetics, Cancer Genetics,
DOI 10.1007/978-1-4419-0449-2_5, © Springer Science+Business Media, LLC 2010

gene located at 17p12 encoding a protein with a poorly defined function (Tavtigian et al. 2001), the putative tumor suppressor gene *RNASEL* located at 1q24–q25 (Carpten et al. 2002), and the *MSR1* gene located at 8p22–23 (Xu et al. 2002). However, no functional study has clearly shown that they have a clear role as susceptibility genes and thus further investigations are needed. These issues are discussed in detail in the chapters of Lange, and Eeles and colleagues.

5.2   Genetic Instability

Genetic instability is an important molecular mechanism during the development of malignancies (Cahill et al. 1999). Two types of genetic instability are the hallmark of adult epithelial malignant diseases and have been proposed as a necessary component for initiation and progression of the malignant phenotype (Loeb 1991; DeMarzo et al. 2003). Although uncommon in prostate cancer (DeMarzo et al. 2003), microsatellite instability is related to defects in genes encoding DNA mismatch repair enzymes (Karran and Bignami 1994). The other type of instability involves numerous and complex structural changes to whole chromosomes and is much common in solid tumors such as prostate cancer, however the underlying molecular mechanisms remain largely unknown. Defective telomeres have been implicated in these mechanisms (Counter et al. 1992; Hackett and Greider 2002). Telomeres are multiple repeats of a 6-base-pair motif (TTAGGG), complexed with binding proteins. They protect chromosome ends from fusing with other chromosome ends or other chromosomes containing double-strand breaks (McClintock 1941). However, in the absence of compensatory mechanisms, telomeric DNA is subject to loss due to cell division and possibly oxidative damage (Rubin and De Marzo 2004). Telomere shortening leads to chromosomal instability that causes an increased cancer incidence in mouse models (Rubin and De Marzo 2004). This may be the result of chromosome fusions, subsequent breakage, and rearrangement (Blasco et al. 1997; Artandi et al. 2000). In human carcinomas, telomeres are often found to be abnormally shortened. The telomeres from prostate cancer cells were shown to be significantly shorter than those from cells in the adjacent normal tissue (Sommerfeld et al. 1996; Donaldson et al. 1999). Telomere shortening was demonstrated in high-grade prostate intraepithelial neoplasia (PIN) lesions, which is considered to be the precursor to prostate cancer (Meeker et al. 2002). Moreover proliferating cells need to stabilize their telomeres so that they can prevent massive chromosomal instability and cell death. This is usually achieved by activating telomerase (Hackett and Greider 2002). Indeed telomerase is active in prostate cancer but generally not in benign prostatic hyperplasia (BPH) or normal prostate tissue (Sommerfeld et al. 1996). Thus, telomere shortening can be considered as a nonspecific biomarker in human prostate neoplasia, occurring early in the process of prostate carcinogenesis.

5.3 Cytogenetics: Chromosomal Aberrations

Chromosomal aberrations in prostate cancer are usually detected by traditional cytogenetics (G-banding), analysis of loss of heterozygosity (LOH), and comparative genomic hybridization (CGH) (Porkka and Visakorpi 2004). Since prostate cancer cells do not grow well in vitro, the first method has not provided with much information. Moreover, only a few whole genome-wide LOH studies have been conducted. Thus CGH remains the most informative tool. CGH studies have revealed two main features characteristic of prostate cancer (Visakorpi et al. 1995b). Firstly, losses of the genetic material are much more common than gains or amplifications, indicating that tumor or metastasis suppressor genes, which are believed to be located in frequently deleted regions, probably play an important role in the tumorigenesis of the prostate. Secondly, many of the chromosomal losses can be detected already in the early stages of prostate cancer, whereas gains and amplifications are mostly seen in hormone-refractory tumors, suggesting that oncogenes become activated at the late stage of the disease. The chromosomal regions (Fig. 5.1) most commonly showing losses in prostate cancers are 6q, 8p, 10q, 13q, 16q, 18q, and Y. The regions 7p/q, 8q, and Xq are the chromosomal regions that most commonly show gains in hormone-refractory and metastatic tumors (Elo and Visakorpi 2001).

The most common losses in prostate cancer occur on the short arm of chromosome 8 (8p) (seen in 48% of tumors) and on the long arm of chromosome 13 (13q) (55%) (Alers et al. 2000). These two chromosomal regions are also most frequently lost in PIN (Nupponen and Visakorpi 2000). Further analysis of chromosome 8 deletions revealed two different loci located at 8p12–p21 and 8p22 (Bova et al. 1993; Trapman et al. 1994; Emmertbuck et al. 1995), containing several genes that are candidate tumor suppressors in prostate, such as *MSR1, NKX3.1, N33* (Bookstein et al. 1997; He et al. 1997), *FEZ1*, and *PRTLS* (Elo and Visakorpi 2001) (Table 5.1). Although the 13q loss is already seen in PIN lesions, it is nevertheless associated with clinical aggressiveness of prostate cancer (Elo and Visakorpi 2001). At least three different loci (13q14, 13q21–22, and 13q33) and some genes have been identified on this chromosome arm (Hyytinen et al. 1999). The retinoblastoma *RB1* tumor suppressor gene (located at 13q14) is often deleted in early prostatic tumorigenesis (Phillips et al. 1994), but *RB1* mutations seem to be very rare in prostate cancer (Elo and Visakorpi 2001; Takaku et al. 2003). Another putative suppressor gene is the endothelin B receptor gene *EDNRB* at 13q21, which has been shown to be hypermethylated and downregulated in prostate cancer (Nelson et al. 1997), but further studies have shown that *EDNRB* is not located in the minimal region of deletion (Hyytinen et al. 1999).

Deletions at 10q (Fig. 5.1) have also been reported (Nupponen et al. 1998; Cher et al. 1996); these regions encode suppressors such as *MXI1* (Eagle et al. 1995) and *PTEN* (Cairns et al. 1997a; Feilotter et al. 1998; Pesche et al. 1998) (Table 5.1).

Regions of chromosomal gain are more often found in advanced prostate cancer. The most common chromosomal alteration detected in hormone-refractory and

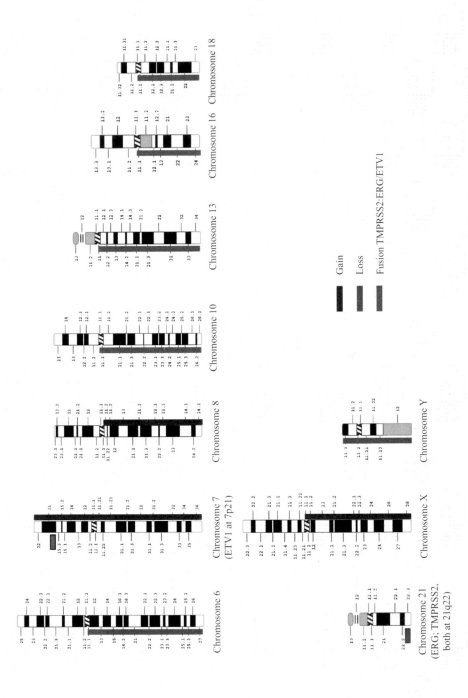

Fig. 5.1 Main regions of chromosomic alterations detected in prostate cancer

Table 5.1 Genes whose expression is modified during prostate cancer progression

Gene	Location	Encoded protein	Function	Alteration in prostate cancer
AMACR	5p13	α-methylacyl-CoA racemase	Implicated in β-oxidation of dietary branched-chain fatty acids	Overexpression
ANXA7	10q21.1–q21.2	Annexin A7	Member of the annexin family of calcium-dependent phospholipid-binding proteins	Loss of heterozygosity
AR	Xq11.2–q12	Androgen receptor	Transcription factor	Overexpression, mutations, activation of ligand-independent AR signaling pathways, change in expression coactivators
ATBF1	16q22.3–q23.1	ATBF1	Homeodomain transcription factor	Missense mutations
BCAR1	16q22–q23	Breast cancer antiestrogen resistance 1	Implicated in cell migration	Overexpression
BCL2	18q21.3	BCL2	Antiapoptotic factor	Overexpression
BMRS1	11q13–q13.2	Breast-cancer metastasis suppressor 1 (BMRS1)	Component of the mSin3a family of histone deacetylase complexes	Loss of expression
CD44	11p13	Cluster of differentiation 44 (CD44)	Implicated in cell–cell interactions, cell adhesion and migration	Hypermethylation

(continued)

Table 5.1 (continued)

Gene	Location	Encoded protein	Function	Alteration in prostate cancer
CD9	12p13.3	Cluster of differentiation 9 (CD9)	Implicated in tissue differentiation, egg-sperm fusion, tumor-cell metastasis, cell adhesion and motility	Decreased expression
CDH1	16q22.1	E-cadherin	Implicated in calcium-dependent cell–cell adhesion	Hypermethylation
CDKN1B	12p13.1–p12	p27kip1	Cell cycle inhibitor	Loss of heterozygosity, downregulation at the protein level
COL7A1	3p21.1	Collagen VII	Major protein of connective tissue in animals	Loss of expression
CTNNB1	3p21	β-catenin	Implicated in E-cadherin-associated cell junction	Mutations
EIF3S3	8q24.11	Eukaryotic translation initiation factor 3, subunit 3 gamma	Translation initiation factor	Overexpression
EDNRB	13q22	Endothelin receptor type B	G-protein-coupled receptor	Hypermethylation
ERG and ETV1/TMPRSS2	21q22.3 – 7p21.3/21q22.3	Fusion oncoprotein ERG and ETV1/TMPRSS2	ERG and ETV1: transcription factorsTMPRSS2: serine protease	Fusion, overexpression
ER-α and ER-β	6q25.1 and 6q24	Estrogen receptors α and β	DNA-binding transcription factors	Hypermethylation
EZH2	7q35–q36	Enhancer of zeste homolog 2	Developmental regulator	Overexpression
FAS	10q24.1	Fatty acid synthetase (FAS)	Implicated in the biosynthesis of hormones and other important molecules	Overexpression

Gene	Location	Name	Function	Alteration
GSTP1	11q13	Glutathione-S-transferase π1 (GSTP1)	Protection from oxidative damage	Hypermethylation
HPN	19q11–q13.2	Hepsin	Putative trypsin-like transmembrane serine protease	Overexpression
ITGB4	17q25	β4-integrin	Interacts with the extracellular matrix, defines cellular shape, mobility, and regulates the cell cycle	Loss of expression
KAI1	11p11.2	Cluster of differentiation 82 (CD82)	Leukocyte surface glycoprotein	Loss of expression
KCNMA1	10q22.3	Large conductance calcium-activated potassium channel alpha subunit	Implicated in control of smooth muscle tone and neuronal excitability	Overexpression
KFL6	10p15	Kruppel-like zinc finger transcription factor (KFL6)	Transcription factor	Loss of heterozygosity, mutations
KIAA0196	8q24.13	Strumpellin	Unknown	Overexpression
KISS1	1q32	Kisspeptin	G-protein-coupled receptor ligand	Loss of expression
LAMA5	20q13.2–q13.3	Laminin 5	Major noncollagenous component of the basal lamina	Loss of expression
MAP2K4	17p11.2	Mitogen-activated protein kinase kinase 4	Ser/Thr protein kinase, activator of MAP kinases in response to various environmental stresses or mitogenic stimuli	Loss of expression
MAP3K7	6q16.1–q16.3	Mitogen-activated protein kinase kinase 7	Transcription and apoptosis regulator	Deletion

(continued)

Table 5.1 (continued)

Gene	Location	Encoded protein	Function	Alteration in prostate cancer
MSR1	8p22	Macrophage scavenger receptor 1 (MSR1)	Protection from oxidative stress	Truncating mutation
MYC	8q24.21	MYC	Implicated in cell cycle progression, apoptosis, and cellular transformation	Overexpression
NKX3.1	8p21	NKX3.1	Homeobox gene	Loss of heterozygosity
NM23	17q21.3	Non metastatic cells 1 protein	Nucleoside diphosphate kinase	Loss of expression
PRC17	17q12	PRC17	RAB GTPase signaling and vesicle trafficking	Overexpression
PSCA	8q24.2	Prostate stem cell antigen (PSCA)	Glycosylphosphatidylinositol-anchored cell membrane glycoprotein	Overexpression
PSGR2	11p15.4	PSGR2	G-protein-coupled receptor	Overexpression
PTEN	10q23.3	Phosphatase and tensin homolog (PTEN)	Inactivates AKT pathway, leading to apoptosis and to decreased cell proliferation	Loss of heterozygosity, hypermethylation
RAD21	8q24	RAD21	Implicated in DNA double-strand break repair and chromatid cohesion during mitosis	Overexpression
RASSF1A	3p21.3	Ras association (RalGDS/AF-6) domain family member 1	Implicated in apoptotic signaling, microtubule stabilization, and mitotic progression	Loss of heterozygosity
RB1	13q14.2	Retinoblastoma	Cell cycle regulator	Rare mutations
SERPINB5	18q21.3	Maspin	Serin peptidase inhibitor	Loss of expression
SNORD50A	6q14.3	SNORD50A	Small nucleolar RNA, C/D box 50A	Mutation

TCEB1	8q21.11	Elongin C	Subunit of a transcription factor	Overexpression
TLOC1/SEC62	3q26.2	TLOC1/SEC62	Component of the endoplasmic reticulum protein translocation machinery	Overexpression
TP53	17p13.1	Tumor protein p53	Apoptosis inducer, cell cycle arrest activator	Mutations
TRPS1	8q24.12	Trichorhinophalangeal syndrome I protein (TRPS1)	Transcription factor	Overexpression

metastatic prostate carcinomas by CGH is gain of 8q. Indeed almost 90% of the advanced tumors show the gain of 8q, whereas only 5% of primary tumors do (Visakorpi et al. 1995b; Nupponen et al. 1998; Cher et al. 1996). The region most commonly amplified is the entire long arm, but two distinct regions 8q21 and 8q23–q24 have been identified (Nupponen et al. 1999) (Fig. 5.1). The *MYC* oncogene, located at 8q24, has been associated with aggressive disease (Cher et al. 1996; Nupponen et al. 1998). Four other genes seem to be overexpressed in hormone-refractory prostate carcinomas: *TCEB1* located at 8q21, *EIF3S3*, *KIAA0196*, and *RAD21* at 8q23–q24 (Nupponen et al. 1999; Porkka et al. 2002, 2004; Porkka and Visakorpi 2004) (Table 5.1). The amplification of EIF3S3 is associated with high Gleason score and advanced clinical stage of the disease (Saramaki et al. 2001). Other proposed target genes for 8q amplification include prostate stem cell antigen (*PSCA*) (Reiter et al. 1998) and *TRPS1* (Chang et al. 2000).

The region Xq11–13 (Fig. 5.1), which encodes the androgen receptor (*AR*), is also commonly amplified in advanced disease. Indeed, 30% of hormone-refractory prostate cancers have been shown to have such an amplification (Koivisto et al. 1997; Visakorpi et al. 1995a).

5.4 Changes in Gene Expression

5.4.1 Loss of Function: Tumor and Metastasis Suppressor Genes

Loss of chromosomal regions, which are associated with a decrease in gene expression, often affects tumor or metastasis suppressor genes. A tumor suppressor gene is defined as a gene whose function when heritably downregulated or otherwise compromised, promotes cancer development or progression (DeMarzo et al. 2003). As in other malignancies, the spread of prostate cancer cells requires the invasion of the stroma, the penetration of the vasculature, the implantation at distant sites (mainly lymph nodes and bones), and the ability to survive at these sites. Changes of adhesion are crucial for tumor cell invasion and metastasis. Invasion and metastasis suppressors are defined as genes that do not affect the growth of primary tumor cells, but can inhibit the development of distant metastasis. Accordingly, decreased (or loss of) expression of metastasis suppressor genes is involved in the spreading of tumor cells to other organs.

Initial downregulation of suppressor genes is often accompanied by modifications of the second allele such as mutation, methylation of the promoter, or modification to the protein product. Although hypermethylation of a promoter is not a loss of genetic material per se, it mediates the loss of function of a gene, by silencing its expression. Since in many cases, the inactivation of both alleles, often by different mechanisms, is required for cancer progression, suppressor gene mutations are considered recessive. However, in some cases such as in haploinsufficiency (discussed later), the inactivation of only one allele is sufficient to promote the disease.

Even if the loss of chromosomal regions is a good indication of the presence of a suppressor gene, confirmation of the suppressive property of such gene requires evidence that the wild-type gene does suppress growth or metastatic potential of tumor cells (DeMarzo et al. 2003). In absence of identification of specific genes, microcell-mediated chromosome transfer has been used to provide functional evidence that suppressor genes are present in these regions. This technique allows introduction of normal human chromosomes or chromosome fragments (usually from foreskin fibroblasts) into cancer cells. The tumorigenic properties of these microcell hybrids are then assessed in vitro (anchorage independence growth in soft agar) and in vivo (subcutaneous or orthotopic cell injections in athymic nude mice). Almost all human chromosomes have been transferred in different tumors; we will mention later the results of such transfers in prostate cancer cells. Although genes implicated in prostate cancer progression located on the long arm of chromosome 18 have not yet been identified, many others located in regions of frequent allelic loss (Table 5.1 and Fig. 5.1) have been characterized and are summarized as follows.

5.4.1.1   Chromosome 3

Although chromosome 3 regions are often lost in human cancer, its introduction has no effect on the in vivo tumorigenicity of prostate cancer cells (Berube et al. 1994). However decreased expression of chromosome 3 genes has been reported.

RASSF1A

RASSF1A is located on the small arm of chromosome 3 (3p21), which commonly undergoes LOH in human cancer (Kok et al. 1997). It is involved in apoptotic signaling, microtubule stabilization, and mitotic progression. Aberrant methylation of the *RASSF1A* promoter region is one of the most frequent epigenetic inactivation events detected in human cancer and leads to silencing of the gene (Dammann et al. 2005). Thus hypermethylation has been observed in a variety of primary tumors, including prostate cancer. Inactivation of *RASSF1A* has been associated with advance tumor stage in prostate cancer. The tumor suppressor RASSF1A may act as a negative RAS effector inhibiting cell growth and inducing cell death.

5.4.1.2   Chromosome 6

SNORD50A

SNORD50A, located at 6q14, is the only mutated gene in the commonly deleted 6q14–q22 region in prostate cancer (Dong et al. 2008). *SNORD50A* is transcriptionally downregulated in tumors while its exogenous expression inhibits colony formation of prostate cancer cells. In few prostate cancer cases, the mutation is a homozygous 2-basepair deletion that abolishes the function of the protein. Although this deletion is also present as a single copy at a similar ratio in healthy individuals, its homozygosity was significantly associated with more advanced prostate cancer. Thus *SNORD50A* is a candidate tumor suppressor gene in prostate cancer.

MAP3K7

Located at 6q16, *MAP3K7* is also included in the commonly deleted region (6q14–22) and encodes a mitogen-activated protein kinase. This gene is deleted in one-third of prostate tumors (Liu et al. 2007). The deletion is associated with higher-grade prostate cancers, occurring in 61% of tumors with Gleason score higher than 8, but only in 22% of tumors with Gleason score below 7.

5.4.1.3 Chromosome 8

Microcell hybrids generated upon the transfer of portions of human chromosome 8 into a rat prostate cancer cell line showed reduced metastatic ability (Nihei et al. 1996), suggesting that one of the metastasis suppressor genes on this chromosome may play a role in the progression of prostate cancer. However, no suppression of the in vivo growth rate or tumorigenicity was observed (Ichikawa et al. 1994).

NKX3.1

NKX3.1 is a homeobox gene with prostate-specific expression. It is located in the region 8p21, which undergoes LOH as an early event in up to 85% of prostate cancers (He et al. 1997; Bhatia-Gaur et al. 1999; Voeller et al. 1997; Vocke et al. 1996). *NKX3.1* is located centrally within the minimally deleted region (Swalwell et al. 2002). Although it does not undergo somatic mutation in human prostate cancer (Voeller et al. 1997; Ornstein et al. 2001), complete loss of NKX3.1 expression has been shown to be associated with hormone-refractory disease and advanced tumor stage (Bowen et al. 2000). The lack of mutations in the remaining *NKX3.1* allele has raised the possibility of haploinsufficiency as the mechanism to abolish the tumor-suppressive activity of NKX3.1 (Porkka and Visakorpi 2004). In early stage disease, reduced NKX3.1 expression correlates with allelic loss, limited promoter methylation, or both (Asatiani et al. 2005). Mice heterozygous for *Nkx3.1* develop prostatic hyperplasia and dysplasia similar to the homozygous *Nkx3.1* deletion mice but with longer latency, suggesting the pathogenic effect of reduced NKX3.1 expression (Bhatia-Gaur et al. 1999; Magee et al. 2003; Abdulkadir et al.

2002). Thus one of the first permanent genetic lesions in an important proportion of human prostate cancer is inactivation of an *NKX3.1* allele causing reduced protein expression (Shand and Gelmann 2006). A germline missense mutation in the *NKX3.1* homeodomain that segregates with the phenotype of early prostate cancer was found to decrease the binding of mutant NKX3.1 to DNA (Zheng et al. 2006), supporting the pathogenic role of this protein.

MSR1

Oxidative damage may be enhanced through decreased macrophage activity due to inactivation of the macrophage scavenger receptor 1 gene *MSR1,* located at 8p22. The MSR1 protein is active as a cell surface trimer to bind a broad range of polyanionic ligands including oxidized low-density lipoprotein (Kodama et al. 1990; Platt and Gordon 2001). When its function is altered, the prostate is under increased oxidative stress resulting from attenuated macrophage function. A truncating mutation in *MSR1* that codes for a protein with dominant negative effects on receptor assembly has been found in African-Americans with prostate cancer (Miller et al. 2003). However some studies failed to identify an association between *MSR1* and prostate cancer risk (Seppala et al. 2003; Wang et al. 2003a).

5.4.1.4 Chromosome 10

The transfer of chromosome 10 into human prostate cancer cells decreased their tumorigenicity in athymic nude mice and reduced their capability to form colonies in soft agar (Murakami et al. 1996), indicating that a tumor suppressor gene associated with prostate cancer is located on this chromosome. Moreover this transfer also suppressed the ability of these hybrids to metastasize to the lung (Nihei et al. 1995), suggesting that this chromosome could also contain a metastasis suppressor gene for prostate cancer. Such properties could have resulted from exogenous expression of PTEN.

PTEN

The phosphatase and tensin homolog *PTEN* is a tumor suppressor gene. It is located at 10q23, which is a common target for deletion and downregulation in prostate cancers (Feilotter et al. 1998; Pesche et al. 1998; Li et al. 1997; Dong et al. 1998, 2001; Orikasa et al. 1998; Wang et al. 1998). *PTEN* codes for a lipid phosphatase that suppresses the effects of phosphatidylinositol-3-kinase by dephosphorylating phosphatidylinositol-3,4,5-tris phosphate (PIP3), a lipid anchor at the inner plasma membrane (Myers et al. 1998). PIP3 is a second messenger that is produced after activation of PIP3 kinase in response to ligation of several growth factor receptors such as IGF-I (DeMarzo et al. 2003). PIP3 activates AKT, whose signaling leads to inhibition of apoptosis and to increased cell proliferation (Vivanco and Sawyers 2002). AKT can phosphorylate p27 (encoded by the *CDKN1B* gene), resulting in cytoplasmic retention of p27 and prevents it from arresting the cell cycle in G1 (Fujita et al. 2002). As for the *NKX3.1* gene, the loss of tumor suppressor activity of *PTEN* may be due to haploinsufficiency (Kwabi-Addo et al. 2001). *PTEN* is also hypermethylated in prostate cancer (Whang et al. 1998). Loss of PTEN expression correlates with advanced stage and high grade (McMenamin et al. 1999). Indeed only a small fraction of primary prostate cancers have *PTEN* deletions and mutations, while more than half of all metastatic lesions have *PTEN* gene alterations (Cairns et al 1997b; Suzuki et al. 1998). Accordingly, exogenous expression of PTEN in PC-3 cells reduced tumor size and completely abolished their metastatic potential in nude mice (Davies et al. 2002). Deletion of *Pten* in mice results in PIN, supporting the role of *PTEN* loss in prostate transformation (Kwabi-Addo et al. 2001; Wang et al. 2003b). Besides, in the mouse, Pten can also collaborate with either Nkx3.1 or p27 in increasing the frequency and extent of high-grade PIN lesions and perhaps early cancer (Di Cristofano et al. 2001; Kim et al. 2002). Furthermore, loss of both *Nkx3.1* and *Pten* results in more aggressive prostate cancer as compared to loss of *Pten* alone (Abate-Shen et al. 2003; Kim et al. 2002).

KLF6

The Kruppel-like zinc finger transcription factor 6 *KLF6* gene is located at 10p15 and undergoes LOH and mutations in about half of primary prostate cancers (Narla et al. 2001). Transfected wild-type KLF6 was shown to reduce cell proliferation and to upregulate p21 expression in a p53-dependent manner, whereas mutated KLF6 proteins did not show this activity (Chen et al. 2003). *KLF6* point mutations and reduced protein expression were found in a small subset of high-grade prostate cancers (Chen et al. 2003), but this finding was not confirmed in another study (Muhlbauer et al. 2003). A *KLF6* germline polymorphism has been shown to affect alternate splicing preferences and to be associated with increased risk of prostate cancer (Narla et al. 2005a). *KLF6* and its splice variants have opposite effects on cell proliferation (Narla et al. 2005b). Further studies are needed to confirm that *KLF6* is a tumor suppressor for prostate cancer.

ANXA7

ANXA7, a putative tumor suppressor gene located at 10q21, encodes a member of the annexin family of calcium-dependent phospholipid-binding proteins. Loss of ANXA7 expression is significantly higher in metastatic and local recurrences of hormone-refractory prostate cancer as compared with primary tumors (Srivastava et al. 2001). About one-third of prostate tumors show LOH at this locus.

5.4.1.5 Chromosome 11

Introduction of human chromosome 11 in rat prostate cancer cells suppressed the metastatic ability without affecting the in vivo growth rate or tumorigenicity of the hybrids (Ichikawa et al. 1992). Thus this chromosome contained a metastasis suppressor gene for prostate cancer, which was identified as *KAI1*.

CD44

The gene encoding the cluster of differentiation 44 (*CD44*) is located at 11p13. CD44 is a cell-surface glycoprotein involved in cell–cell interactions, cell adhesion and migration. *CD44* is downregulated in high-grade prostate cancer and metastases and is considered as a metastasis suppressor gene in a rat model (Gao et al. 1997). Its decreased expression could result from hypermethylation of *CD44* promoter (Lou et al. 1999). CD44 is a prostate epithelial stem cells marker and is associated with poor prognosis in prostate cancer patients (Hurt et al. 2008).

KAI1

KAI1, located at 11p11, encodes the cluster of differentiation 82 (CD82) and is a member of the tetraspanin superfamily. Members of this protein family associate with each other and with other proteins to form multimolecular complexes forming a tetraspanin web (Rubinstein et al. 1996). These proteins serve as molecular facilitators on the cell surface and provide a dynamic network for molecular interactions (Boucheix and Rubinstein 2001; Maecker et al. 1997; Hemler 2001). Significant decrease in KAI1 expression was originally seen by comparing normal prostate tissues to localized and to metastatic prostate cancer (Dong et al. 1996). In primary prostate cancer, KAI1 expression was also inversely correlated with Gleason score and clinical stage (Ueda et al. 1996). Moreover, further analysis in primary prostate cancer indicated that KAI1 overexpression could restrain tumor progression, while KAI1 downregulation was associated with more aggressive tumors (Bouras and Frauman 1999). When introduced in rat prostate cancer cells, KAI1 was able to suppress their metastatic phenotype (Dong et al. 1995; Kauffman et al. 2003). Taken together, these results indicate strongly that *KAI1* could be considered a metastasis suppressor gene.

GSTP1

Oxidative damage has been suggested as a frequent mechanism to initiate prostate carcinogenesis. Oxidative damage may be linked to dietary factors or to atrophic changes that accompany the aging process (Nelson et al. 2003). Susceptibility to oxidative damage may be enhanced by methylation of genes that confer protection against oxidation. The glutathione-*S*-transferase π1 *GSTP1* gene, located at 11q13, encodes an enzyme involved in catalyzing the transfer of protons from reduced glutathione to oxidants, thereby protecting cells from carcinogenic factors. *GSTP1* is a target for promoter hypermethylation (Shand and Gelmann 2006) and is one of the most commonly altered genes in prostate cancer (DeMarzo et al. 2003; Elo and Visakorpi 2001). Somatic hypermethylation of the *GSTP1* promoter is related to decreased expression of GSTP1 protein in almost all prostate cancers (Miller et al. 1999; Lin et al. 2001; DeMarzo et al. 2003; De Marzo et al. 2003; Lee et al. 1994; Santourlidis et al. 1999; Woodson et al. 2003). Silencing of *GSTP1* by hypermethylation was found in 90–95% of prostate carcinoma, 70% of PIN, and 6% of prostatic intraepithelial atrophy (PIA), hence emerging as a marker for the transition of normal prostate epithelium to PIN (Nakayama et al. 2003; Lee et al. 1994). Moreover *GSTP1* methylation can be used to analyze urinary sediment (Cairns et al. 2001; Gonzalgo et al. 2003) or other bodily fluids (Goessl et al. 2000) for evidence of premalignant or malignant prostatic epithelium.

5.4.1.6   Chromosome 12

The transfer of a portion of chromosome 12 (12pter-12q13) suppressed tumorigenicity in athymic nude mice (Berube et al. 1994), suggesting that one or more genes on this chromosome may be tumor suppressor genes in prostate cancer.

CDKN1B

CDKN1B is located at 12p13–12, a region of LOH that is found in 50% of prostate cancer cases (Kibel et al. 1998, 1999). The *CDKN1B* gene encodes the cyclin-dependent kinase inhibitor p27, a member of the Cip/Kip family of cell cycle inhibitors (Shand and Gelmann 2006). Haploinsufficiency inactivates p27 tumor-suppressive functions (Fero et al. 1998); accordingly reintroduction of p27 has been shown to have tumor suppressor properties in model systems (Philipp-Staheli et al. 2001). The p27 protein is expressed at high level in normal prostate epithelium, but is downregulated in most high-grade PIN and prostate cancer lesions (Guo et al. 1997; De Marzo et al. 1998). Loss of p27 also correlates with poor prognosis and reduced disease-free survival (Cote et al. 1998; Yang et al. 1998; Guo et al. 1997). In prostate cancer, the mechanism responsible for the decreased of p27 expression may also involve translational or post-translational regulation (DeMarzo et al. 2003). PI3K pathway activation decreases p27 expression, this effect being blocked by PTEN, whose suppression of AKT activation increases levels of p27 (Nakamura et al. 2000). *PTEN* and *CDKN1* alterations have also been shown to cosegregate in prostate-cancer families, suggesting their interaction in prostate cancer risk (Xu et al. 2004).

CD9

The cluster of differentiation 9 (CD9), also referred to as MRP-1 (motility-related protein 1), is another member of the tetraspanin superfamily (Boucheix and Rubinstein 2001). The CD9 protein has been implicated in many cellular processes such as egg-sperm fusion (Le Naour et al. 2000; Miyado et al. 2000), cell adhesion and motility (Yanez-Mo et al. 2001). Transfection of *CD9* reduces metastasis in vivo and this has been related to the suppression of tumor cell growth and motility (Ikeyama et al. 1993). Although the mechanism responsible for CD9 protein downregulation is unknown, its decreased expression has been implicated in progression of breast (Miyake et al. 1995), nonsmall cell lung (Higashiyama et al. 1995), and colon cancers (Cajot et al. 1997). Decreased CD9 expression also correlated with poor prognosis in several human cancers, such as colon (Hashida et al. 2002), lung (Higashiyama et al. 1997), breast (Miyake et al. 1995, 1996), and ovarian carcinomas (Houle et al. 2002). We have shown that CD9 expression is greatly reduced and even lost as tumors become less differentiated and more advanced in stage. Conversely, CD9 expression is inversely correlated with prostatic carcinoma progression and metastasis (Wang et al. 2007). Moreover overexpression of CD9 induces mitotic catastrophe (a death pathway induced by irradiation) in human prostate cancer cells (Zvereff et al. 2007), further indicating that CD9 may be a tumor suppressor gene in prostate cancer.

5.4.1.7   Chromosome 13

Although microcell-mediated transfer of chromosome 13 in rat prostate cancer cells had no effect on the tumorigenic properties of the hybrids, it suppressed lung metastasis (Hosoki et al. 2002), suggesting that this chromosome contains one or more metastasis suppressor gene.

RB1

The retinoblastoma gene *RB1* located at 13q14 is the strongest tumor suppressor gene candidate for the 13q loss (Porkka and Visakorpi 2004). RB1 is a negative regulator of the cell cycle. The encoded protein also stabilizes constitutive heterochromatin to maintain the overall chromatin structure (Gonzalo et al. 2005). The active hypophosphorylated form of the protein binds and inactivates transcription factor E2F1, while phosphorylation of RB releases an activated E2F1. Defects in this gene are a cause of childhood cancer retinoblastoma (RB), bladder cancer, and osteogenic sarcoma. However mutations in the *RB1* gene are very rare in prostate cancer (Takaku et al. 2003; Elo and Visakorpi 2001).

5.4.1.8   Chromosome 16

Similar to chromosome 13, introduction of chromosome 16 in rat prostate cancer cells decreased the number of metastatic lesions to the lung (Mashimo et al. 1998), demonstrating that this chromosome also contains metastatic suppressor genes important for the progression of prostate cancer.

ATBF1

ATBF1 located at 16q22 was identified by LOH analysis. ATBF1 is a multiple homeodomain transcription factor that interacts with the MYB oncoprotein (Kaspar et al. 1999) and regulates expression of α-fetoprotein (Yasuda et al. 1994). Missense mutations likely to inactivate the protein function have been found in one-third of prostate tumors.

CDH1

The E-cadherin gene *CDH1*, located at 16q22, is a member of the transmembrane glycoprotein family and mediates calcium-dependent cell to cell adhesion. The cadherins govern epithelial morphogenesis in the embryo and maintain adult epithelial tissue differentiation and structural integrity (DeMarzo et al. 2003). Abnormal or reduced expression of E-cadherin has been correlated with advanced stage and poor clinical outcome in human prostate cancer (Umbas et al. 1994). Loss of the 16q arm is often seen in advanced prostate cancer, but no somatic mutations in *CDH1* have been found (Suzuki et al. 1996). Hypermethylation of the *CDH1* promoter was originally proposed to be responsible for the decreased expression of *CDH1* (Graff et al. 1995), but this has not been confirmed (Woodson et al. 2003).

5.4.1.9   Chromosome 17

Upon chromosome 17 introduction in human prostate cancer cells, the hybrids showed a reduced capability to form colony in soft agar and decreased tumorigenicity in athymic nude mice, (Murakami et al. 1995), likely resulting from the expression of tumor suppressor genes (such as TP53) located on this chromosome

TP53

The tumor suppressor gene *TP53* is the most commonly mutated gene in human cancers. *TP53* encodes the tumor protein p53, which is a key regulator of the cell cycle by controlling the transition from the G1 phase to the S phase (Porkka and Visakorpi 2004). When DNA is damaged, TP53 can either induce apoptosis or a cell cycle arrest to allow DNA repair. Mutated TP53 protein has a prolonged half-life leading to nuclear accumulation of the abnormal protein, which has been shown to be associated with poor prognosis (Visakorpi et al. 1992). Mutations in the *TP53* gene are rare in early localized prostate cancer, whereas in advanced prostate carcinomas they are found in about 20–40% of cases (Bookstein et al. 1993; Visakorpi et al. 1992; Navone et al. 1993). Mutated TP53 has potent anti-apoptotic activity and could be responsible for bypassing cell cycle checkpoints allowing sustained proliferation and the accumulation of additional genetic changes (DeMarzo et al. 2003).

5.4.1.10   Other Downregulated Genes

Modern molecular techniques such as microarrays and comparative genomic hybridization (CGH) have identified genes whose expression is decreased during prostate cancer progression. Table 5.1 lists many of these genes. For example, loss of laminin 5 (*LAMA5* at 20q13.2–q13.3), collagen VII (*COL7A1* at 3p21.1), and β4-integrin (*ITGB4* at 17q25) protein expression has been shown in prostate cancer (Nagle et al. 1995). The promoter of other genes such as *EDNRB* (at 13q22) encoding the endothelin B receptor (Nelson et al. 1997), *ER-α* (at 6q25.1) encoding the estrogen receptor α (Li et al. 2000; Sasaki et al. 2002), and *ER-β* (at 6q24) encoding the estrogen receptor β (Sasaki et al. 2002) is methylated in prostate cancers. Other putative metastasis suppressor genes have also been identified, such as *NM23* (at 17q21.3), *SERPINB5* (at 18q21.3), *BMRS1* (at 11q13), *KISS1* (at 1q31), and *MAP2K4* (at 17p11.2) (Jaeger et al. 2001). For many of those, functional analysis in prostate cancer cells and tissues is still needed to confirm their implication in disease progression.

5.4.2   Gain of Function: Oncogenes

Although loss of chromosomal regions is an important feature of prostate cancer cells, some amplifications of genetic material, resulting in increased expression of the encoded proteins, have also been noticed in these tumors. Moreover, overexpression of specific proteins, sometimes in absence of gain of genetic material, has been reported. Such gain of function is associated with expression of oncogenes, whose encoded proteins promote tumor progression. Since such overexpression could come from one allele only, the mutations responsible for these are considered dominant. Table 5.1 lists many of these, including the following.

5.4.2.1 Chromosome 3

CTNNB1

CTNNB1, located at 3p21, encodes β-catenin, which is an E-cadherin-associated cell junction protein. *CTNNB1* is mutated in 5% of prostate carcinomas (Voeller et al. 1998). Mutations stabilize the protein, leading to its nuclear accumulation. β-catenin is an activator of Tcf/Lef transcription but has also been suggested to function as an androgen receptor coactivator (Truica et al. 2000).

TLOC1/SEC62

Located at 3q26, *TLOC1/SEC62* encodes a protein being a component of the endoplasmic reticulum protein translocation machinery. This gene is highly amplified in prostate cancer. These additional copies of this gene are accompanied by an overexpression of both its mRNA and its protein (Jung et al. 2006). Such changes are seen in prostate tumors from patients having a lower risk and a longer time to progression following radical prostatectomy.

5.4.2.2 Chromosome 5

Microcell-mediated transfer of chromosome 5 in prostate cancer cells demonstrated the tumor-suppressive ability of this chromosome (Ewing et al. 1995). However no suppressor gene has been identified yet.

AMACR

AMACR located at 5p13 encodes α-methylacyl-CoA racemase, which is upregulated at both mRNA and protein levels in prostate cancer, and could thus be used as a marker (Jiang et al. 2001; Rubin et al. 2002; Luo et al. 2002). AMACR also labels high-grade PIN glands and occasional benign glands. AMACR has a key role in β-oxidation of dietary branched-chain fatty acids.

5.4.2.3 Chromosome 7

The introduction of human chromosome 7 in rat prostate cancer cells suppresses the metastatic ability of the resulting hybrids, whereas no suppression of tumorigenicity is observed (Nihei et al. 1999), suggesting that this chromosome contains a metastasis suppressor gene. Although extra copies of regions of both arms of this chromosome are commonly seen in hormone-refractory and metastatic tumors (Elo and Visakorpi 2001), no gene has been identified so far.

5.4.2.4   Chromosome 8

MYC

Amplification of genetic material on the long arm of chromosome 8 correlates with aggressiveness of tumors (Savinainen et al. 2004). The 8q24 region encodes the *MYC* oncogene whose specific amplification correlated with a worse prognosis in prostate cancer (Savinainen et al. 2004). *MYC* is a well-known oncogene that is activated upon amplification or translocation in many human cancers (Pelengaris et al. 2002). *MYC* mRNAs have been reported to be at abnormally high levels in prostate cancer (DeMarzo et al. 2003).

PSCA

Although its function is not clearly understood, the prostate stem cell antigen *PSCA*, located at 8q24, is a cell surface marker whose protein product is overexpressed in prostate cancer (Reiter et al. 2000; Gu et al. 2000).

Other genes are also present in the 8q amplification. The *TCEB1* gene located at 8q21, the *EIF3S3*, *KIAA0196*, as well as *RAD21* and *TRPS1* genes at 8q23–q24 are overexpressed and amplified in 20–30% of the hormone-refractory prostate carcinomas (Nupponen et al. 1999; Porkka et al. 2002; Porkka and Visakorpi 2004; Chang et al. 2000).

5.4.2.5   Chromosome 10

KCNMA1

KCNMA1, located at 10q22, encodes the large conductance calcium-activated potassium channel alpha subunit. KCNMA1 is amplified in late-stage human prostate cancers, whereas the amplification is absent in most normal tissues, precursor lesions, and clinically organ-confined prostate cancers (Bloch et al. 2007). The amplification is associated with mRNA and protein overexpression, leading to cell proliferation.

5.4.2.6   Chromosome 11

PSGR2

PSGR2, located at 11p15, encodes a G-protein-coupled receptor, which is highly overexpressed in prostate cancer (Weng et al. 2006). The expression of PSGR2 is prostate specific and it significantly increases in human high-grade PIN and prostate cancers as compared to normal and BPH tissues.

5.4.2.7 Chromosome 16

BCAR1

The breast-cancer antiestrogen resistance 1 gene (*BCAR1*) is located at 16q23. *BCAR1* increased expression is associated with disease progression. Indeed, BCAR1 is present in about 25% of localized prostate cancer, mainly in high Gleason score tumors, as well as in 60% of lymph node metastasis and 80% of hormone-refractory prostate cancer (Fromont et al. 2007).

5.4.2.8 Chromosome 17

PRC17

Located at 17q12, the prostate cancer gene 17 (*PRC17*) induces tumorigenic properties in vitro and in vivo in a mouse model (Pei et al. 2002). The gene is amplified in 15% of prostate cancers and is overexpressed in about half of metastatic prostate tumors, suggesting a potent oncogenic activity.

5.4.2.9 Chromosome 18

Introducing chromosome 18 in prostate cancer cells greatly reduced the tumorigenic phenotype, showing that chromosome 18 may encode one or more tumor suppressor genes (Gagnon et al. 2006). Moreover the transfer of chromosome 18 significantly reduced tumor burden in extraskeletal sites in mice (Padalecki et al. 2003).

BCL2

The antiapoptotic gene *BCL2* is located at 18q21. BCL2 is expressed mostly in prostate basal cells in healthy prostate tissue but is upregulated at two stages of prostate cancer progression: BCL2 is overexpressed within the luminal epithelium in high-grade PIN lesions, but is absent in most low-to-intermediate grade carcinomas. BCL2 also accumulates in many androgen-independent prostate cancers (DiPaola et al. 2001). Overexpression of BCL2 is observed in 30–60% of prostate cancer (Liu et al. 2003).

5.4.2.10 Chromosome 21

ERG and ETV1/TMPRSS2

The ETS transcription family members ETG and ETV1 were shown to be over-expressed in an important proportion of prostate cancer tissues. A bioinformatics approach has been used to discover candidate oncogenic chromosomal aberrations and has allowed to identify a translocation implicating these genes (Tomlins et al. 2005). Either *ERG* located at 21q22 or *ETV1* located at 7p21 is activated by a TMPRSS2:ERG or TMPRSS2:ETV1 chromosomal translocation that fuses the 3′ end of either gene to the 5′ end of the androgen-regulated *TMPRSS2* gene located at 21q22 to generate an androgen-responsive fusion oncoprotein (Tomlins et al. 2005). *TMPRSS2* encodes a prostate-specific cell-surface serine protease that is overexpressed in many cancers (Lin et al. 1999; Paoloni-Giacobino et al. 1997). Fusion of *ETG* or *ETV1* with *TMPRSS2* was found in most cases, indicating that the fusion is the most likely cause for such overexpression (Tomlins et al. 2005). Observed in close to 80% of tumor analyzed, this translocation event is likely to be the most common rearrangement present in prostate cancer. A mutated form of *TMPRSS2* has been found in one case of aggressive prostate cancer (Vaarala et al. 2001).

5.4.2.11 Chromosome X

AR

The development of prostate cancer has been considered for half a century to be dependent on androgens (Huggins and Hodges 2002). These hormones are needed for growth and development of the prostate, and they are the essential survival factor for prostate epithelial cells (Kokontis and Liao 1999). The androgen receptor (AR) is a member of the steroid and thyroid hormone receptor gene superfamily and is encoded by a gene located at Xq11–12. This nuclear receptor exerts its action by binding hormone in the cytoplasm, translocating to the nucleus where it dimerizes and binds to DNA to initiate the formation of a transcriptional complex at an androgen-responsive gene promoter (Shang et al. 2002). It has been known for many years that withdrawal of androgens leads to a rapid decline in prostate cancer growth. But this response is transitory and despite an initial beneficial response, prostate cancers inevitably stop responding as they progress to an androgen-independent state (Amler et al. 2000; Mousses et al. 2001). During prostate cancer progression, there seems to be several molecular mechanisms involved in order to achieve AR function in the absence of classic ligands (DeMarzo et al. 2003).

The N-terminal transcriptional-activating domain of the protein is coded by the first exon of the *AR* gene, which contains a trinucleotide CAG repeat that varies in length and codes for a polyglutamine stretch. There is an inverse relationship between the length of the CAG repeat and AR transcriptional activity (Sartor et al. 1999; Bennett et al. 2002). Shorter CAG repeat length has been associated with a greater risk of developing both primary and advanced prostate cancer (Heinlein and Chang 2004; Tayeb et al. 2004; Tsujimoto et al. 2004; Giovannucci et al. 1997; Kantoff et al. 1998; Hsing et al. 2000). Reduced CAG repeats also predisposes to prostate cancer recurrence and early disease onset

(Nam et al. 2000; Bratt et al. 1999; Hardy et al. 1996). In some androgen-independent prostate cancers, truncation or fragmentation of the repeat causes hyperactivation of the receptor (Alvarado et al. 2005; Buchanan et al. 2004; Schoenberg et al. 1994).

AR mutations are rare in untreated or castrated prostate cancer patients (Culig et al. 2001; Wallen et al. 1999). However, *AR* mutations are present in 20–25% of patients treated with antiandrogens, such as flutamide and bicalutamide (Taplin et al. 1995; Haapala et al. 2001). Some mutations may alter the ligand specificity of the AR and the receptor may be paradoxically activated by antiandrogens (Haapala et al. 2001; Hara et al. 2003). AR may be activated by missense mutations (Bentel and Tilley 1996; Buchanan et al. 2001; Culig et al. 1997; Marcelli et al. 2000; Newmark et al. 1992; Suzuki et al. 1993; Tilley et al. 1996; Wallen et al. 1999; Taplin et al. 1995, 1999, 2003) that broaden the scope of hormone specificity and/ or enhanced hormonal response (Tan et al. 1997; Veldscholte et al. 1990a; Veldscholte et al. 1990b).

The *AR* gene is amplified in 30% of hormone-refractory prostate carcinomas from patients treated with androgen withdrawal (Visakorpi et al. 1995a; Elo and Visakorpi 2001). AR expression is sustained throughout the clinical phases of androgen-independent disease (Heinlein and Chang 2004). No amplifications were found in untreated tumors (Palmberg et al. 2000). This suggests that androgen withdrawal selects the gene amplification and that tumors with *AR* gene amplification may be androgen hypersensitive instead of independent. Patients with AR gene amplification respond better to the second-line maximal androgen blockade than patients without *AR* amplification (Palmberg et al. 2000). The amplification leads to the overexpression of the gene, but surprisingly almost all hormone-refractory prostate carcinomas express high levels of AR (Linja et al. 2001). The mechanisms for the AR overexpression in tumors not containing the gene amplification remain unknown. Her-2/neu has been suggested to activate AR, especially when androgen levels are low, as this is the case with androgen withdrawal. Besides, transactivation of the *AR* gene is regulated by coregulators which could be involved in prostate tumorigenesis (Visakorpi 2003), such as p160 family members (Slagsvold et al. 2001) and β-catenin (Pawlowski et al. 2002; Mulholland et al. 2002; Yang et al. 2002).

5.4.2.12 Other Overexpressed genes

As mentioned in Table 5.1, there are other genes whose expression is increased during the progression of the disease. Fatty acid synthetase (*FAS* at 10q24.1) has been found to be overexpressed in prostate cancer (Shurbaji et al. 1992; Swinnen et al. 2002). Hepsin (*HPN*, at 19q11–q13.2) is a putative trypsin-like transmembrane serine protease overexpressed in prostate cancer (Rhodes et al. 2002; Swinnen et al. 2002). *EZH2* at 7q35–q36 is a developmental regulatory gene that is a transcriptional repressor and is found in higher concentrations in metastatic prostate cancers than in primary tumors (Varambally et al. 2002).

5.5 Conclusions

The knowledge of genetic alterations in prostate cancer has significantly increased during the last decade. Multiple genes seem to be involved in the neoplastic process. Although some alterations (such as the TMPRSS2/ERG translocations) are frequently seen in tumors, it is unlikely that the same set(s) of genes will be implicated in all prostate cancers. The identification of the genes inactivated (suppressor) or activated (oncogenes) in a given patient will likely predict the response to specific therapies. Indeed, some of these genes have become the basis of new targeted treatment strategies.

Acknowledgments Laure Humbert received studentships from the McGill Urology Division and from the Research Institute of the McGill University Health Centre. The work from Mario Chevrette's laboratory (CD9 section) was funded by the Cancer Research Society, Inc. A special thanks to David Adler, Ph.D., Department of Pathology, University of Washington, Seattle for the use of Idiogram Albums and for having the vision of creating a web site devoted to cytogenetics.

References

Abate-Shen C, Banach-Petrosky WA, Sun X, Economides KD, Desai N, Gregg JP, Borowsky AD, Cardiff RD, Shen MM (2003) Nkx3.1; Pten mutant mice develop invasive prostate adenocarcinoma and lymph node metastases. Cancer Res 63:3886–3890

Abdulkadir SA, Magee JA, Peters TJ, Kaleem Z, Naughton CK, Humphrey PA, Milbrandt J (2002) Conditional loss of Nkx3.1 in adult mice induces prostatic intraepithelial neoplasia. Mol Cell Biol 22:1495–1503

Alers JC, Rochat J, Krijtenburg PJ, Hop WC, Kranse R, Rosenberg C, Tanke HJ, Schroder FH, van Dekken H (2000) Identification of genetic markers for prostatic cancer progression. Lab Invest 80:931–942

Alvarado C, Beitel LK, Sircar K, Aprikian A, Trifiro M, Gottlieb B (2005) Somatic mosaicism and cancer: a micro-genetic examination into the role of the androgen receptor gene in prostate cancer. Cancer Res 65:8514–8518

Amler LC, Agus DB, LeDuc C, Sapinoso ML, Fox WD, Kern S, Lee D, Wang V, Leysens M, Higgins B, Martin J, Gerald W, Dracopoli N, Cordon-Cardo C, Scher HI, Hampton GM (2000) Dysregulated expression of androgen-responsive and nonresponsive genes in the androgen-independent prostate cancer xenograft model CWR22–R1. Cancer Res 60:6134–6141

Artandi SE, Chang S, Lee SL, Alson S, Gottlieb GJ, Chin L, DePinho RA (2000) Telomere dysfunction promotes non-reciprocal translocations and epithelial cancers in mice. Nature 406:641–645

Asatiani E, Huang WX, Wang A, Ortner ER, Cavalli LR, Haddad BR, Gelmann EP (2005) Deletion, methylation, and expression of the NKX3.1 suppressor gene in primary human prostate cancer. Cancer Res 65:1164–1173

Balk SP, Ko YJ, Bubley GJ (2003) Biology of prostate-specific antigen. J Clin Oncol 21:383–391

Bennett CL, Price DK, Kim S, Liu D, Jovanovic BD, Nathan D, Johnson ME, Montgomery JS, Cude K, Brockbank JC, Sartor O, Figg WD (2002) Racial variation in CAG repeat lengths within the androgen receptor gene among prostate cancer patients of lower socioeconomic status. J Clin Oncol 20:3599–3604

Bentel JM, Tilley WD (1996) Androgen receptors in prostate cancer. J Endocrinol 151:1–11

Berube NG, Speevak MD, Chevrette M (1994) Suppression of tumorigenicity of human prostate cancer cells by introduction of human chromosome del(12)(q13). Cancer Res 54: 3077–3081

Bhatia-Gaur R, Donjacour AA, Sciavolino PJ, Kim M, Desai N, Young P, Norton CR, Gridley T, Cardiff RD, Cunha GR, Abate-Shen C, Shen MM (1999) Roles for Nkx3.1 in prostate development and cancer. Genes Dev 13:966–977

Blasco MA, Lee HW, Hande MP, Samper E, Lansdorp PM, DePinho RA, Greider CW (1997) Telomere shortening and tumor formation by mouse cells lacking telomerase RNA. Cell 91:25–34

Bloch M, Ousingsawat J, Simon R, Schraml P, Gasser TC, Mihatsch MJ, Kunzelmann K, Bubendorf L (2007) KCNMA1 gene amplification promotes tumor cell proliferation in human prostate cancer. Oncogene 26:2525–2534

Bookstein R, MacGrogan D, Hilsenbeck SG, Sharkey F, Allred DC (1993) p53 is mutated in a subset of advanced-stage prostate cancers. Cancer Res 53:3369–3373

Bookstein R, Bova GS, MacGrogan D, Levy A, Isaacs WB (1997) Tumour-suppressor genes in prostatic oncogenesis: a positional approach. Br J Urol 79:28–36

Boucheix C, Rubinstein E (2001) Tetraspanins. Cell Mol Life Sci 58:1189–1205

Bouras T, Frauman AG (1999) Expression of the prostate cancer metastasis suppressor gene KAI1 in primary prostate cancers: a biphasic relationship with tumour grade. J Pathol 188: 382–388

Bova GS, Carter BS, Bussemakers MJG, Emi M, Fujiwara Y, Kyprianou N, Jacobs SC, Robinson JC, Epstein JI, Walsh PC, Isaacs WB (1993) Homozygous deletion and frequent allelic loss of chromosome-8P22 loci in human prostate-cancer. Cancer Res 53:3869–3873

Bowen C, Bubendorf L, Voeller HJ, Slack R, Willi N, Sauter G, Gasser TC, Koivisto P, Lack EE, Kononen J, Kallioniemi OP, Gelmann EP (2000) Loss of NKX3.1 expression in human prostate cancers correlates with tumor progression. Cancer Res 60:6111–6115

Bratt O, Borg A, Kristoffersson U, Lundgren R, Zhang QX, Olsson H (1999) CAG repeat length in the androgen receptor gene is related to age at diagnosis of prostate cancer and response to endocrine therapy, but not to prostate cancer risk. Br J Cancer 81:672–676

Buchanan G, Greenberg NM, Scher HI, Harris JM, Marshall VR, Tilley WD (2001) Collocation of androgen receptor gene mutations in prostate cancer. Clin Cancer Res 7:1273–1281

Buchanan G, Yang M, Cheong A, Harris JM, Irvine RA, Lambert PF, Moore NL, Raynor M, Neufing PJ, Coetzee GA, Tilley WD (2004) Structural and functional consequences of glutamine tract variation in the androgen receptor. Hum Mol Genet 13:1677–1692

Cahill DP, Kinzler KW, Vogelstein B, Lengauer C (1999) Genetic instability and darwinian selection in tumours (Reprinted from Trends Biochem Sci 12 (1999)). Trends Cell Biol 9:M57–M60

Cairns P, Okami K, Halachmi S, Halachmi N, Esteller M, Herman JG, Isaacs WB, Bova GS, Sidransky D (1997a) Frequent inactivation of PTEN/MMAC1 in primary prostate cancer. Cancer Res 57:4997–5000

Cairns P, Okami K, Halachmi S, Halachmi N, Esteller M, Herman JG, Jen J, Isaacs WB, Bova GS, Sidransky D (1997b) Frequent inactivation of PTEN/MMAC1 in primary prostate cancer. Cancer Res 57:4997–5000

Cairns P, Esteller M, Herman JG, Schoenberg M, Jeronimo C, Sanchez-Cespedes M, Chow NH, Grasso M, Wu L, Westra WB, Sidransky D (2001) Molecular detection of prostate cancer in urine by GSTP1 hypermethylation. Clin Cancer Res 7:2727–2730

Cajot JF, Sordat I, Silvestre T, Sordat B (1997) Differential display cloning identifies motility-related protein (MRP1/CD9) as highly expressed in primary compared to metastatic human colon carcinoma cells. Cancer Res 57:2593–2597

Carpten J, Nupponen N, Isaacs S, Sood R, Robbins C, Xu J, Faruque M, Moses T, Ewing C, Gillanders E, Hu P, Buinovszky P, Makalowska I, Baffoe-Bonnie A, Faith D, Smith J, Stephan D, Wiley K, Brownstein M, Gildea D, Kelly B, Jenkins R, Hostetter G, Matikainen M, Schleutker J, Klinger K, Connors T, Xiang Y, Wang Z, De Marzo A, Papadopoulos N,

Kallioniemi OP, Burk R, Meyers D, Gronberg H, Meltzer P, Silverman R, Bailey-Wilson J, Walsh P, Isaacs W, Trent J (2002) Germline mutations in the ribonuclease L gene in families showing linkage with HPC1. Nat Genet 30:181–184

Carter BS, Bova GS, Beaty TH, Steinberg GD, Childs B, Isaacs WB, Walsh PC (1993) Hereditary prostate-cancer – epidemiologic and clinical-features. J Urol 150:797–802

Chang GTG, Steenbeek M, Schippers E, Blok LJ, van Weerden WM, van Alewijk DCJG, Eussen BHJ, van Steenbrugge GJ, Brinkmann AO (2000) Characterization of a zinc-finger protein and its association with apoptosis in prostate cancer cells. J Natl Cancer Inst 92:1414–1421

Chen C, Hyytinen ER, Sun X, Helin HJ, Koivisto PA, Frierson HF Jr, Vessella RL, Dong JT (2003) Deletion, mutation, and loss of expression of KLF6 in human prostate cancer. Am J Pathol 162:1349–1354

Cher ML, Bova GS, Moore DH, Small EJ, Carroll PR, Pin SS, Epstein JI, Isaacs WB, Jensen RH (1996) Genetic alterations in untreated metastases and androgen-independent prostate cancer detected by comparative genomic hybridization and allelotyping. Cancer Res 56: 3091–3102

Cote RJ, Shi Y, Groshen S, Feng AC, Cordon-Cardo C, Skinner D, Lieskovosky G (1998) Association of p27Kip1 levels with recurrence and survival in patients with stage C prostate carcinoma. J Natl Cancer Inst 90:916–920

Counter CM, Avilion AA, Lefeuvre CE, Stewart NG, Greider CW, Harley CB, Bacchetti S (1992) Telomere shortening associated with chromosome instability is arrested in immortal cells which express telomerase activity. EMBO J 11:1921–1929

Culig Z, Hobisch A, Hittmair A, Cronauer MV, Radmayr C, Bartsch G, Klocker H (1997) Androgen receptor gene mutations in prostate cancer. Implications for disease progression and therapy. Drugs Aging 10:50–58

Culig Z, Klocker H, Bartsch G, Hobisch A (2001) Androgen receptor mutations in carcinoma of the prostate: significance for endocrine therapy. Am J Pharmacogenomics 1:241–249

Dammann R, Schagdarsurengin U, Seidel C, Strunnikova M, Rastetter M, Baier K, Pfeifer GP (2005) The tumor suppressor RASSF1A in human carcinogenesis: an update. Histol Histopathol 20:645–663

Davies MA, Kim SJ, Parikh NU, Dong Z, Bucana CD, Gallick GE (2002) Adenoviral-mediated expression of MMAC/PTEN inhibits proliferation and metastasis of human prostate cancer cells. Clin Cancer Res 8:1904–1914

De Marzo AM, Meeker AK, Epstein JI, Coffey DS (1998) Prostate stem cell compartments: expression of the cell cycle inhibitor p27Kip1 in normal, hyperplastic, and neoplastic cells. Am J Pathol 153:911–919

De Marzo AM, Meeker AK, Zha S, Luo J, Nakayama M, Platz EA, Isaacs WB, Nelson WG (2003) Human prostate cancer precursors and pathobiology. Urology 62:55–62

DeMarzo AM, Nelson WG, Isaacs WB, Epstein JI (2003) Pathological and molecular aspects of prostate cancer. Lancet 361:955–964

Di Cristofano A, De Acetis M, Koff A, Cordon-Cardo C, Pandolfi PP (2001) Pten and p27KIP1 cooperate in prostate cancer tumor suppression in the mouse. Nat Genet 27:222–224

DiPaola RS, Patel J, Rafi MM (2001) Targeting apoptosis in prostate cancer. Hematol Oncol Clin North Am 15:509–524

Donaldson L, Fordyce C, Gilliland F, Smith A, Feddersen R, Joste N, Moyzis R, Griffith J (1999) Association between outcome and telomere DNA content in prostate cancer. J Urol 162:1788–1792

Dong JT, Lamb PW, Rinker-Schaeffer CW, Vukanovic J, Ichikawa T, Isaacs JT, Barrett JC (1995) KAI1, a metastasis suppressor gene for prostate cancer on human chromosome 11p11.2. Science 268:884–886

Dong JT, Suzuki H, Pin SS, Bova GS, Schalken JA, Isaacs WB, Barrett JC, Isaacs JT (1996) Down-regulation of the KAI1 metastasis suppressor gene during the progression of human prostatic cancer infrequently involves gene mutation or allelic loss. Cancer Res 56:4387–4390

Dong JT, Sipe TW, Hyytinen ER, Li CL, Heise C, McClintock DE, Grant CD, Chung LWK, Frierson HF (1998) PTEN/MMAC1 is infrequently mutated in pT2 and pT3 carcinomas of the prostate. Oncogene 17:1979–1982

Dong JT, Li CL, Sipe TW, Frierson HF (2001) Mutations of PTEN/MMAC1 in primary prostate cancers from Chinese patients. Clin Cancer Res 7:304–308

Dong XY, Rodriguez C, Guo P, Sun X, Talbot JT, Zhou W, Petros J, Li Q, Vessella RL, Kibel AS, Stevens VL, Calle EE, Dong JT (2008) SnoRNA U50 is a candidate tumor-suppressor gene at 6q14.3 with a mutation associated with clinically significant prostate cancer. Hum Mol Genet 17:1031–1042

Eagle LR, Yin XY, Brothman AR, Williams BJ, Atkin NB, Prochownik EV (1995) Mutation of the Mxi1 gene in prostate-cancer. Nat Genet 9:249–255

Elo JP, Visakorpi T (2001) Molecular genetics of prostate cancer. Ann Med 33:130–141

Emmertbuck MR, Vocke CD, Pozzatti RO, Duray PH, Jennings SB, Florence CD, Zhuang ZP, Bostwick DG, Liotta LA, Linehan WM (1995) Allelic loss on chromosome 8P12–21 in micro-dissected prostatic intraepithelial neoplasia. Cancer Res 55:2959–2962

Ewing CM, Ru N, Morton RA, Robinson JC, Wheelock MJ, Johnson KR, Barrett JC, Isaacs WB (1995) Chromosome 5 suppresses tumorigenicity of PC3 prostate cancer cells: correlation with re-expression of alpha-catenin and restoration of E-cadherin function. Cancer Res 55:4813–4817

Feilotter HE, Nagai MA, Boag AH, Eng C, Mulligan LM (1998) Analysis of PTEN and the 10q23 region in primary prostate carcinomas. Oncogene 16:1743–1748

Fero ML, Randel E, Gurley KE, Roberts JM, Kemp CJ (1998) The murine gene p27Kip1 is haplo-insufficient for tumour suppression. Nature 396:177–180

Fromont G, Vallancien G, Validire P, Levillain P, Cussenot O (2007) BCAR1 expression in prostate cancer: association with 16q23 LOH status, tumor progression and EGFR/KAI1 staining. Prostate 67:268–273

Fujita N, Sato S, Katayama K, Tsuruo T (2002) Akt-dependent phosphorylation of p27Kip1 promotes binding to 14-3-3 and cytoplasmic localization. J Biol Chem 277:28706–28713

Gagnon A, Ripeau JS, Zvieriev V, Chevrette M (2006) Chromosome 18 suppresses tumori-genic properties of human prostate cancer cells. Genes Chromosomes Cancer 45:220–230

Gao AC, Lou W, Dong JT, Isaacs JT (1997) CD44 is a metastasis suppressor gene for prostatic cancer located on human chromosome 11p13. Cancer Res 57:846–849

Giovannucci E, Stampfer MJ, Krithivas K, Brown M, Dahl D, Brufsky A, Talcott J, Hennekens CH, Kantoff PW (1997) The CAG repeat within the androgen receptor gene and its relation-ship to prostate cancer. Proc Natl Acad Sci USA 94:3320–3323

Goessl C, Krause H, Muller M, Heicappell R, Schrader M, Sachsinger J, Miller K (2000) Fluorescent methylation-specific polymerase chain reaction for DNA-based detection of pros-tate cancer in bodily fluids. Cancer Res 60:5941–5945

Gonzalgo ML, Pavlovich CP, Lee SM, Nelson WG (2003) Prostate cancer detection by GSTP1 methylation analysis of postbiopsy urine specimens. Clin Cancer Res 9:2673–2677

Gonzalo S, Garcia-Cao M, Fraga MF, Schotta G, Peters AH, Cotter SE, Eguia R, Dean DC, Esteller M, Jenuwein T, Blasco MA (2005) Role of the RB1 family in stabilizing histone methylation at constitutive heterochromatin. Nat Cell Biol 7:420–428

Graff JR, Herman JG, Lapidus RG, Chopra H, Xu R, Jarrard DF, Isaacs WB, Pitha PM, Davidson NE, Baylin SB (1995) E-cadherin expression is silenced by DNA hypermethylation in human breast and prostate carcinomas. Cancer Res 55:5195–5199

Gronberg H, Isaacs SD, Smith JR, Carpten JD, Bova GS, Freije D, Xu JF, Meyers DA, Collins FS, Trent JM, Walsh PC, Isaacs WB (1997) Characteristics of prostate cancer in families potentially linked to the hereditary prostate cancer 1 (HPC1) locus. JAMA 278:1251–1255

Gu Z, Thomas G, Yamashiro J, Shintaku IP, Dorey F, Raitano A, Witte ON, Said JW, Loda M, Reiter RE (2000) Prostate stem cell antigen (PSCA) expression increases with high gleason score, advanced stage and bone metastasis in prostate cancer. Oncogene 19: 1288–1296

Guo Y, Sklar GN, Borkowski A, Kyprianou N (1997) Loss of the cyclin-dependent kinase inhibitor p27(Kip1) protein in human prostate cancer correlates with tumor grade. Clin Cancer Res 3:2269–2274

Haapala K, Hyytinen ER, Roiha M, Laurila M, Rantala I, Helin HJ, Koivisto PA (2001) Androgen receptor alterations in prostate cancer relapsed during a combined androgen blockade by orchiectomy and bicalutamide. Lab Invest 81:1647–1651

Hackett JA, Greider CW (2002) Balancing instability: dual roles for telomerase and telomere dysfunction in tumorigenesis. Oncogene 21:619–626

Hara T, Miyazaki J, Araki H, Yamaoka M, Kanzaki N, Kusaka M, Miyamoto M (2003) Novel mutations of androgen receptor: a possible mechanism of bicalutamide withdrawal syndrome. Cancer Res 63:149–153

Hardy DO, Scher HI, Bogenreider T, Sabbatini P, Zhang ZF, Nanus DM, Catterall JF (1996) Androgen receptor CAG repeat lengths in prostate cancer: correlation with age of onset. J Clin Endocrinol Metab 81:4400–4405

Hashida H, Takabayashi A, Tokuhara T, Taki T, Kondo K, Kohno N, Yamaoka Y, Miyake M (2002) Integrin alpha3 expression as a prognostic factor in colon cancer: association with MRP-1/CD9 and KAI1/CD82. Int J Cancer 97:518–525

He WW, Sciavolino PJ, Wing J, Augustus M, Hudson P, Meissner PS, Curtis RT, Shell BK, Bostwick DG, Tindall DJ, Gelmann EP, AbateShen C, Carter KC (1997) A novel human prostate-specific, androgen-regulated homeobox gene (NKX3.1) that maps to 8p21, a region frequently deleted in prostate cancer. Genomics 43:69–77

Heinlein CA, Chang C (2004) Androgen receptor in prostate cancer. Endocr Rev 25:276–308

Hemler ME (2001) Specific tetraspanin functions. J Cell Biol 155:1103–1107

Higashiyama M, Taki T, Ieki Y, Adachi M, Huang CL, Koh T, Kodama K, Doi O, Miyake M (1995) Reduced motility related protein-1 (MRP-1/CD9) gene expression as a factor of poor prognosis in non-small cell lung cancer. Cancer Res 55:6040–6044

Higashiyama M, Doi O, Kodama K, Yokouchi H, Adachi M, Huang CL, Taki T, Kasugai T, Ishiguro S, Nakamori S, Miyake M (1997) Immunohistochemically detected expression of motility-related protein-1 (MRP-1/CD9) in lung adenocarcinoma and its relation to prognosis. Int J Cancer 74:205–211

Hosoki S, Ota S, Ichikawa Y, Suzuki H, Ueda T, Naya Y, Akakura K, Igarashi T, Oshimura M, Nihei N, Barrett JC, Ichikawa T, Ito H (2002) Suppression of metastasis of rat prostate cancer by introduction of human chromosome 13. Asian J Androl 4:131–136

Houle CD, Ding XY, Foley JF, Afshari CA, Barrett JC, Davis BJ (2002) Loss of expression and altered localization of KAI1 and CD9 protein are associated with epithelial ovarian cancer progression. Gynecol Oncol 86:69–78

Hsing AW, Gao YT, Wu G, Wang X, Deng J, Chen YL, Sesterhenn IA, Mostofi FK, Benichou J, Chang C (2000) Polymorphic CAG and GGN repeat lengths in the androgen receptor gene and prostate cancer risk: a population-based case-control study in China. Cancer Res 60:5111–5116

Huggins C, Hodges CV (2002) Studies on prostatic cancer: I. The effect of castration, of estrogen and of androgen injection on serum phosphatases in metastatic carcinoma of the prostate. J Urol 168:9–12

Hurt EM, Kawasaki BT, Klarmann GJ, Thomas SB, Farrar WL (2008) CD44+ CD24(-) prostate cells are early cancer progenitor/stem cells that provide a model for patients with poor prognosis. Br J Cancer 98:756–765

Hyytinen ER, Frierson HF, Boyd JC, Chung LWK, Dong JT (1999) Three distinct regions of allelic loss at 13q14, 13q21–22, and 13q33 in prostate cancer. Genes Chromosomes Cancer 25:108–114

Ichikawa T, Ichikawa Y, Dong J, Hawkins AL, Griffin CA, Isaacs WB, Oshimura M, Barrett JC, Isaacs JT (1992) Localization of metastasis suppressor gene(s) for prostatic cancer to the short arm of human chromosome 11. Cancer Res 52:3486–3490

Ichikawa T, Nihei N, Suzuki H, Oshimura M, Emi M, Nakamura Y, Hayata I, Isaacs JT, Shimazaki J (1994) Suppression of metastasis of rat prostatic cancer by introducing human chromosome 8. Cancer Res 54:2299–2302

Ikeyama S, Koyama M, Yamaoko M, Sasada R, Miyake M (1993) Suppression of cell motility and metastasis by transfection with human motility-related protein (MRP-1/CD9) DNA. J Exp Med 177:1231–1237

Jaeger EB, Samant RS, Rinker-Schaeffer CW (2001) Metastasis suppression in prostate cancer. Cancer Metastasis Rev 20:279–286

Jiang Z, Woda BA, Rock KL, Xu Y, Savas L, Khan A, Pihan G, Cai F, Babcook JS, Rathanaswami P, Reed SG, Xu J, Fanger GR (2001) P504S: a new molecular marker for the detection of prostate carcinoma. Am J Surg Pathol 25:1397–1404

Johns LE, Houlston RS (2003) A systematic review and meta-analysis of familial prostate cancer risk. BJU Int 91:789–794

Jung V, Kindich R, Kamradt J, Jung M, Muller M, Schulz WA, Engers R, Unteregger G, Stockle M, Zimmermann R, Wullich B (2006) Genomic and expression analysis of the 3q25–q26 amplification unit reveals TLOC1/SEC62 as a probable target gene in prostate cancer. Mol Cancer Res 4:169–176

Kantoff P, Giovannucci E, Brown M (1998) The androgen receptor CAG repeat polymorphism and its relationship to prostate cancer. Biochim Biophys Acta 1378:C1–C5

Karran P, Bignami M (1994) DNA damage tolerance, mismatch repair and genome instability. Bioessays 16:833–839

Kaspar P, Dvorakova M, Kralova J, Pajer P, Kozmik Z, Dvorak M (1999) Myb-interacting protein, ATBF1, represses transcriptional activity of Myb oncoprotein. J Biol Chem 274:14422–14428

Kauffman EC, Robinson VL, Stadler WM, Sokoloff MH, Rinker-Schaeffer CW (2003) Metastasis suppression: the evolving role of metastasis suppressor genes for regulating cancer cell growth at the secondary site. J Urol 169:1122–1133

Kibel AS, Schutte M, Kern SE, Isaacs WB, Bova GS (1998) Identification of 12p as a region of frequent deletion in advanced prostate cancer. Cancer Res 58:5652–5655

Kibel AS, Freije D, Isaacs WB, Bova GS (1999) Deletion mapping at 12p12–13 in metastatic prostate cancer. Genes Chromosomes Cancer 25:270–276

Kim MJ, Cardiff RD, Desai N, Banach-Petrosky WA, Parsons R, Shen MM, Abate-Shen C (2002) Cooperativity of Nkx3.1 and Pten loss of function in a mouse model of prostate carcinogenesis. Proc Natl Acad Sci USA 99:2884–2889

Kodama T, Freeman M, Rohrer L, Zabrecky J, Matsudaira P, Krieger M (1990) Type I macrophage scavenger receptor contains alpha-helical and collagen-like coiled coils. Nature 343:531–535

Koivisto P, Kononen J, Palmberg C, Tammela T, Hyytinen E, Isola J, Trapman J, Cleutjens K, Noordzij A, Visakorpi T, Kallioniemi OP (1997) Androgen receptor gene amplification: a possible molecular mechanism for androgen deprivation therapy failure in prostate cancer. Cancer Res 57:314–319

Kok K, Naylor SL, Buys CH (1997) Deletions of the short arm of chromosome 3 in solid tumors and the search for suppressor genes. Adv Cancer Res 71:27–92

Kokontis JM, Liao S (1999) Molecular action of androgen in the normal and neoplastic prostate. Vitam Horm 55:219–307

Kwabi-Addo B, Giri D, Schmidt K, Podsypanina K, Parsons R, Greenberg N, Ittmann M (2001) Haploinsufficiency of the Pten tumor suppressor gene promotes prostate cancer progression. Proc Natl Acad Sci USA 98:11563–11568

Langeberg WJ, Isaacs WB, Stanford JL (2007) Genetic etiology of hereditary prostate cancer. Front Biosci 12:4101–4110

Le Naour F, Rubinstein E, Jasmin C, Prenant M, Boucheix C (2000) Severely reduced female fertility in CD9-deficient mice. Science 287:319–321

Lee WH, Morton RA, Epstein JI, Brooks JD, Campbell PA, Bova GS, Hsieh WS, Isaacs WB, Nelson WG (1994) Cytidine methylation of regulatory sequences near the pi-class glutathione

S-transferase gene accompanies human prostatic carcinogenesis. Proc Natl Acad Sci USA 91:11733–11737

Li J, Yen C, Liaw D, Podsypanina K, Bose S, Wang SI, Puc J, Miliaresis C, Rodgers L, McCombie R, Bigner SH, Giovanella BC, Ittmann M, Tycko B, Hibshoosh H, Wigler MH, Parsons R (1997) PTEN, a putative protein tyrosine phosphatase gene mutated in human brain, breast, and prostate cancer. Science 275:1943–1947

Li LC, Chui R, Nakajima K, Oh BR, Au HC, Dahiya R (2000) Frequent methylation of estrogen receptor in prostate cancer: correlation with tumor progression. Cancer Res 60:702–706

Lichtenstein P, Holm NV, Verkasalo PK, Iliadou A, Kaprio J, Koskenvuo M, Pukkala E, Skytthe A, Hemminki K (2000) Environmental and heritable factors in the causation of cancer – analyses of cohorts of twins from Sweden, Denmark, and Finland. N Engl J Med 343:78–85

Lin B, Ferguson C, White JT, Wang S, Vessella R, True LD, Hood L, Nelson PS (1999) Prostate-localized and androgen-regulated expression of the membrane-bound serine protease TMPRSS2. Cancer Res 59:4180–4184

Lin X, Tascilar M, Lee WH, Vles WJ, Lee BH, Veeraswamy R, Asgari K, Freije D, van Rees B, Gage WR, Bova GS, Isaacs WB, Brooks JD, DeWeese TL, De Marzo AM, Nelson WG (2001) GSTP1 CpG island hypermethylation is responsible for the absence of GSTP1 expression in human prostate cancer cells. Am J Pathol 159:1815–1826

Linja MJ, Savinainen KJ, Saramaki OR, Tammela TL, Vessella RL, Visakorpi T (2001) Amplification and overexpression of androgen receptor gene in hormone-refractory prostate cancer. Cancer Res 61:3550–3555

Liu W, Bulgaru A, Haigentz M, Stein CA, Perez-Soler R, Mani S (2003) The BCL2-family of protein ligands as cancer drugs: the next generation of therapeutics. Curr Med Chem Anticancer Agents 3:217–223

Liu W, Chang BL, Cramer S, Koty PP, Li T, Sun J, Turner AR, Kap-Herr C, Bobby P, Rao J, Zheng SL, Isaacs WB, Xu J (2007) Deletion of a small consensus region at 6q15, including the MAP3K7 gene, is significantly associated with high-grade prostate cancers. Clin Cancer Res 13:5028–5033

Loeb LA (1991) Mutator phenotype may be required for multistage carcinogenesis. Cancer Res 51:3075–3079

Lou W, Krill D, Dhir R, Becich MJ, Dong JT, Frierson HF Jr, Isaacs WB, Isaacs JT, Gao AC (1999) Methylation of the CD44 metastasis suppressor gene in human prostate cancer. Cancer Res 59:2329–2331

Luo J, Zha S, Gage WR, Dunn TA, Hicks JL, Bennett CJ, Ewing CM, Platz EA, Ferdinandusse S, Wanders RJ, Trent JM, Isaacs WB, De Marzo AM (2002) Alpha-methylacyl-CoA racemase: a new molecular marker for prostate cancer. Cancer Res 62:2220–2226

Maecker HT, Todd SC, Levy S (1997) The tetraspanin superfamily: molecular facilitators. FASEB J 11:428–442

Magee JA, Abdulkadir SA, Milbrandt J (2003) Haploinsufficiency at the Nkx3.1 locus: a paradigm for stochastic, dosage-sensitive gene regulation during tumor initiation. Cancer Cell 3:273–283

Marcelli M, Ittmann M, Mariani S, Sutherland R, Nigam R, Murthy L, Zhao Y, DiConcini D, Puxeddu E, Esen A, Eastham J, Weigel NL, Lamb DJ (2000) Androgen receptor mutations in prostate cancer. Cancer Res 60:944–949

Mashimo T, Watabe M, Cuthbert AP, Newbold RF, Rinker-Schaeffer CW, Helfer E, Watabe K (1998) Human chromosome 16 suppresses metastasis but not tumorigenesis in rat prostatic tumor cells. Cancer Res 58:4572–4576

McClintock B (1941) The stability of broken ends of chromosomes in zea mays. Genetics 26:234–282

McMenamin ME, Soung P, Perera S, Kaplan I, Loda M, Sellers WR (1999) Loss of PTEN expression in paraffin-embedded primary prostate cancer correlates with high Gleason score and advanced stage. Cancer Res 59:4291–4296

Meeker AK, Hicks JL, Platz EA, March GE, Bennett CJ, Delannoy MJ, De Marzo AM (2002) Telomere shortening is an early somatic DNA alteration in human prostate tumorigenesis. Cancer Res 62:6405–6409

Miller JR, Hocking AM, Brown JD, Moon RT (1999) Mechanism and function of signal transduction by the Wnt/beta-catenin and Wnt/Ca2+ pathways. Oncogene 18:7860–7872

Miller DC, Zheng SL, Dunn RL, Sarma AV, Montie JE, Lange EM, Meyers DA, Xu J, Cooney KA (2003) Germ-line mutations of the macrophage scavenger receptor 1 gene: association with prostate cancer risk in African-American men. Cancer Res 63:3486–3489

Miyado K, Yamada G, Yamada S, Hasuwa H, Nakamura Y, Ryu F, Suzuki K, Kosai K, Inoue K, Ogura A, Okabe M, Mekada E (2000) Requirement of CD9 on the egg plasma membrane for fertilization. Science 287:321–324

Miyake M, Nakano K, Ieki Y, Adachi M, Huang CL, Itoi S, Koh T, Taki T (1995) Motility related protein 1 (MRP-1/CD9) expression: inverse correlation with metastases in breast cancer. Cancer Res 55:4127–4131

Miyake M, Nakano K, Itoi SI, Koh T, Taki T (1996) Motility-related protein-1 (MRP-1/CD9) reduction as a factor of poor prognosis in breast cancer. Cancer Res 56:1244–1249

Mousses S, Wagner U, Chen Y, Kim JW, Bubendorf L, Bittner M, Pretlow T, Elkahloun AG, Trepel JB, Kallioniemi OP (2001) Failure of hormone therapy in prostate cancer involves systematic restoration of androgen responsive genes and activation of rapamycin sensitive signaling. Oncogene 20:6718–6723

Muhlbauer KR, Grone HJ, Ernst T, Grone E, Tschada R, Hergenhahn M, Hollstein M (2003) Analysis of human prostate cancers and cell lines for mutations in the TP53 and KLF6 tumour suppressor genes. Br J Cancer 89:687–690

Mulholland DJ, Cheng H, Reid K, Rennie PS, Nelson CC (2002) The androgen receptor can promote beta-catenin nuclear translocation independently of adenomatous polyposis coli. J Biol Chem 277:17933–17943

Murakami YS, Brothman AR, Leach RJ, White RL (1995) Suppression of malignant phenotype in a human prostate cancer cell line by fragments of normal chromosomal region 17q. Cancer Res 55:3389–3394

Murakami YS, Albertsen H, Brothman AR, Leach RJ, White RL (1996) Suppression of the malignant phenotype of human prostate cancer cell line PPC-1 by introduction of normal fragments of human chromosome 10. Cancer Res 56:2157–2160

Myers MP, Pass I, Batty IH, Van der Kaay J, Stolarov JP, Hemmings BA, Wigler MH, Downes CP, Tonks NK (1998) The lipid phosphatase activity of PTEN is critical for its tumor suppressor function. Proc Natl Acad Sci USA 95:13513–13518

Nagle RB, Hao J, Knox JD, Dalkin BL, Clark V, Cress AE (1995) Expression of hemidesmosomal and extracellular matrix proteins by normal and malignant human prostate tissue. Am J Pathol 146:1498–1507

Nakamura N, Ramaswamy S, Vazquez F, Signoretti S, Loda M, Sellers WR (2000) Forkhead transcription factors are critical effectors of cell death and cell cycle arrest downstream of PTEN. Mol Cell Biol 20:8969–8982

Nakayama M, Bennett CJ, Hicks JL, Epstein JI, Platz EA, Nelson WG, De Marzo AM (2003) Hypermethylation of the human glutathione S-transferase-pi gene (GSTP1) CpG island is present in a subset of proliferative inflammatory atrophy lesions but not in normal or hyperplastic epithelium of the prostate: a detailed study using laser-capture microdissection. Am J Pathol 163:923–933

Nam RK, Elhaji Y, Krahn MD, Hakimi J, Ho M, Chu W, Sweet J, Trachtenberg J, Jewett MA, Narod SA (2000) Significance of the CAG repeat polymorphism of the androgen receptor gene in prostate cancer progression. J Urol 164:567–572

Narla G, Heath KE, Reeves HL, Li D, Giono LE, Kimmelman AC, Glucksman MJ, Narla J, Eng FJ, Chan AM, Ferrari AC, Martignetti JA, Friedman SL (2001) KLF6, a candidate tumor suppressor gene mutated in prostate cancer. Science 294:2563–2566

Narla G, Difeo A, Reeves HL, Schaid DJ, Hirshfeld J, Hod E, Katz A, Isaacs WB, Hebbring S, Komiya A, McDonnell SK, Wiley KE, Jacobsen SJ, Isaacs SD, Walsh PC, Zheng SL, Chang

BL, Friedrichsen DM, Stanford JL, Ostrander EA, Chinnaiyan AM, Rubin MA, Xu J, Thibodeau SN, Friedman SL, Martignetti JA (2005a) A germline DNA polymorphism enhances alternative splicing of the KLF6 tumor suppressor gene and is associated with increased prostate cancer risk. Cancer Res 65:1213–1222

Narla G, Difeo A, Yao S, Banno A, Hod E, Reeves HL, Qiao RF, Camacho-Vanegas O, Levine A, Kirschenbaum A, Chan AM, Friedman SL, Martignetti JA (2005b) Targeted inhibition of the KLF6 splice variant, KLF6 SV1, suppresses prostate cancer cell growth and spread. Cancer Res 65:5761–5768

Navone NM, Troncoso P, Pisters LL, Goodrow TL, Palmer JL, Nichols WW, von Eschenbach AC, Conti CJ (1993) p53 protein accumulation and gene mutation in the progression of human prostate carcinoma. J Natl Cancer Inst 85:1657–1669

Nelson JB, Lee WH, Nguyen SH, Jarrard DF, Brooks JD, Magnuson SR, Opgenorth TJ, Nelson WG, Bova GS (1997) Methylation of the 5' CpG island of the endothelin B receptor gene is common in human prostate cancer. Cancer Res 57:35–37

Nelson WG, De Marzo AM, Isaacs WB (2003) Prostate cancer. N Engl J Med 349:366–381

Newmark JR, Hardy DO, Tonb DC, Carter BS, Epstein JI, Isaacs WB, Brown TR, Barrack ER (1992) Androgen receptor gene mutations in human prostate cancer. Proc Natl Acad Sci USA 89:6319–6323

Nihei N, Ichikawa T, Kawana Y, Kuramochi H, Kugo H, Oshimura M, Killary AM, Rinker-Schaeffer CW, Barrett JC, Isaacs JT (1995) Localization of metastasis suppressor gene(s) for rat prostatic cancer to the long arm of human chromosome 10. Genes Chromosomes Cancer 14:112–119

Nihei N, Ichikawa T, Kawana Y, Kuramochi H, Kugoh H, Oshimura M, Hayata I, Shimazaki J, Ito H (1996) Mapping of metastasis suppressor gene(s) for rat prostate cancer on the short arm of human chromosome 8 by irradiated microcell-mediated chromosome transfer. Genes Chromosomes Cancer 17:260–268

Nihei N, Ohta S, Kuramochi H, Kugoh H, Oshimura M, Barrett JC, Isaacs JT, Igarashi T, Ito H, Masai M, Ichikawa Y, Ichikawa T (1999) Metastasis suppressor gene(s) for rat prostate cancer on the long arm of human chromosome 7. Genes Chromosomes Cancer 24:1–8

Nupponen NN, Visakorpi T (2000) Molecular cytogenetics of prostate cancer. Microsc Res Tech 51:456–463

Nupponen NN, Kakkola L, Koivisto P, Visakorpi T (1998) Genetic alterations in hormone-refractory recurrent prostate carcinomas. Am J Pathol 153:141–148

Nupponen NN, Porkka K, Kakkola L, Tanner M, Persson K, Borg K, Isola J, Visakorpi T (1999) Amplification and overexpression of p40 subunit of eukaryotic translation initiation factor 3 in breast and prostate cancer. Am J Pathol 154:1777–1783

Orikasa K, Fukushige S, Hoshi S, Orikasa S, Kondo K, Miyoshi Y, Kubota Y, Horii A (1998) Infrequent genetic alterations of the PTEN gene in Japanese patients with sporadic prostate cancer. J Hum Genet 43:228–230

Ornstein DK, Cinquanta M, Weiler S, Duray PH, Emmert-Buck MR, Vocke CD, Linehan WM, Ferretti JA (2001) Expression studies and mutational analysis of the androgen regulated homeobox gene NKX3.1 in benign and malignant prostate epithelium. J Urol 165:1329–1334

Padalecki SS, Weldon KS, Reveles XT, Buller CL, Grubbs B, Cui Y, Yin JJ, Hall DC, Hummer BT, Weissman BE, Dallas M, Guise TA, Leach RJ, Johnson-Pais TL (2003) Chromosome 18 suppresses prostate cancer metastases. Urol Oncol 21:366–373

Palmberg C, Koivisto P, Kakkola L, Tammela TL, Kallioniemi OP, Visakorpi T (2000) Androgen receptor gene amplification at primary progression predicts response to combined androgen blockade as second line therapy for advanced prostate cancer. J Urol 164:1992–1995

Paoloni-Giacobino A, Chen H, Peitsch MC, Rossier C, Antonarakis SE (1997) Cloning of the TMPRSS2 gene, which encodes a novel serine protease with transmembrane, LDLRA, and SRCR domains and maps to 21q22.3. Genomics 44:309–320

Pawlowski JE, Ertel JR, Allen MP, Xu M, Butler C, Wilson EM, Wierman ME (2002) Liganded androgen receptor interaction with beta-catenin: nuclear co-localization and modulation of transcriptional activity in neuronal cells. J Biol Chem 277:20702–20710

Pei L, Peng Y, Yang Y, Ling XB, Van Eyndhoven WG, Nguyen KC, Rubin M, Hoey T, Powers S, Li J (2002) PRC17, a novel oncogene encoding a Rab GTPase-activating protein, is amplified in prostate cancer. Cancer Res 62:5420–5424

Pelengaris S, Khan M, Evan G (2002) c-MYC: more than just a matter of life and death. Nat Rev Cancer 2:764–776

Pesche S, Latil A, Muzeau F, Cussenot O, Fournier G, Longy M, Eng C, Lidereau R (1998) PTEN/MMAC1/TEP1 involvement in primary prostate cancers. Oncogene 16:2879–2883

Philipp-Staheli J, Payne SR, Kemp CJ (2001) p27(Kip1): regulation and function of a haploinsufficient tumor suppressor and its misregulation in cancer. Exp Cell Res 264:148–168

Phillips SMA, Barton CM, Lee SJ, Morton DG, Wallace DMA, Lemoine NR, Neoptolemos JP (1994) Loss of the Retinoblastoma Susceptibility Gene (Rb1) Is A Frequent and Early Event in Prostatic Tumorigenesis. Br J Cancer 70:1252–1257

Platt N, Gordon S (2001) Is the class A macrophage scavenger receptor (SR-A) multifunctional? – The mouse's tale. J Clin Invest 108:649–654

Porkka KP, Visakorpi T (2004) Molecular mechanisms of prostate cancer. Eur Urol 45:683–691

Porkka K, Saramaki O, Tanner M, Visakorpi T (2002) Amplification and overexpression of elongin C gene discovered in prostate cancer by cDNA microarrays. Lab Invest 82:629–637

Porkka KP, Tammela TL, Vessella RL, Visakorpi T (2004) RAD21 and KIAA0196 at 8q24 are amplified and overexpressed in prostate cancer. Genes Chromosomes Cancer 39:1–10

Reiter RE, Gu ZN, Watabe T, Thomas G, Szigeti K, Davis E, Wahl M, Nisitani S, Yamashiro J, Le Beau MM, Loda M, Witte ON (1998) Prostate stem cell antigen: a cell surface marker overexpressed in prostate cancer. Proc Natl Acad Sci USA 95:1735–1740

Reiter RE, Sato I, Thomas G, Qian J, Gu Z, Watabe T, Loda M, Jenkins RB (2000) Coamplification of prostate stem cell antigen (PSCA) and MYC in locally advanced prostate cancer. Genes Chromosomes Cancer 27:95–103

Rhodes DR, Barrette TR, Rubin MA, Ghosh D, Chinnaiyan AM (2002) Meta-analysis of microarrays: interstudy validation of gene expression profiles reveals pathway dysregulation in prostate cancer. Cancer Res 62:4427–4433

Rubin MA, De Marzo AM (2004) Molecular genetics of human prostate cancer. Modern Pathology 17:380–388

Rubin MA, Zhou M, Dhanasekaran SM, Varambally S, Barrette TR, Sanda MG, Pienta KJ, Ghosh D, Chinnaiyan AM (2002) alpha-Methylacyl coenzyme A racemase as a tissue biomarker for prostate cancer. JAMA 287:1662–1670

Rubinstein E, Le Naour F, Lagaudriere-Gesbert C, Billard M, Conjeaud H, Boucheix C (1996) CD9, CD63, CD81, and CD82 are components of a surface tetraspan network connected to HLA-DR and VLA integrins. Eur J Immunol 26:2657–2665

Santourlidis S, Florl A, Ackermann R, Wirtz HC, Schulz WA (1999) High frequency of alterations in DNA methylation in adenocarcinoma of the prostate. Prostate 39:166–174

Saramaki O, Willi N, Bratt O, Gasser TC, Koivisto P, Nupponen NN, Bubendorf L, Visakorpi T (2001) Amplification of EIF3S3 gene is associated with advanced stage in prostate cancer. Am J Pathol 159:2089–2094

Sartor O, Zheng Q, Eastham JA (1999) Androgen receptor gene CAG repeat length varies in a race-specific fashion in men without prostate cancer. Urology 53:378–380

Sasaki M, Tanaka Y, Perinchery G, Dharia A, Kotcherguina I, Fujimoto S, Dahiya R (2002) Methylation and inactivation of estrogen, progesterone, and androgen receptors in prostate cancer. J Natl Cancer Inst 94:384–390

Savinainen KJ, Linja MJ, Saramaki OR, Tammela TL, Chang GT, Brinkmann AO, Visakorpi T (2004) Expression and copy number analysis of TRPS1, EIF3S3 and MYC genes in breast and prostate cancer. Br J Cancer 90:1041–1046

Schaid DJ, McDonnell SK, Blute ML, Thibodeau SN (1998) Evidence for autosomal dominant inheritance of prostate cancer. Am J Hum Genet 62:1425–1438

Schoenberg MP, Hakimi JM, Wang S, Bova GS, Epstein JI, Fischbeck KH, Isaacs WB, Walsh PC, Barrack ER (1994) Microsatellite mutation (CAG24 gt;18) in the androgen receptor gene in human prostate cancer. Biochem Biophys Res Commun 198:74–80

Seppala EH, Ikonen T, Autio V, Rokman A, Mononen N, Matikainen MP, Tammela TL, Schleutker J (2003) Germ-line alterations in MSR1 gene and prostate cancer risk. Clin Cancer Res 9:5252–5256

Shand RL, Gelmann ER (2006) Molecular biology of prostate-cancer pathogenesis. Curr Opin Urol 16:123–131

Shang Y, Myers M, Brown M (2002) Formation of the androgen receptor transcription complex. Mol Cell 9:601–610

Shurbaji MS, Kuhajda FP, Pasternack GR, Thurmond TS (1992) Expression of oncogenic antigen 519 (OA-519) in prostate cancer is a potential prognostic indicator. Am J Clin Pathol 97:686–691

Slagsvold T, Kraus I, Fronsdal K, Saatcioglu F (2001) DNA binding-independent transcriptional activation by the androgen receptor through triggering of coactivators. J Biol Chem 276:31030–31036

Sommerfeld HJ, Meeker AK, Piatyszek MA, Bova GS, Shay JW, Coffey DS (1996) Telomerase activity: a prevalent marker of malignant human prostate tissue. Cancer Res 56:218–222

Srivastava M, Bubendorf L, Srikantan V, Fossom L, Nolan L, Glasman M, Leighton X, Fehrle W, Pittaluga S, Raffeld M, Koivisto P, Willi N, Gasser TC, Kononen J, Sauter G, Kallioniemi OP, Srivastava S, Pollard HB (2001) ANX7, a candidate tumor suppressor gene for prostate cancer. Proc Natl Acad Sci USA 98:4575–4580

Suzuki H, Sato N, Watabe Y, Masai M, Seino S, Shimazaki J (1993) Androgen receptor gene mutations in human prostate cancer. J Steroid Biochem Mol Biol 46:759–765

Suzuki H, Komiya A, Emi M, Kuramochi H, Shiraishi T, Yatani R, Shimazaki J (1996) Three distinct commonly deleted regions of chromosome arm 16q in human primary and metastatic prostate cancers. Genes Chromosomes Cancer 17:225–233

Suzuki H, Freije D, Nusskern DR, Okami K, Cairns P, Sidransky D, Isaacs WB, Bova GS (1998) Interfocal heterogeneity of PTEN/MMAC1 gene alterations in multiple metastatic prostate cancer tissues. Cancer Res 58:204–209

Swalwell JI, Vocke CD, Yang YF, Walker JR, Grouse L, Myers SH, Gillespie JW, Bostwick DG, Duray PH, Linehan WM, Emmert-Buck MR (2002) Determination of a minimal deletion Interval on chromosome band 8p21 in sporadic prostate cancer. Genes Chromosomes Cancer 33:201–205

Swinnen JV, Roskams T, Joniau S, Van Poppel H, Oyen R, Baert L, Heyns W, Verhoeven G (2002) Overexpression of fatty acid synthase is an early and common event in the development of prostate cancer. Int J Cancer 98:19–22

Takaku H, Minagawa A, Takagi M, Nashimoto M (2003) A candidate prostate cancer suscepti-bility gene encodes tRNA 3′ processing endoribonuclease. Nucleic Acids Res 31:2272–2278

Tan J, Sharief Y, Hamil KG, Gregory CW, Zang DY, Sar M, Gumerlock PH, deVere White RW, Pretlow TG, Harris SE, Wilson EM, Mohler JL, French FS (1997) Dehydroepiandrosterone activates mutant androgen receptors expressed in the androgen-dependent human prostate cancer xenograft CWR22 and LNCaP cells. Mol Endocrinol 11:450–459

Taplin ME, Bubley GJ, Shuster TD, Frantz ME, Spooner AE, Ogata GK, Keer HN, Balk SP (1995) Mutation of the androgen-receptor gene in metastatic androgen-independent prostate cancer. N Engl J Med 332:1393–1398

Taplin ME, Bubley GJ, Ko YJ, Small EJ, Upton M, Rajeshkumar B, Balk SP (1999) Selection for androgen receptor mutations in prostate cancers treated with androgen antagonist. Cancer Res 59:2511–2515

Taplin ME, Rajeshkumar B, Halabi S, Werner CP, Woda BA, Picus J, Stadler W, Hayes DF, Kantoff PW, Vogelzang NJ, Small EJ (2003) Androgen receptor mutations in androgen-independent prostate cancer: Cancer and Leukemia Group B Study 9663. J Clin Oncol 21:2673–2678

Tavtigian SV, Simard J, Teng DHF, Abtin V, Baumgard M, Beck A, Camp NJ, Carillo AR, Chen Y, Dayananth P, Desrochers M, Dumont M, Farnham JM, Frank D, Frye C, Ghaffari S, Gupte JS, Hu R, Iliev D, Janecki T, Kort EN, Laity KE, Leavitt A, Leblanc G, McArthur-Morrison J, Pederson A, Penn B, Peterson KT, Reid JE, Richards S, Schroeder M, Smith R, Snyder SC, Swedlund B, Swensen J, Thomas A, Tranchant M, Woodland AM, Labrie F, Skolnick MH, Neuhausen S, Rommens J, Cannon-Albright LA (2001) A candidate prostate cancer susceptibility gene at chromosome 17p. Nat Genet 27:172–180

Tayeb MT, Clark C, Murray GI, Sharp L, Haites NE, McLeod HL (2004) Length and somatic mosaicism of CAG and GGN repeats in the androgen receptor gene and the risk of prostate cancer in men with benign prostatic hyperplasia. Ann Saudi Med 24:21–26

Tilley WD, Buchanan G, Hickey TE, Bentel JM (1996) Mutations in the androgen receptor gene are associated with progression of human prostate cancer to androgen independence. Clin Cancer Res 2:277–285

Tomlins SA, Rhodes DR, Perner S, Dhanasekaran SM, Mehra R, Sun XW, Varambally S, Cao X, Tchinda J, Kuefer R, Lee C, Montie JE, Shah RB, Pienta KJ, Rubin MA, Chinnaiyan AM (2005) Recurrent fusion of TMPRSS2 and ETS transcription factor genes in prostate cancer. Science 310:644–648

Trapman J, Sleddens HFBM, Vanderweiden MM, Dinjens WNM, Konig JJ, Schroder FH, Faber PW, Bosman FT (1994) Loss of heterozygosity of chromosome-8 microsatellite loci implicates a candidate tumor-suppressor gene between the loci D8S87 and D8S133 in human prostate-cancer. Cancer Res 54:6061–6064

Truica CI, Byers S, Gelmann EP (2000) Beta-catenin affects androgen receptor transcriptional activity and ligand specificity. Cancer Res 60:4709–4713

Tsujimoto Y, Takakuwa T, Takayama H, Nishimura K, Okuyama A, Aozasa K, Nonomura N (2004) In situ shortening of CAG repeat length within the androgen receptor gene in prostatic cancer and its possible precursors. Prostate 58:283–290

Ueda T, Ichikawa T, Tamaru J, Mikata A, Akakura K, Akimoto S, Imai T, Yoshie O, Shiraishi T, Yatani R, Ito H, Shimazaki J (1996) Expression of the KAI1 protein in benign prostatic hyperplasia and prostate cancer. Am J Pathol 149:1435–1440

Umbas R, Isaacs WB, Bringuier PP, Schaafsma HE, Karthaus HF, Oosterhof GO, Debruyne FM, Schalken JA (1994) Decreased E-cadherin expression is associated with poor prognosis in patients with prostate cancer. Cancer Res 54:3929–3933

Vaarala MH, Porvari K, Kyllonen A, Lukkarinen O, Vihko P (2001) The TMPRSS2 gene encoding transmembrane serine protease is overexpressed in a majority of prostate cancer patients: detection of mutated TMPRSS2 form in a case of aggressive disease. Int J Cancer 94:705–710

Varambally S, Dhanasekaran SM, Zhou M, Barrette TR, Kumar-Sinha C, Sanda MG, Ghosh D, Pienta KJ, Sewalt RG, Otte AP, Rubin MA, Chinnaiyan AM (2002) The polycomb group protein EZH2 is involved in progression of prostate cancer. Nature 419:624–629

Veldscholte J, Ris-Stalpers C, Kuiper GG, Jenster G, Berrevoets C, Claassen E, van Rooij HC, Trapman J, Brinkmann AO, Mulder E (1990a) A mutation in the ligand binding domain of the androgen receptor of human LNCaP cells affects steroid binding characteristics and response to anti-androgens. Biochem Biophys Res Commun 173:534–540

Veldscholte J, Voorhorst-Ogink MM, Bolt-de Vries J, van Rooij HC, Trapman J, Mulder E (1990b) Unusual specificity of the androgen receptor in the human prostate tumor cell line LNCaP: high affinity for progestagenic and estrogenic steroids. Biochim Biophys Acta 1052:187–194

Visakorpi T (2003) The molecular genetics of prostate cancer. Urology 62:3–10

Visakorpi T, Kallioniemi OP, Heikkinen A, Koivula T, Isola J (1992) Small subgroup of aggressive, highly proliferative prostatic carcinomas defined by p53 accumulation. J Natl Cancer Inst 84:883–887

Visakorpi T, Hyytinen E, Koivisto P, Tanner M, Keinanen R, Palmberg C, Palotie A, Tammela T, Isola J, Kallioniemi OP (1995a) In vivo amplification of the androgen receptor gene and progression of human prostate-cancer. Nat Genet 9:401–406

Visakorpi T, Kallioniemi AH, Syvanen AC, Hyytinen ER, Karhu R, Tammela T, Isola JJ, Kallioniemi OP (1995b) Genetic changes in primary and recurrent prostate-cancer by comparative genomic hybridization. Cancer Res 55:342–347

Vivanco I, Sawyers CL (2002) The phosphatidylinositol 3-Kinase AKT pathway in human cancer. Nat Rev Cancer 2:489–501

Vocke CD, Pozzatti RO, Bostwick DG, Florence CD, Jennings SB, Strup SE, Duray PH, Liotta LA, Emmertbuck MR, Linehan WM (1996) Analysis of 99 microdissected prostate carcinomas reveals a high frequency of allelic loss on chromosome 8p12–21. Cancer Res 56:2411–2416

Voeller HJ, Augustus M, Madike V, Bova GS, Carter KC, Gelmann EP (1997) Coding region of NKX3.1, a prostate-specific homeobox gene on 8p21, is not mutated in human prostate cancers. Cancer Res 57:4455–4459

Voeller HJ, Truica CI, Gelmann EP (1998) Beta-catenin mutations in human prostate cancer. Cancer Res 58:2520–2523

Wallen MJ, Linja M, Kaartinen K, Schleutker J, Visakorpi T (1999) Androgen receptor gene mutations in hormone-refractory prostate cancer. J Pathol 189:559–563

Wang SI, Parsons R, Ittmann M (1998) Homozygous deletion of the PTEN tumor suppressor gene in a subset of prostate adenocarcinomas. Clin Cancer Res 4:811–815

Wang L, McDonnell SK, Cunningham JM, Hebbring S, Jacobsen SJ, Cerhan JR, Slager SL, Blute ML, Schaid DJ, Thibodeau SN (2003a) No association of germline alteration of MSR1 with prostate cancer risk. Nat Genet 35:128–129

Wang S, Gao J, Lei Q, Rozengurt N, Pritchard C, Jiao J, Thomas GV, Li G, Roy-Burman P, Nelson PS, Liu X, Wu H (2003b) Prostate-specific deletion of the murine Pten tumor suppressor gene leads to metastatic prostate cancer. Cancer Cell 4:209–221

Wang JC, Begin LR, Berube NG, Chevalier S, Aprikian AG, Gourdeau H, Chevrette M (2007) Down-regulation of CD9 expression during prostate carcinoma progression is associated with CD9 mRNA modifications. Clin Cancer Res 13:2354–2361

Weng J, Wang J, Hu X, Wang F, Ittmann M, Liu M (2006) PSGR2, a novel G-protein coupled receptor, is overexpressed in human prostate cancer. Int J Cancer 118:1471–1480

Whang YE, Wu X, Suzuki H, Reiter RE, Tran C, Vessella RL, Said JW, Isaacs WB, Sawyers CL (1998) Inactivation of the tumor suppressor PTEN/MMAC1 in advanced human prostate cancer through loss of expression. Proc Natl Acad Sci USA 95:5246–5250

Woodson K, Hayes R, Wideroff L, Villaruz L, Tangrea J (2003) Hypermethylation of GSTP1, CD44, and E-cadherin genes in prostate cancer among US Blacks and Whites. Prostate 55:199–205

Xu JF, Zheng SL, Komiya A, Mychaleckyj JC, Isaacs SD, Hu JJ, Sterling D, Lange EM, Hawkins GA, Turner A, Ewing CM, Faith DA, Johnson JR, Suzuki H, Bujnovszky P, Wiley KE, DeMarzo AM, Bova GS, Chang BL, Hall MC, McCullough DL, Partin AW, Kassabian VS, Carpten JD, Bailey-Wilson JE, Trent JM, Ohar J, Bleecker ER, Walsh PC, Isaacs WB, Meyers DA (2002) Germline mutations and sequence variants of the macrophage scavenger receptor 1 gene are associated with prostate cancer risk. Nat Genet 32:321–325

Xu J, Langefeld CD, Zheng SL, Gillanders EM, Chang BL, Isaacs SD, Williams AH, Wiley KE, Dimitrov L, Meyers DA, Walsh PC, Trent JM, Isaacs WB (2004) Interaction effect of PTEN and CDKN1B chromosomal regions on prostate cancer linkage. Hum Genet 115:255–262

Yanez-Mo M, Tejedor R, Rousselle P, Madrid F (2001) Tetraspanins in intercellular adhesion of polarized epithelial cells: spatial and functional relationship to integrins and cadherins. J Cell Sci 114:577–587

Yang RM, Naitoh J, Murphy M, Wang HJ, Phillipson J, deKernion JB, Loda M, Reiter RE (1998) Low p27 expression predicts poor disease-free survival in patients with prostate cancer. J Urol 159:941–945

Yang F, Li X, Sharma M, Sasaki CY, Longo DL, Lim B, Sun Z (2002) Linking beta-catenin to androgen-signaling pathway. J Biol Chem 277:11336–11344

Yasuda H, Mizuno A, Tamaoki T, Morinaga T (1994) ATBF1, a multiple-homeodomain zinc finger protein, selectively down-regulates AT-rich elements of the human alpha-fetoprotein gene. Mol Cell Biol 14:1395–1401

Zheng SL, Ju JH, Chang BL, Ortner E, Sun JL, Isaacs SD, Sun JS, Wiley KE, Liu WN, Zemedkun M, Walsh PC, Ferretti J, Gruschus J, Isaacs WB, Gelmann EP, Xu JF (2006) Germ-line mutation of NKX3.1 cosegregates with hereditary prostate cancer and alters the homeodomain structure and function. Cancer Res 66:69–77

Zvereff V, Wang JC, Shun K, Lacoste J, Chevrette M (2007) Colocalisation of CD9 and mortalin in CD9-induced mitotic catastrophe in human prostate cancer cells. Br J Cancer 97:941–948

Chapter 6
Molecular Genetics of Testicular Germ Cell Tumor

Katherine L. Nathanson

6.1 Introduction

The term "germ cell tumor" encompasses both male and female tumors that arise from germ cells with subtypes differentiated based on chromosomal changes and imprinting status. While five subtypes of germ cell tumors are described (Oosterhuis and Looijenga 2005) only three arise in the male testis – pediatric germ cell tumors (generally yolk sac), adolescent and adult testicular germ cell tumors, and spermatocytic seminoma. Of those, the most frequent are testicular germ cell tumors (TGCT), which are the most common cancer in men aged 20–40 (Ries et al. 2007). The incidence of TGCT in the United States has steadily risen from 3.2 in 100,000 in 1973 to 5.3 per 100,000 in 2004 (54%) (Ries et al. 2007), mainly limited to the white population. However, TGCT is still relatively rare, accounting for only 2% of male malignancies. In 2007, it is estimated that 7,920 men will be diagnosed with TGCT in the United States (Ries et al. 2007). TGCT has been described as "a model for a curable neoplasm," since most patients will be cured and become long-term survivors.

Currently, the prognosis and treatment of patients with TGCT is based upon the histology of the tumor and stage at presentation. There are two major histologic subtypes of TGCT: seminomas and nonseminomas (also known as nonseminomatous germ cell tumor); each subtype constitutes ~50% of TGCT diagnoses. Standard pathological analysis is used mainly to discriminate between seminoma and nonseminoma. However, immunohistochemical markers are a very useful adjunct to characterize the different subtypes of nonseminoma, embryonal carcinoma, teratoma, yolk sac tumor and choriocarcinoma, and seminoma. A panel of PLAP (placental-like alkaline phosphatase), Oct3/4, CD30, cytokeratin, AFP (alphafetoprotein), and HCG (human chorionic gonadotropin) can be used to identify the

K.L. Nathanson
Department of Medicine, Division of Medical Genetics, University of Pennsylvania School of Medicine, 513 BRB2/3, 421 Curie Blvd., Philadelphia, PA, 19104, USA
e-mail: knathans@mail.med.upenn.edu

W.D. Foulkes and K.A. Cooney (eds.), *Male Reproductive Cancers:*
Epidemiology, Pathology and Genetics, Cancer Genetics,
DOI 10.1007/978-1-4419-0449-2_6, © Springer Science+Business Media, LLC 2010

different types of TGCT. Seminomas are positive for PLAP and Oct3/4, embryonal carcinoma PLAP, Oct3/4, CD30 and cytokeratin, yolk sac tumor cytokeratin and AFP, and choriocarcinoma HCG.

Both seminomas and nonseminomas are postulated to arise from primordial germ cells (PGCs) and go through a precursor stage, intratubular germ cell neoplasia undifferentiated (ITGCNU) (Oosterhuis and Looijenga 2005). ITGCNU appears to develop from undifferentiated PGCs based on evidence from studies demonstrating their similarity in cellular ultrastructure, patterns of imprinting, and gene expression (van Gurp et al. 1994, Rajpert-De Meyts et al. 2003, Almstrup et al. 2004). All ITGCNU appear to develop into TGCT, i.e., there is no spontaneous regression (Hoei-Hansen et al. 2004). Several lines of evidence link delayed maturation of PGCs to increased risk of TGCT. Among patients with intersex conditions and abnormalities of chromosomal number, delayed differentiation of PGCs has been associated with development of ITNGCU (Rajpert-De Meyts et al. 1998, Cools et al. 2005). Recent data suggest that the increased risk of TGCT in Down syndrome males is due to delayed and potentially abnormal maturation of PGCs (Satge et al. 1997, Cools et al. 2006). These data implicate PGCs as the progenitor cells of TGCT and potentially conditions that delay their maturation as increasing risk of TGCT. The pathology of these tumors is discussed in detail in Chap. 4

Treatment of TGCT is based on histology (semimona vs. nonseminoma), stage, and serum markers. The vast majority of patients with seminoma present with disease localized to the testis. Seminomas are radiosensitive and have a more indolent natural history. Stage I seminoma is treated with radical orchiectomy, and either active surveillance, low-intensity chemotherapy, or radiation therapy (Neill et al. 2007, de Wit and Fizazi 2006). Stage I nonseminomas are treated with radical orchiectomy followed by active surveillance, retroperitoneal lymph node dissection, or low-intensity chemotherapy (Choueiri et al. 2007). For patients with metastatic disease, cisplatin-based chemotherapy is administered with curative intent (Feldman et al. 2008). These patients are classified into good-, intermediate-, and poor-prognosis categories based upon a number of clinical factors including the TGCT subtype (seminoma versus nonseminoma), the site of the primary (gonadal/retroperitoneal versus mediastinal), the degree of serum tumor marker elevation, and whether visceral disease is present. The International Germ Cell Cancer Collaborative Group (IGCCCG) classification of the individual patient with metastatic disease predicts prognosis and determines the choice of chemotherapy regimen and the number of chemotherapy cycles administered (International Germ Cell Cancer Collaborative Group, 1997, Schmoll et al. 2004).

While somatic genetic changes within TGCTs have been investigated extensively, only recently have studies begun to correlate these changes with prognosis or response to therapy. The lack of studies is in part due to the paucity of tumors that do not respond to treatment, so that accruing enough tumors to examine the question of prognosis is difficult. In addition, as the presence of nonseminoma within a predominantly seminomatous TGCT can impact patient treatment, the majority of the tumor can be needed for diagnostic purposes and thus not available for research studies. However, there is a strong rationale for and interest in understanding the genetic changes important in TGCTs and correlating these changes with clinical outcome. If there are genetic changes that differentiate which patients with metastatic disease likely will not be cured with standard cisplatin-based chemotherapy, more intensive and/or novel therapies could be targeted specifically for this poor prognosis population.

6.2   Single Gene Changes in TGCT

Several genetic changes have been examined in multiple TGCT studies, predominant among them, *KIT* and *TP53*. However, point mutations may be relatively infrequent in TGCT, as compared to chromosomal aberrations. Based on their survey of 518 genes of the kinase family in 13 TGCTs (7 seminomas, 6 nonseminomas), Stratton and colleagues predict that there are few somatic mutations in TGCT (Bignell et al. 2006). They identified only a single mutation in *STK10*; no additional mutations in *STK10* were identified after screening an additional 40 cases. While they did not identify any mutations in *KIT* in the initial series of TGCT, they were able to detect three mutations in their confirmation series. The lack of somatic mutations is consistent with the chemosensitivity of TGCT, which may be due to ineffective DNA damage response in conjunction with intact cell cycle checkpoints (Masters and Koberle 2003).

The most common somatic point mutations in TGCT are in *KIT*, which regulates primordial germ cell migration, proliferation, and apoptosis (Mauduit et al. 1999, Przygodzki et al. 2002, Sakuma et al. 2003, Kemmer et al. 2004). Recent genome wide association studies have implicated variation at the KIT ligand (KITLG) as the most significant risk factor for TGCT, with a per allele relative risk of 3.1 (95% CI 2.29, 4.13), reinforcing the importance of this pathway in TGCT development (Kanetsky et al. 2009, Rapley et al. 2009). A review of the data from COSMIC (http://www.sanger.ac.uk/genetics/CGP/cosmic/) reveals 9% of TGCT (49/510) with mutations, which mainly occur in seminomas (47/211, 22%) (Forbes et al. 2006). In addition, *KIT* mutations are observed in 26% (15/56) of extragonadal TGCTs, again principally in seminomas (15/41, 36%). A number of studies have examined the frequency of *KIT* mutations in TGCT, with varying results. The vast majority of activating mutations have been found in the activation loop (exon 17), predominantly at exon 816, with very few mutations observed in exon 11 (Kemmer et al. 2004). An initial report of *KIT* mutations studied activating mutations at nucleotide 816 and found a very high frequency in 61 TGCTs from 46 men with bilateral disease (93%), but a much lower frequency in 224 unilateral TGCTs (1.3%) (Looijenga et al. 2003). These data suggest that the mutation occurs before the primordial germ cell divided, and migrated to the testes, and that the presence of the mutation could be predictive of bilateral disease. The latter is important as it would indicate which patients may need more aggressive clinical follow-up. However, additional studies did not confirm as high a rate in bilateral TGCTs (28%), although it was higher than that seen in unilateral disease (2.6%) (Rapley et al. 2004). McIntyre et al. also did not identify an increased rate of *KIT* mutations in bilateral disease, but only evaluated a small number of tumors (McIntyre et al. 2005b). Two more recent studies have examined larger series of tumors. In 155 unilateral and 22 bilateral TGCTs, Biermann and colleagues found a significantly higher frequency of exon 17 *KIT* mutations in bilateral disease (14/22, 63.6%) compared to unilateral disease (10/155, 6.4%) (Biermann et al. 2007). However, in 170 unilateral and 32 bilateral TGCTs from the UK, there was no significant difference in mutation frequency with 5.1% (9/175) and 3.1% (1/32) (Coffey et al. 2008). Thus, the question of whether there is increased *KIT* mutation frequency in bilateral TGCT has not been completely resolved.

Overexpression and amplification of *KIT* also has been demonstrated. The identification of *KIT* amplification came through array-based comparative genomic hybridization (aCGH) studies identifying an amplicon at 4q12 and finding that *KIT* was the only gene amplified in a number of seminomas (Rodriguez et al. 2003, Goddard et al. 2007). Amplification of *KIT* alone was found in 17% and as part of a larger region in an additional 7% of seminomas (McIntyre et al. 2005a). However, there was not a correlation between amplification and expression levels.

c-KIT also has been hypothesized to play a role in TGCT progression and therapeutic resistance. Using IHC, one study has shown a reduction in levels in seminomas compared to IGCNUs ($p < 0.006$) (Biermann et al. 2007). Using IHC, Kollmannsberger et al. stained for the presence of KIT, the EGFR family and HER-2/neu amplification in 22 patients with chemoresistant TGCTs and compared them to 12 chemosensitive tumors, with the goal of determining whether patients' chemoresistant TGCTs might be candidates for currently available targeted therapies (Kollmannsberger et al. 2002). They did not observe any difference in IHC staining patterns between the chemoresistant and sensitive tumors, and positive staining was limited in both cases. Madani and colleagues examined KIT and EGFR in 23 chemotherapy refractory nonseminomas (15 late relapses and 8 transformed seminomas) (Madani et al. 2003). In contrast to the findings by Kollmansberger, they reported c-KIT and EGFR expression in 48% and 65% of patients, respectively. Mandani observed c-KIT expression outside the nonseminomatous elements of the tumor, which may imply that targeted therapy would be useful for transformed TGCTs based on the cellular origin of the transformed elements. However, there are two case reports of patients with dissemminated seminoma with KIT overexpression that have responded to imatinib (Pectasides et al. 2008, Pedersini et al. 2007). They did not identify any *KIT* mutations, consistent with earlier observations of mutations predominantly in seminomas.

After *KIT*, the most commonly mutated gene in TGCT is *KRAS*. Activating mutations in *KRAS* have been found in 5% (11/216) of TGCTs cataloged in the COSMIC database (Forbes et al. 2006). All the mutations are missense mutations at codon 12. Again, most of the mutations have been found in seminomas (8/107), without the same prevalence as for *KIT*, but the numbers tested have been smaller (Moul et al. 1992, Olie et al. 1995, Sommerer et al. 2005). *KRAS* is located within most consistently amplified region in TGCT on 12p, discussed in detail in Section 6.6. Overexpression and mutation of *KRAS* appear to be mutually exclusive events in TGCT (McIntyre et al. 2005b). V600E mutations in *BRAF* have been found in only a few nonseminomas (McIntyre et al. 2005b, Sommerer et al. 2005). Finally, loss of PTEN protein expression through IHC was identified in 86% and 56% of nonseminoma and seminomas; loss of heterozygosity and mutations in *PTEN* is found in 36% and 9%, respectively (Di Vizio et al. 2005). Based on the data on *KIT* and *NRAS* activation, occasional *BRAF* mutations, and *PTEN* loss, the MAP kinase signaling and PI3K pathways appear to be activated in TGCT. Activated ERK, as assessed by IHC, has been observed in TGCT, further confirming the activation of the MAPK pathway in TGCT (Sommerer et al. 2005).

Multiple studies have examined whether changes in TP53 are present in TGCT, either though IHC or through mutational screening of tumors (Kersemaekers et al. 2002). IHC of TP53 shows a high level of wild-type protein in TGCTs as compared to normal testis; however, many studies report less than 10% of nuclei within the TGCTs as staining positive (Schenkman et al. 1995, Kersemaekers et al. 2002). Mutations in *TP53* are extremely infrequent in sporadic TGCT (Heimdal et al. 1993, Peng et al. 1993, Schenkman et al. 1995, Petitjean et al. 2007). Houldsworth and colleagues suggested that *TP53* mutations may correlate with resistance to chemotherapy, based on their identification of four *TP53* mutations (17%) in 23 tumors associated with chemoresistance and a decreased apoptotic response to cisplatin in a TGCT cell line with a P53 mutation (Houldsworth et al. 1998). The association of TP53 status with therapeutic response in TGCT cell lines has been further reinforced by expression profiling studies, which have shown upregulation of TP53 targets following exposure to cisplatin (Kerley-Hamilton et al. 2005). TP53-independent pathways also have been implicated in the sensitivity of TGCT cell lines to cisplatin, and specifically upregulation of the MAPK signaling pathway, as discussed earlier, is thought to allow apoptosis (Schweyer et al. 2004).

In contrast, 18 tumors associated with chemoresistance were evaluated with TP53 staining by IHC; none of the tumor had decreases in protein or mutations in *TP53* (Kersemaekers et al. 2002). TP53 was studied, among a large group of proteins using IHC in unselected patients, in metastatic patients who had achieved remission and chemoresistant TGCTs; while the presence of wild-type TP53 did correlate with apoptotic index (r(s) = 0.66, $p < 0.001$), it was not different between groups (Mayer et al. 2003b). Using IHC of TP53 and Ki67, apoptosis (assayed by TUNEL), HCG and AFP, Mazumdar et al. used cluster analysis to differentiate prognostic subgroups within nonseminomas (Mazumdar et al. 2003). They identified a cluster that was associated with a better prognosis at 5 years of 94% (95% CI 86–100%), which included good-, intermediate-, and poor-risk patients. Cluster affiliation was an independent predictor of outcome ($p = 0.04$), but not as powerful as IGCCCG risk status ($p = 0.005$). In general, the clustered TGCTs had lower TP53 expression, apoptotic indexes, HCG levels, and higher Ki67 expression and AFP levels. While this study did not examine *TP53* mutation status as a marker of prognosis, the necessity of including multiple markers in the cluster analysis to predict outcome suggests that even if each plays a role, it is not the definitive one.

Based on the relative infrequency of *TP53* mutations in TGCT, other methods of silencing the TP53 pathway have been sought. A screen for miRNAs that act as oncogenes revealed two microRNAs (miRNAs) that act within the TP53 pathway, miR-372 and miR-373, permitting cellular proliferation in the presence of intact TP53 (Voorhoeve et al. 2006). These miRNAs were identified using a miRNA library to transduce fibroblasts immortalized with hTERT, which were subsequently transduced with a RAS^{V12} vector. miRNAs that allowed growth, which of necessity meant lack of functional P53, were identified; these miRNAs permitted cellular transformation resembling TP53 knockdown. In response to ionizing radiation, the cells containing the miRNAs underwent cell cycle arrest, as opposed to cells with suppressed TP53 expression. The expression of the miRNAs prevents CDK inhibition. Thus, the phenotype associated with miRNAs recapitulates loss of wild-type TP53, but maintains an intact response to DNA damage. As TGCTs contain intact TP53 and are sensitive to DNA-damaging agents, they hypothesized that the miRNAs would be overexpressed, in TGCT which was found in several types, including ITGNU, seminoma, and embryonal carcinoma (Looijenga et al. 2007). Additional miRNAs also have been identified in germ cell tumors which appear to differentially express them based on their level of differentiation which further substantiated the initial report (Gillis et al. 2007). The miRNAs are thought to interact with LATS2 (Large Tumor Suppressor homolog 2), a serine-theorine kinase, which interacts with Aurora A in spindle formation at the onset of mitosis and interacts with a negative regulator of TP53 (Yabuta et al. 2007). Thus miR-372 and miR-373 are thought to substitute for loss of TP53 in TGCT.

6.3   Microsatellite Instability in TGCT

Microsatellite instability in tumors is caused by deficiency of any of the mismatch repair (MMR) enzymes, including hMSH2, hMLH1, hMSH6, hPMS2. Normal MMR is directed at excising nucleotides that are incorrectly paired with the nucleotide on the opposite DNA strand. Mismatched base pairing most frequently happens after DNA replication. A reduction in MMR efficiency leads to genetic instability, in particular the expansion or contraction of short repetitive stretches of DNA sequence such as dinucleotide repeat sequences (microsatellites). Microsatellite instability (MSI) has been observed in sporadic human tumors due to somatic loss of function of MMR genes; these tumors remain diploid but have deleterious mutations, particularly changes in the length of repeated nucleotides (Liu et al. 1995). Germline mutations in the MMR genes are associated with the Hereditary Nonpolyposis Colorectal Cancer syndrome (HNPCC) (Peltomaki et al. 1993a, Nystrom-Lahti et al. 1994); TGCT is not a component tumor of HNPCC.

Microsatellite instability (MSI) has been observed in a subset of TGCTs ranging from 0 to 29% in several small studies of TGCTs (Lothe et al. 1993, Peltomaki et al. 1993b, Murty et al. 1994, Huddart et al. 1995, Faulkner and Friedlander 2000, Devouassoux-Shisheboran et al. 2001). In the studies finding evidence of MSI, it was not a widespread phenomenon but limited to only a one or a few microsatellites (Murty et al. 1994, Huddart et al. 1995, Faulkner and Friedlander 2000, Devouassoux-Shisheboran et al. 2001). These studies all concluded that MSI does not play a significant role in TGCT pathogenesis. Several studies have reported higher rates of instability in tri- and tetranucleotide than dinucleotide repeat sequences (Huddart et al. 1995, Faulkner and Friedlander 2000).

Microsatellite instability has been postulated to be a marker of chemoresistant disease. Mayer et al. examined MSI in 111 TGCTs, eleven of which they character-ized as chemoresistant, using eight mono- or dinucleotide markers (Mayer et al. 2002). Only six of the 100 control or chemosensitive TGCTs exhibited a locus of MSI, consistent with previous studies. However, in the 11 chemoresistant tumors, MSI was seen in five cases, four of which had two or more loci of MSI. The chemoresistant tumors that were MSI positive had a longer median progression-free survival ($p=0.05$); however, the numbers were small. As in previous papers, the authors found consistent positive immunohistochemical staining for the MMR proteins MLH1, MSH2, and MSH6, even in tumors that exhibited loci of MSI. Velasco et al. examined 118 TGCTs, 36 of whom had relapsed, for MSI using 10 markers, and found MSI in 30 TGCTs (25%) at 3 or more markers, and a correla-tion with low MSH2 or MLH1 staining (Velasco et al. 2004). Both the high rate of MSI and correlation with immunohistochemistry differed from previous reports. As the markers used were similar to previous studies, changes in those under study would not represent an explanation for the difference in findings (Devouassoux-Shisheboran et al. 2001, Mayer et al. 2002). An alternative explanation for the dif-ference in rates of MSI is the higher rate of chemorefractory patients. MSI and low MSH2 staining were associated with an increased risk of recurrence when com-pared to TGCTs with loss of heterozygosity (LOH) only, at the markers under study for MSI, and high MSH2 staining, independently ($p=0.017$, $p=0.0003$, respec-tively) and together ($p=0.0027$). A smaller study did not find a correlation between MSI and chemoresistance, but may have been underpowered (Olasz et al. 2005). The association of MSI and chemoresistance needs further study with larger sample sets before it can be used in the clinical setting to distinguish between the TGCTs likely to recur and those that will not.

6.4 Epigenetics of TGCT

Epigenetic studies of TGCT, both genome wide and single gene, have demonstrated differences in methylation status among the different TGCT histologies. Seminomas are essentially without methylation, while nonseminomas have levels of methyla-tion comparable to other tumor types (Lind et al. 2007). Furthermore, the level of methylation appears to correlate with the differentiation of the tumor, in that within nonseminomatous germ cell tumors, teratomas have the highest level of methyla-tion and embryonal carcinomas the lowest. As discussed earlier, the TGCTs are thought to develop from primordial germ cells, in which parental imprinting is erased (Hoei-Hansen et al. 2006). The epigenetic profile in TGCT thus can be seen as a parallel to the course of remethylation in development which increases with differentiation.

The initial observation of differences in genome wide methylation status in seminomas and nonseminomas came from a study by Lothe and colleagues, which used restriction landmark genomic screening (Smiraglia et al. 2002). Studies of individual genes by their group and others also support the difference in methylation status between seminomas and nonseminomas (Lind et al. 2006). Various genes have been studied, including *MGMT* and *RASSF1A*, both of which have been found to be hypermethylated in nonseminomas, but not in seminomas (Honorio et al. 2003, Smith-Sorensen et al. 2002, Koul et al. 2004, Lind et al. 2006). Expression profiling of TGCT found that DNMT3B (DNA (cytosine -5-)-methyltransferase 3 beta) and DNMT3L (DNA (cytosine -5-)-methyltransferase 3 like) are overexpressed in nonseminomas as compared to seminomas, consistent with the increased methylation in nonseminomas (Almstrup et al. 2005).

6.5   Expression Profiling Studies in TGCT

Expression profiling of TGCT has focused on two major questions: 1) identifying genes expressed in ITGCNU as initiators of TGCT and 2) subsetting the different types of TGCT for which specific genes can be identified. Several small studies of ITGNU have been done and recently two independent expression profiling datasets examining ITGNU ($n=6$) were combined to identify overexpressed genes. The genes most highly expressed were Oct4 (*POUF5*), *NANOG* and *PDPN*, all of which were over 15-fold increased as compared to normal testes (Hoei-Hansen et al. 2005, Almstrup et al. 2007). The list of genes was put through the EASE software, and enriched gene sets were related to translation and ribosome-related genes. Using the Ingenuity Pathway Analysis software two networks were identified, one focusing on MYC, previously reported to be overexpressed in ITGNU (Shuin et al. 1994) and a second focusing around embryonic development. In general, genes that are found to be overexpressed in ITGCNU are associated with a stem cell phenotype, consistent with the hypothesis that TGCTs develop from PGCs, whereas those with decreased expression are associated with spermatogenesis (Almstrup et al. 2004, Almstrup et al. 2005, Skotheim et al. 2005).

Many of the more recent studies have combined aCGH and expression profiling to identify genes that are concurrently amplified and overexpressed or conversely deleted with lower expression in the different subtypes of TGCT. However, previous studies focused solely on expression profiling as a mechanism to subset and evaluate TGCTs. One of the most striking early findings, reiterated throughout, is the overexpression of genes expressed in embryonic stem cells and associated with stem cell development (Almstrup et al. 2004, Port et al. 2005, Juric et al. 2005). Some of these genes appear to be overexpressed in both seminomas and embryonal carcinomas, such as *POUF5F1* and *NANOG*, while others are only expressed in embryonal carcinomas including *SOX2* and *FGF4*. Many of the genes expressed in ITCNU, and in TGCT, are expressed in embryonic stem cells; however, VASA, a marker of germ cell identity, is only observed in TGCT (Zeeman et al. 2002). *VASA* is a DEAD box protein conserved from *Drosophila* to man. VASA expression is specific to the germ cell linage and mutation has shown it to be essential for germ cell proliferation (Zeeman et al. 2002, Noce et al. 2001, Castrillon et al. 2000).

While many of the expression profiling studies have highlighted the importance of the stem cell genes in TGCT, other interesting findings have emerged as well. In teratomas, the pathway that is more overexpressed centers around *CDKN1A* (p21), *CCND1*, and *CDK6* (Juric et al. 2005). Expression of these genes may overcome p21-mediated cell cycle arrest, which has been postulated as a mechanism of the chemotherapeutic resistance observed in teratomas (Mayer et al. 2003a). Additional expression changes that differentiate seminoma and nonseminomas include upregulated genes, *SLC43A1* and *IGF2*, and downregulated genes, *GRB7* and *PFKP* (Skotheim et al. 2002, Hofer et al. 2005). Many of the genes identified through expression profiling are used in practice to identify TGCT using immunohistochemistry, in particular *PUOF5F1* (Oct4), but those genes found to differentiate seminoma and nonseminoma have not yet been translated into clinical practice.

6.6   Chromosomal Changes in TGCT (Cytogenetics and Comparative Genomic Hybridization)

TGCT are usually triploid to hypotetraploid (Rodriguez et al. 1992). By far the most common genetic change observed in TGCT is amplification of 12p, which occurs in 100% of TGCT, regardless of histology (Rodriguez et al. 2003, von Eyben, 2004). Usually isochromosome 12p [i(12p)] is observed; tandem duplication of 12p can be seen as well. Less frequently (~10%), amplification of smaller regions of 12p have been identified, usually of 12p11.2-p12.1 (Rodriguez et al. 2003, Zafarana et al. 2003). Based on the frequency of 12p amplification, it has been proposed as a cancer-initiating event (Murty and Chaganti 1998). However, studies targeting 12p in ITGCNU have not identified the specific genetic change, suggesting it may be involved in progression rather than initiation (Rosenberg et al. 2000). The region on 12p contains multiple genes postulated to be involved in TGCT, such as Cyclin D2 (*CCND2*), and *STELLAR*, and *NANOG*, which play important roles in stem cell maintenance (Houldsworth et al. 2006). *CCND2* is a member of the group of cyclin genes, which regulate the cell cycle and are overexpressed in all tumor types, except choriocarcinoma (Skotheim et al. 2006, Sicinski et al. 1996). *CCND2* normally is expressed when undifferentiated spermatogonia start to differentiate; homozygous loss of *CCND2* causes both male and female infertility (Beumer et al. 2000). Amplifications of Cyclins D1 and D2, particularly D1, are commonly observed in multiple cancer types, and are thought to serve as oncogenes, driving the cell cycle. *NANOG* and *STELLAR* are pluripotency genes expressed in both primordial germ cells and TGCT similar to *Oct4* (*POU5F1*), which also is overexpressed in TGCT (Hoei-Hansen et al. 2005, Palumbo et al. 2002, Ezeh et al. 2005). All of these genes are likely to play important roles in TGCT tumorigenesis.

The amplified region on 12p has been characterized using expression profiling, in addition to cytogenetic methods (Korkola et al. 2006). Within the region of highest amplification, there is a cluster at 12p13.1 with 86 transcripts found to be overexpressed in at least one subtype of TGCT. The profile of gene overexpression within the cluster appears to vary among TGCT subtypes, with only *SLC2A3* (*GLUT3*), a glucose transporter, and *REA* increased in all (Korkola et al. 2006). *NANOG, DPPA2*, and *GDF3* are overexpressed; they also are coregulated in human embryonic stem cells (Clark et al. 2004, Skotheim et al. 2006). Based on these data, there appears to be no single driver gene for the 12p amplification; however, the region is important for TGCT likely due to both overexpression of *CCND2* and activation of the multiple stem cell genes in the region, each of which leads to increased cell proliferation and tumor maintenance.

Other chromosomal changes have been observed in TGCT, albeit at lower frequency that amplification of 12p. Increases in copy number at 7p21-pter, 7q21-q33, 8q12-23 (seminoma), 12p11-pter, 17q11-q21 (nonseminoma), 21q21-qter, 22q11-qter (seminoma), and Xq have been seen, as well as losses at 4q21-qter, 5q14-qter, 11p11-p15, 11q14-q24, 13q14-q31, and 18q12-qter were observed using cytogenetic techniques (von Eyben 2004). Genomic changes, such as amplification of chromosomes 1, 5, 7, 8, 12q and loss of chromosome 18, have been reported in ITGCNU (Rosenberg et al. 2000). Using conventional comparative genomic hybridization (CGH), amplification of 15p and 22q was associated with seminoma, while amplification of proximal 17q and deletion of 10q were associated with nonseminomas (Kraggerud et al. 2002). Gains of 17q are seen in 70% of TGCTs, with a proximal region of 17q amplified in nonseminomas and a distal region of 17q amplified in seminomas. Using expression profiling looking for overexpressed genes, driver candidates were postulated: *GRB7* and *JUP* in the proximal region and *LLGL2* and *PDE6G* in the distal region (Skotheim et al. 2002). Array-based CGH in 17 TGCTs showed amplifications of 7p15.2 and 21q22.2 and deletions of 4p16.3 and 22q13.3 as additional frequent genomic changes (Skotheim et al. 2006). Using BAC-based arrays (spaced at 1 Mb across the genome) in 74 TGCTS, 13 seminomas and 61 nonseminomas, additional regions of interest (beyond conventional CGH) were identified and previously identified regions were refined (Korkola et al. 2008). The analysis revealed multiple regions that were frequently amplified or deleted across all types of TGCT. Small novel genomic changes were described using this technique, including regions of deletion on 9q, 10q, and 13q. In addition, with this large group of tumors, subtype specific genomic changes could be identified. Seminomas were associated with amplifications of 8q23.3-12 and deletions of 5p33-35.3, 11q23.1-25, and 13q12.11-34; embryonal carcinomas with amplification of 17p11.2-q21.32 and deletion of 2p25.3; and yolk sac tumors with amplification of 1q31.3-42.3, 3p, 14q11.2-32.33 and 20q and deletion of 8q11.1-23.1 (Korkola et al. 2008). All of the TGCTs had expression profiling, so differential expression between tumor types was evaluated for the significantly changed regions using aCGH. Outside of 12p, the most frequent amplification, 7p21.1-31.1, which was observed in 58% of TGCTs, contained four overexpressed genes (*UPP1, ANLN*, two unknown genes). In the 14 deleted regions with loss in more than 40% of TGSTs, only four genes showed downregulation as compared to those without loss in those regions. Within the regions with differential frequencies of amplification and deletion between seminoma and nonseminoma, several genes could be identified. These genes included *SPRY2* (within a region of deletion of chromosome 12) and *SOX17* (amplification of chromosome 8) in seminomas (Korkola et al. 2006). Additionally *EOMES* and *BMP2*, already associated with yolk sac tumors, were observed as overexpressed in this study. However, the target genes in many of these regions of amplification and deletion association with specific subtypes of TGCT remain unidentified.

In one study of 17 tumors from relapse-free patients and 17 chemotherapy-resistant tumors using standard comparative genomic hybridization, high-level amplifications were not detected (outside of 12p) in the chemosensitive tumors, but were detected in the chemoresistant tumors (Rao et al. 1998). Further studies of chromosomal changes in relationship to prognosis and sensitivity to chemotherapeutic agents are needed.

6.7 Other Biomarkers Studied in Association with Prognosis

Several other cancer biomarkers have been studied in conjunction with tumor stage and prognosis. Mandoky and colleagues have examined HER-2/neu and lung resistance-related protein (LRP) expression in TGCTs (Mandoky et al. 2003, Mandoky et al. 2004b, Mandoky et al. 2004a). They assessed HER-2/neu expression in 59 nonseminomas with teratomatous elements, and detected expression in 14 (24%) of specimens, associated with teratoma and choriocarcinoma. HER-2/Neu expression correlated with clinical stage ($p = 0.0004$) and outcome ($p = 0.008$). These findings are consistent with those by Madani et al. who found EGFR positivity in a significant percentage of chemotherapy refractory TGCTs. Mandoky et al. also examined LRP expression in 70 TGCTs using IHC, and found positive staining in 29 (41%) tumors. LRP is a major vault protein that may mediate multidrug resistance by the compartmentalization of drugs away from the intracellular drug targets (Scheffer et al. 1995, Kitazono et al. 1999). The authors substantiated the IHC findings using RT-PCR and Western blotting to examine mRNA and protein levels, respectively. The authors did not identify any relationship between LRP positivity and stage. However, more patients with LRP-negative tumors achieved complete response, ($p = 0.015$) and those with expression of LRP had a shorter overall survival ($p = 0.043$). Neither of these studies has been replicated in other sample sets. A recent study by Hatekeyama et al. identified trophinin expression by IHC in 158 TGCTs (Hatakeyama et al. 2004). Trophinin is a membrane protein that facilitates the invasion of the endometrium by trophoblasts during implantation. The frequency of trophinin staining increased with increasing stage ($p < 0.001$) and was positive in all patients with lung metastasis across tumor types and stages. Trophinin staining correlated with β-hCG levels ($p = 0.004$), suggesting that β-hCG may act to increase trophinin levels. It should be noted that somatic mutations were not directly assessed in any these studies.

Beyond understanding what genetic changes may be linked to TGCT stage and prognosis, there is considerable interest in defining the genetic changes that lead to sensitivity or conversely resistance to cisplatin-based therapy (Masters and Koberle 2003). Understanding what makes TGCTs sensitive to cisplatin may allow us to sensitize other tumors types to cisplatin and improve their cure rates. Thus, it is very important that further genetic changes predictive of prognosis and response to chemotherapy are elucidated in TGCTs.

6.8   Conclusions

TGCTS are thought to develop from the PGC. While the tumor-initiating cell has been well defined, the genetic changes that accompany the progression from germ cell to cancer are not well understood. Amplification of 12p is a consistent feature of TGCTs; the region contains both Cyclin D2 (CCND2) and multiple genes associated with stem cell maintenance, all of which may be important in TGCTs. As in many other cancers, activation of the KIT and MAPK signaling pathways appears to play significant roles in tumorigenesis. *KIT* mutation and amplification is well described, as well as *KRAS* mutations, which activate these pathways. KIT signaling also is known to play a crucial role in the proliferation, differentiation, and migration of germ cells, emphasizing the link between normal and cancer development. The importance of the KIT and MAPK signaling pathways has been reinforced with the identification of variants within them as associated with TGCT susceptibility. Nonetheless, much research remains to be done so that the signaling pathways important in TGCT can be elucidated.

References

Almstrup K, Hoei-Hansen CE, Wirkner U, Blake J, Schwager C, Ansorge W, Nielsen JE, Skakkebaek NE, Rajpert-De Meyts E, Leffers H (2004) Embryonic stem cell-like features of testicular carcinoma in situ revealed by genome-wide gene expression profiling. Cancer Res 64:4736–4743

Almstrup K, Hoei-Hansen CE, Nielsen JE, Wirkner U, Ansorge W, Skakkebaek NE, Rajpert-De Meyts E, Leffers H (2005) Genome-wide gene expression profiling of testicular carcinoma in situ progression into overt tumours. Br J Cancer 92:1934–1941

Almstrup K, Leffers H, Lothe RA, Skakkebaek NE, Sonne SB, Nielsen JE, Rajpert-De Meyts E, Skotheim RI (2007) Improved gene expression signature of testicular carcinoma in situ. Int J Androl 30:292–302 discussion 303

Beumer TL, Roepers-Gajadien HL, Gademan IS, Kal HB, De Rooij DG (2000) Involvement of the D-type cyclins in germ cell proliferation and differentiation in the mouse. Biol Reprod 63:1893–1898

Biermann K, Goke F, Nettersheim D, Eckert D, Zhou H, Kahl P, Gashaw I, Schorle H, Buttner R (2007) c-KIT is frequently mutated in bilateral germ cell tumours and down-regulated during progression from intratubular germ cell neoplasia to seminoma. J Pathol 213:311–318

Bignell G, Smith R, Hunter C, Stephens P, Davies H, Greenman C, Teague J, Butler A, Edkins S, Stevens C, O'Meara S, Parker A, Avis T, Barthorpe S, Brackenbury L, Buck G, Clements J, Cole J, Dicks E, Edwards K, Forbes S, Gorton M, Gray K, Halliday K, Harrison R, Hills K, Hinton J, Jones D, Kosmidou V, Laman R, Lugg R, Menzies A, Perry J, Petty R, Raine K, Shepherd R, Small A, Solomon H, Stephens Y, Tofts C, Varian J, Webb A, West S, Widaa S, Yates A, Gillis AJ, Stoop HJ, van Gurp RJ, Oosterhuis JW, Looijenga LH, Futreal PA, Wooster R, Stratton MR (2006) Sequence analysis of the protein kinase gene family in human testicular germ-cell tumors of adolescents and adults. Genes Chromosomes Cancer 45:42–46

Bowles J, Knight D, Smith C, Wilhelm D, Richman J, Mamiya S, Yashiro K, Chawengsaksophak K, Wilson MJ, Rossant J, Hamada H, Koopman P (2006) Retinoid signaling determines germ cell fate in mice. Science 312:596–600

Castrillon DH, Quade BJ, Wang TY, Quigley C, Crum CP (2000) The human VASA gene is specifically expressed in the germ cell lineage. Proc Natl Acad Sci U S A 97:9585–9590

Choueiri TK, Stephenson AJ, Gilligan T, Klein EA (2007) Management of clinical stage I non-seminomatous germ cell testicular cancer. Urol Clin N Am 34:137–148 abstract viii

Clark AT, Rodriguez RT, Bodnar MS, Abeyta MJ, Cedars MI, Turek PJ, Firpo MT, Reijo Pera RA (2004) Human STELLAR, NANOG, and GDF3 genes are expressed in pluripotent cells and map to chromosome 12p13, a hotspot for teratocarcinoma. Stem Cells 22:169–179

Coffey J, Linger R, Pugh J, Dudakia D, Sokal M, Easton DF, Timothy Bishop D, Stratton M, Huddart R, Rapley EA (2008) Somatic KIT mutations occur predominantly in seminoma germ cell tumors and are not predictive of bilateral disease: report of 220 tumors and review of literature. Genes Chromosomes Cancer 47:34–42

Cools M, van Aerde K, Kersemaekers AM, Boter M, Drop SL, Wolffenbuttel KP, Steyerberg EW, Oosterhuis JW, Looijenga LH (2005) Morphological and immunohistochemical differences between gonadal maturation delay and early germ cell neoplasia in patients with undervirilization syndromes. J Clin Endocrinol Metab 90:5295–5303

Cools M, Honecker F, Stoop H, Veltman JD, de Krijger RR, Steyerberg E, Wolffenbuttel KP, Bokemeyer C, Lau YF, Drop SL, Looijenga LH (2006) Maturation delay of germ cells in fetuses with trisomy 21 results in increased risk for the development of testicular germ cell tumors. Hum Pathol 37:101–111

de Wit R, Fizazi K (2006) Controversies in the management of clinical stage I testis cancer. J Clin Oncol 24:5482–5492

Devouassoux-Shisheboran M, Mauduit C, Bouvier R, Berger F, Bouras M, Droz JP, Benahmed M (2001) Expression of hMLH1 and hMSH2 and assessment of microsatellite instability in testicular and mediastinal germ cell tumours. Mol Hum Reprod 7:1099–1105

Di Vizio D, Cito L, Boccia A, Chieffi P, Insabato L, Pettinato G, Motti ML, Schepis F, D'Amico W, Fabiani F, Tavernise B, Venuta S, Fusco A, Viglietto G (2005) Loss of the tumor suppressor gene PTEN marks the transition from intratubular germ cell neoplasias (ITGCN) to invasive germ cell tumors. Oncogene 24:1882–1894

Ezeh UI, Turek PJ, Reijo RA, Clark AT (2005) Human embryonic stem cell genes OCT4, NANOG, STELLAR, and GDF3 are expressed in both seminoma and breast carcinoma. Cancer 104:2255–2265

Faulkner SW, Friedlander ML (2000) Microsatellite instability in germ cell tumors of the testis and ovary. Gynecol Oncol 79:38–43

Feldman DR, Bosl GJ, Sheinfeld J, Motzer RJ (2008) Medical treatment of advanced testicular cancer. JAMA 299:672–684

Forbes S, Clements J, Dawson E, Bamford S, Webb T, Dogan A, Flanagan A, Teague J, Wooster R, Futreal PA, Stratton MR (2006) COSMIC 2005. Br J Cancer 94:318–322

Gillis AJ, Stoop HJ, Hersmus R, Oosterhuis JW, Sun Y, Chen C, Guenther S, Sherlock J, Veltman I, Baeten J, van der Spek PJ, de Alarcon P, Looijenga LH (2007) High-throughput microRNAome analysis in human germ cell tumours. J Pathol 213:319–328

Goddard NC, McIntyre A, Summersgill B, Gilbert D, Kitazawa S, Shipley J (2007) KIT and RAS signaling pathways in testicular germ cell tumours: new data and a review of the literature. Int J Androl 30:337–348 discussion 349

Hatakeyama S, Ohyama C, Minagawa S, Inoue T, Kakinuma H, Kyan A, Arai Y, Suga T, Nakayama J, Kato T, Habuchi T, Fukuda MN (2004) Functional correlation of trophinin expression with the malignancy of testicular germ cell tumor. Cancer Res 64:4257–4262

Heimdal K, Lothe RA, Lystad S, Holm R, Fossa SD, Borresen AL (1993) No germline TP53 mutations detected in familial and bilateral testicular cancer. Genes Chromosomes Cancer 6:92–97

Hoei-Hansen CE, Nielsen JE, Almstrup K, Hansen MA, Skakkebaek NE, Rajpert-Demeyts E, Leffers H (2004) Identification of genes differentially expressed in testes containing carcinoma in situ. Mol Hum Reprod 10:423–431

Hoei-Hansen CE, Almstrup K, Nielsen JE, Brask Sonne S, Graem N, Skakkebaek NE, Leffers H, Rajpert-De Meyts E (2005) Stem cell pluripotency factor NANOG is expressed in human fetal gonocytes, testicular carcinoma in situ and germ cell tumours. Histopathology 47:48–56

Hoei-Hansen CE, Sehested A, Juhler M, Lau YF, Skakkebaek NE, Laursen H, Rajpert-De Meyts E (2006) New evidence for the origin of intracranial germ cell tumours from primordial germ cells: expression of pluripotency and cell differentiation markers. J Pathol 209:25–33

Hofer MD, Browne TJ, He L, Skotheim RI, Lothe RA, Rubin MA (2005) Identification of two molecular groups of seminomas by using expression and tissue microarrays. Clin Cancer Res 11:5722–5729

Honorio S, Agathanggelou A, Wernert N, Rothe M, Maher ER, Latif F (2003) Frequent epigenetic inactivation of the RASSF1A tumour suppressor gene in testicular tumours and distinct methylation profiles of seminoma and nonseminoma testicular germ cell tumours. Oncogene 22:461–466

Houldsworth J, Xiao H, Murty VV, Chen W, Ray B, Reuter VE, Bosl GJ, Chaganti RS (1998) Human male germ cell tumor resistance to cisplatin is linked to TP53 gene mutation. Oncogene 16:2345–2349

Houldsworth J, Korkola JE, Bosl GJ, Chaganti RS (2006) Biology and genetics of adult male germ cell tumors. J Clin Oncol 24:5512–5518

Huddart RA, Wooster R, Horwich A, Cooper CS (1995) Microsatellite instability in human testicular germ cell tumours. Br J Cancer 72:642–645

International Germ Cell Cancer Collaborative Group (1997) International Germ Cell Consensus Classification: a prognostic factor-based staging system for metastatic germ cell cancers. J Clin Oncol 15:594–603

Jaruzelska J, Kotecki M, Kusz K, Spik A, Firpo M, Reijo Pera RA (2003) Conservation of a Pumilio–Nanos complex from Drosophila germ plasm to human germ cells. Dev Genes Evol 213:120–126

Juric D, Sale S, Hromas RA, Yu R, Wang Y, Duran GE, Tibshirani R, Einhorn LH, Sikic BI (2005) Gene expression profiling differentiates germ cell tumors from other cancers and defines subtype-specific signatures. Proc Natl Acad Sci U S A 102:17763–17768

Kanetsky PA, Mitra N, Vardhanabhuti S, Li M, Vaughn DJ, Letrero R, Ciosek SL, Doody DR, Smith LM, Weaver J, Albano A, Chen C, Starr JR, Rader DJ, Godwin AK, Reilly MP, Hakonarson H, Schwartz SM, Nathanson KL (2009) Common variation in KITLG and at 5q31.3 predisposes to testicular germ cell cancer. Nat Genet 41 (7): 811–5

Kemmer K, Corless CL, Fletcher JA, Mcgreevey L, Haley A, Griffith D, Cummings OW, Wait C, Town A, Heinrich MC (2004) KIT mutations are common in testicular seminomas. Am J Pathol 164:305–313

Kerley-Hamilton JS, Pike AM, Li N, Direnzo J, Spinella MJ (2005) A p53-dominant transcriptional response to cisplatin in testicular germ cell tumor-derived human embryonal carcinoma. Oncogene 24:6090–6100

Kersemaekers AM, Mayer F, Molier M, van Weeren PC, Oosterhuis JW, Bokemeyer C, Looijenga LH (2002) Role of P53 and MDM2 in treatment response of human germ cell tumors [see comment]. J Clin Oncol 20:1551–1561

Kitazono M, Sumizawa T, Takebayashi Y, Chen ZS, Furukawa T, Nagayama S, Tani A, Takao S, Aikou T, Akiyama S (1999) Multidrug resistance and the lung resistance-related protein in human colon carcinoma SW-620 cells [see comment]. J Natl Cancer Inst 91:1647–1653

Kollmannsberger C, Mayer F, Pressler H, Koch S, Kanz L, Oosterhuis JW, Looijenga LH, Bokemeyer C (2002) Absence of c-KIT and members of the epidermal growth factor receptor family in refractory germ cell cancer [see comment]. Cancer 95:301–308

Korkola JE, Houldsworth J, Chadalavada RS, Olshen AB, Dobrzynski D, Reuter VE, Bosl GJ, Chaganti RS (2006) Down-regulation of stem cell genes, including those in a 200-kb gene cluster at 12p13.31, is associated with in vivo differentiation of human male germ cell tumors. Cancer Res 66:820–827

Korkola JE, Heck S, Olshen AB, Reuter VE, Bosl GJ, Houldsworth J, Chaganti RS (2008) In vivo differentiation and genomic evolution in adult male germ cell tumors. Genes Chromosomes Cancer 47:43–55

Koubova J, Menke DB, Zhou Q, Capel B, Griswold MD, Page DC (2006) Retinoic acid regulates sex-specific timing of meiotic initiation in mice. Proc Natl Acad Sci U S A 103:2474–2479

Koul S, Mckiernan JM, Narayan G, Houldsworth J, Bacik J, Dobrzynski DL, Assaad AM, Mansukhani M, Reuter VE, Bosl GJ, Chaganti RS, Murty VV (2004) Role of promoter hypermethylation in Cisplatin treatment response of male germ cell tumors. Mol Cancer 3:16

Kraggerud SM, Skotheim RI, Szymanska J, Eknaes M, Fossa SD, Stenwig AE, Peltomaki P, Lothe RA (2002) Genome profiles of familial/bilateral and sporadic testicular germ cell tumors. Genes Chromosomes Cancer 34:168–174

Lind GE, Skotheim RI, Fraga MF, Abeler VM, Esteller M, Lothe RA (2006) Novel epigenetically deregulated genes in testicular cancer include homeobox genes and SCGB3A1 (HIN-1). J Pathol 210:441–449

Lind GE, Skotheim RI, Lothe RA (2007) The epigenome of testicular germ cell tumors. APMIS 115:1147–1160

Liu B, Nicolaides NC, Markowitz S, Willson JK, Parsons RE, Jen J, Papadopolous N, Peltomaki P, de la Chapelle A, Hamilton SR, Kinzler KW, Vogelstein B (1995) Mismatch repair gene defects in sporadic colorectal cancers with microsatellite instability. Nat Genet 9:48–55

Looijenga LH, de Leeuw H, van Oorschot M, van Gurp RJ, Stoop H, Gillis AJ, de Gouveia Brazao CA, Weber RF, Kirkels WJ, van Dijk T, von Lindern M, Valk P, Lajos G, Olah E, Nesland JM, Fossa SD, Oosterhuis JW (2003) Stem cell factor receptor (c-KIT) codon 816 mutations predict development of bilateral testicular germ-cell tumors. Cancer Res 63:7674–7678

Looijenga LH, Gillis AJ, Stoop H, Hersmus R, Oosterhuis JW (2007) Relevance of microRNAs in normal and malignant development, including human testicular germ cell tumours. Int J Androl 30:304–314 discussion 314–315

Lothe RA, Peltomaki P, Meling GI, Aaltonen LA, Nystrom-Lahti M, Pylkkanen L, Heimdal K, Andersen TI, Moller P, Rognum TO, Fossa SD, Haldorsen T, Langmark F, Brogger A, de la Chapelle A, Borresen A-L (1993) Genomic instability in colorectal cancer: relationship to clinicopathological variables and family history. Cancer Res 53:5849–5852

Madani A, Kemmer K, Sweeney C, Corless C, Ulbright T, Heinrich M, Einhorn L (2003) Expression of KIT and epidermal growth factor receptor in chemotherapy refractory non-seminomatous germ-cell tumors. Ann Oncol 14:873–880

Mandoky L, Geczi L, Bodrogi I, Toth J, Bak M (2003) Expression of HER-2/neu in testicular tumors. Anticancer Res 23:3447–3451

Mandoky L, Geczi L, Bodrogi I, Toth J, Csuka O, Kasler M, Bak M (2004a) Clinical relevance of HER-2/neu expression in germ-cell testicular tumors. Anticancer Res 24:2219–2224

Mandoky L, Geczi L, Doleschall Z, Bodrogi I, Csuka O, Kasler M, Bak M (2004b) Expression and prognostic value of the lung resistance-related protein (LRP) in germ cell testicular tumors. Anticancer Res 24:1097–1104

Masters JR, Koberle B (2003) Curing metastatic cancer: lessons from testicular germ-cell tumours. Nat Rev Cancer 3:517–525

Mauduit C, Hamamah S, Benahmed M (1999) Stem cell factor/c-kit system in spermatogenesis. Hum Reprod Update 5:535–545

Mayer F, Gillis AJ, Dinjens W, Oosterhuis JW, Bokemeyer C, Looijenga LH (2002) Microsatellite instability of germ cell tumors is associated with resistance to systemic treatment. Cancer Res 62:2758–2760

Mayer F, Honecker F, Looijenga LH, Bokemeyer C (2003a) Towards an understanding of the biological basis of response to cisplatin-based chemotherapy in germ-cell tumors. Ann Oncol 14:825–832

Mayer F, Stoop H, Scheffer GL, Scheper R, Oosterhuis JW, Looijenga LH, Bokemeyer C (2003b) Molecular determinants of treatment response in human germ cell tumors. Clin Cancer Res 9:767–773

Mazumdar M, Bacik J, Tickoo SK, Dobrzynski D, Donadio A, Bajorin D, Motzer R, Reuter V, Bosl GJ (2003) Cluster analysis of p53 and Ki67 expression, apoptosis, alpha-fetoprotein, and human chorionic gonadotrophin indicates a favorable prognostic subgroup within the embryonal carcinoma germ cell tumor. J Clin Oncol 21:2679–2688

McIntyre A, Summersgill B, Grygalewicz B, Gillis AJ, Stoop J, van Gurp RJ, Dennis N, Fisher C, Huddart R, Cooper C, Clark J, Oosterhuis JW, Looijenga LH, Shipley J (2005a) Amplification and overexpression of the KIT gene is associated with progression in the seminoma subtype of testicular germ cell tumors of adolescents and adults. Cancer Res 65:8085–8089

Mcintyre A, Summersgill B, Spendlove HE, Huddart R, Houlston R, Shipley J (2005b) Activating mutations and/or expression levels of tyrosine kinase receptors GRB7, RAS, and BRAF in testicular germ cell tumors. Neoplasia 7:1047–1052

Moul JW, Theune SM, Chang EH (1992) Detection of RAS mutations in archival testicular germ cell tumors by polymerase chain reaction and oligonucleotide hybridization. Genes Chromosomes Cancer 5:109–118

Murty VV, Chaganti RS (1998) A genetic perspective of male germ cell tumors. Semin Oncol 25:133–144

Murty VV, Li RG, Mathew S, Reuter VE, Bronson DL, Bosl GJ, Chaganti RS (1994) Replication error-type genetic instability at 1q42–43 in human male germ cell tumors. Cancer Res 54:3983–3985

Neill M, Warde P, Fleshner N (2007) Management of low-stage testicular seminoma. Urol Clin N Am 34:127–136 abstract vii–viii

Noce T, Okamoto-Ito S, Tsunekawa N (2001) Vasa homolog genes in mammalian germ cell development. Cell Struct Funct 26:131–136

Nystrom-Lahti M, Parsons R, Sistonen P, Pylkkanen L, Aaltonen LA, Leach FS, Hamilton SR, Watson P, Bronson E, Fusaro R, Cavalieri J, Lynch J, Lanspa SJ, Smyrk T, Lynch P, Drouhard T, Kinzler KW, Vogelstein B, Lynch HT, de la Chapelle A, Peltomaki P (1994) Mismatch repair genes on chromosomes 2p and 3p account for a major share of hereditary nonpolyposis colorectal cancer families evaluable by linkage. Am J Hum Genet 55:659–665

Olasz J, Mandoky L, Geczi L, Bodrogi I, Csuka O, Bak M (2005) Influence of hMLH1 methylation, mismatch repair deficiency and microsatellite instability on chemoresistance of testicular germ-cell tumors. Anticancer Res 25:4319–4324

Olie RA, Looijenga LH, Boerrigter L, Top B, Rodenhuis S, Langeveld A, Mulder MP, Oosterhuis JW (1995) N- and KRAS mutations in primary testicular germ cell tumors: incidence and possible biological implications. Genes Chromosomes Cancer 12:110–116

Oosterhuis JW, Looijenga LH (2005) Testicular germ-cell tumours in a broader perspective. Nat Rev Cancer 5:210–222

Palumbo C, van Roozendaal K, Gillis AJ, van Gurp RH, de Munnik H, Oosterhuis JW, van Zoelen EJ, Looijenga LH (2002) Expression of the PDGF alpha-receptor 1.5 kb transcript, OCT-4, and c-KIT in human normal and malignant tissues. Implications for the early diagnosis of testicular germ cell tumours and for our understanding of regulatory mechanisms. J Pathol 196:467–477

Pectasides D, Nikolaou M, Pectasides E, Koumarianou A, Valavanis C, Economopoulos T (2008) Complete response after imatinib mesylate administration in a patient with chemoresistant stage IV seminoma. Anticancer Res 28 (4C):2317–20

Pedersini R, Vattemi E, Mazzoleni G, Graiff C (2007) Complete response after treatment with imatinib in pretreated disseminated testicular seminoma with overexpression of c-KIT. Lancet Oncol 8 (11):1039–40

Peltomaki P, Aaltonen L, Sistonen P, Pylkkanen L, Mecklin J-P, Jarvinen H, Green JS, Jass JR, Weber JL, Leach FS, Petersen GM, Hamilton SR, de la Chapelle A, Vogelstein B (1993a) Genetic mapping of a locus predisposing to human colorectal cancer. Science 260:810–812

Peltomaki P, Lothe RA, Aaltonen LA, Pylkkanen L, Nystrom-Lahti M, Seruca R, David L, Holm R, Ryberg D, Haugen A, Et AL (1993b) Microsatellite instability is associated with tumors that characterize the hereditary non-polyposis colorectal carcinoma syndrome. Cancer Res 53:5853–5855

Peng HQ, Hogg D, Malkin D, Bailey D, Gallie BL, Bulbul M, Jewett M, Buchanan J, Goss PE (1993) Mutations of the p53 gene do not occur in testis cancer. Cancer Res 53:3574–3578

Petitjean A, Mathe E, Kato S, Ishioka C, Tavtigian SV, Hainaut P, Olivier M (2007) Impact of mutant p53 functional properties on TP53 mutation patterns and tumor phenotype: lessons from recent developments in the IARC TP53 database. Hum Mutat 28:622–629

Port M, Schmelz HU, Stockinger M, Sparwasser C, Albers P, Pottek T, Abend M (2005) Gene expression profiling in seminoma and nonseminoma. J Clin Oncol 23:58–69

Przygodzki RM, Hubbs AE, Zhao FQ, O'Leary TJ (2002) Primary mediastinal seminomas: evidence of single and multiple KIT mutations. Lab Invest 82:1369–1375

Rajpert-De Meyts E, Jorgensen N, Brondum-Nielsen K, Muller J, Skakkebaek NE (1998) Developmental arrest of germ cells in the pathogenesis of germ cell neoplasia. APMIS 106:198–204 discussion 204–206

Rajpert-De Meyts E, Bartkova J, Samson M, Hoei-Hansen CE, Frydelund-Larsen L, Bartek J, Skakkebaek NE (2003) The emerging phenotype of the testicular carcinoma in situ germ cell. APMIS 111:267–278 discussion 278–279

Rao PH, Houldsworth J, Palanisamy N, Murty VV, Reuter VE, Motzer RJ, Bosl GJ, Chaganti RS (1998) Chromosomal amplification is associated with cisplatin resistance of human male germ cell tumors. Cancer Res 58:4260–4263

Rapley EA, Hockley S, Warren W, Johnson L, Huddart R, Crockford G, Forman D, Leahy MG, Oliver DT, Tucker K, Friedlander M, Phillips KA, Hogg D, Jewett MA, Lohynska R, Daugaard G, Richard S, Heidenreich A, Geczi L, Bodrogi I, Olah E, Ormiston WJ, Daly PA, Looijenga LH, Guilford P, Aass N, Fossa SD, Heimdal K, Tjulandin SA, Liubchenko L, Stoll H, Weber W, Einhorn L, Weber BL, McMaster M, Greene MH, Bishop DT, Easton D, Stratton MR (2004) Somatic mutations of KIT in familial testicular germ cell tumours. Br J Cancer 90:2397–2401

Rapley EA, Turnbull C, Al Olama AA, Dermitzakis ET, Linger R, Huddart RA, Renwick A, Hughes D, Hines S, Seal S, Morrison J, Nsengimana J, Deloukas P, Rahman N, Bishop DT, Easton DF, Stratton MR (2009) A genome-wide association study of testicular germ cell tumor. Nat Genet 41 (7):807–10

Reijo RA, Dorfman DM, Slee R, Renshaw AA, Loughlin KR, Cooke H, Page DC (2000) DAZ family proteins exist throughout male germ cell development and transit from nucleus to cytoplasm at meiosis in humans and mice. Biol Reprod 63:1490–1496

Ries LAG, Melbert D, Krapcho M, Mariotto A, Miller BA, Feuer EJ, Clegg L, Horner MJ, Howlader N, Eisner MP, Reichman M, Edwards BK (2007) SEER cancer statistics review, 1975–2004. National Cancer Institute, Bethesda, MD

Rodriguez E, Mathew S, Reuter V, Ilson DH, Bosl GJ, Chaganti RS (1992) Cytogenetic analysis of 124 prospectively ascertained male germ cell tumors. Cancer Res 52:2285–2291

Rodriguez S, Jafer O, Goker H, Summersgill BM, Zafarana G, Gillis AJ, van Gurp RJ, Oosterhuis JW, Lu YJ, Huddart R, Cooper CS, Clark J, Looijenga LH, Shipley JM (2003) Expression profile of genes from 12p in testicular germ cell tumors of adolescents and adults associated with i(12p) and amplification at 12p11.2-p12.1. Oncogene 22:1880–1891

Rosenberg C, van Gurp RJ, Geelen E, Oosterhuis JW, Looijenga LH (2000) Overrepresentation of the short arm of chromosome 12 is related to invasive growth of human testicular seminomas and nonseminomas. Oncogene 19:5858–5862

Sakuma Y, Sakurai S, Oguni S, Hironaka M, Saito K (2003) Alterations of the c-kit gene in tes-
    ticular germ cell tumors. Cancer Sci 94:486–491
Satge D, Sasco AJ, Cure H, Leduc B, Sommelet D, Vekemans MJ (1997) An excess of testicular
    germ cell tumors in Down's syndrome: three case reports and a review of the literature. Cancer
    80:929–935
Scheffer GL, Wijngaard PL, Flens MJ, Izquierdo MA, Slovak ML, Pinedo HM, Meijer CJ, Clevers
    HC, Scheper RJ (1995) The drug resistance-related protein LRP is the human major vault
    protein [see comment]. Nat Med 1:578–582
Schenkman NS, Sesterhenn IA, Washington L, Tong YA, Weghorst CM, Buzard GS, Srivastava
    S, Moul JW (1995) Increased p53 protein does not correlate to p53 gene mutations in micro-
    dissected human testicular germ cell tumors. J Urol 154:617–621
Schmoll HJ, Souchon R, Krege S, Albers P, Beyer J, Kollmannsberger C, Fossa SD, Skakkebaek
    NE, de Wit R, Fizazi K, Droz JP, Pizzocaro G, Daugaard G, de Mulder PH, Horwich A,
    Oliver T, Huddart R, Rosti G, Paz Ares L, Pont O, Hartmann JT, Aass N, Algaba F, Bamberg
    M, Bodrogi I, Bokemeyer C, Classen J, Clemm S, Culine S, de Wit M, Derigs HG,
    Dieckmann KP, Flasshove M, Garcia del Muro X, Gerl A, Germa-Lluch JR, Hartmann M,
    Heidenreich A, Hoeltl W, Joffe J, Jones W, Kaiser G, Klepp O, Kliesch S, Kisbenedek L,
    Koehrmann KU, Kuczyk M, Laguna MP, Leiva O, Loy V, Mason MD, Mead GM, Mueller
    RP, Nicolai N, Oosterhof GO, Pottek T, Rick O, Schmidberger H, Sedlmayer F, Siegert W,
    Studer U, Tjulandin S, von der Maase H, Walz P, Weinknecht S, Weissbach L, Winter E,
    Wittekind C (2004) European consensus on diagnosis and treatment of germ cell cancer: a
    report of the European Germ Cell Cancer Consensus Group (EGCCCG). Ann Oncol
    15:1377–1399
Schweyer S, Soruri A, Meschter O, Heintze A, Zschunke F, Miosge N, Thelen P, Schlott T,
    Radzun HJ, Fayyazi A (2004) Cisplatin-induced apoptosis in human malignant testicular germ
    cell lines depends on MEK/ERK activation. Br J Cancer 91:589–598
Shuin T, Misaki H, Kubota Y, Yao M, Hosaka M (1994) Differential expression of protooncogenes
    in human germ cell tumors of the testis. Cancer 73:1721–1727
Sicinski P, Donaher JL, Geng Y, Parker SB, Gardner H, Park MY, Robker RL, Richards JS,
    Mcginnis LK, Biggers JD, Eppig JJ, Bronson RT, Elledge SJ, Weinberg RA (1996) Cyclin D2
    is an FSH-responsive gene involved in gonadal cell proliferation and oncogenesis. Nature
    384:470–474
Skotheim RI, Monni O, Mousses S, Fossa SD, Kallioniemi OP, Lothe RA, Kallioniemi A (2002)
    New insights into testicular germ cell tumorigenesis from gene expression profiling. Cancer
    Res 62:2359–2364
Skotheim RI, Lind GE, Monni O, Nesland JM, Abeler VM, Fossa SD, Duale N, Brunborg G,
    Kallioniemi O, Andrews PW, Lothe RA (2005) Differentiation of human embryonal carcino-
    mas in vitro and in vivo reveals expression profiles relevant to normal development. Cancer
    Res 65:5588–5598
Skotheim RI, Autio R, Lind GE, Kraggerud SM, Andrews PW, Monni O, Kallioniemi O, Lothe
    RA (2006) Novel genomic aberrations in testicular germ cell tumors by array-CGH, and asso-
    ciated gene expression changes. Cell Oncol 28:315–326
Smiraglia DJ, Szymanska J, Kraggerud SM, Lothe RA, Peltomaki P, Plass C (2002) Distinct
    epigenetic phenotypes in seminomatous and nonseminomatous testicular germ cell tumors.
    Oncogene 21:3909–3916
Smith-Sorensen B, Lind GE, Skotheim RI, Fossa SD, Fodstad O, Stenwig AE, Jakobsen KS,
    Lothe RA (2002) Frequent promoter hypermethylation of the O6-Methylguanine-DNA
    Methyltransferase (MGMT) gene in testicular cancer. Oncogene 21:8878–8884
Sommerer F, Hengge UR, Markwarth A, Vomschloss S, Stolzenburg JU, Wittekind C, Tannapfel
    A (2005) Mutations of BRAF and RAS are rare events in germ cell tumours. Int J Cancer
    113:329–335
Tsuda M, Sasaoka Y, Kiso M, Abe K, Haraguchi S, Kobayashi S, Saga Y (2003) Conserved role
    of nanos proteins in germ cell development. Science 301:1239–1241

van Gurp RJ, Oosterhuis JW, Kalscheuer V, Mariman EC, Looijenga LH (1994) Biallelic expression of the H19 and IGF2 genes in human testicular germ cell tumors. J Natl Cancer Inst 86:1070–1075

Velasco A, Riquelme E, Schultz M, Wistuba II, Villarroel L, Koh MS, Leach FS (2004) Microsatellite instability and loss of heterozygosity have distinct prognostic value for testicular germ cell tumor recurrence. Cancer Biol Ther 3:1152–1158 discussion 1159–1161

von Eyben FE (2004) Chromosomes, genes, and development of testicular germ cell tumors. Cancer Genet Cytogenet 151:93–138

Voorhoeve PM, le Sage C, Schrier M, Gillis AJ, Stoop H, Nagel R, Liu Y-P, van Duijse J, Drost J, Griekspoor A, Zlotorynski E, Yabuta N, De Vita G, Nojima H, Looijenga LH, Agami R (2006) A genetic screen implicates miRNA-372 and miRNA-373 as oncogenes in testicular germ cell tumors. Cell 124:1169–1181

Yabuta N, Okada N, Ito A, Hosomi T, Nishihara S, Sasayama Y, Fujimori A, Okuzaki D, Zhao H, Ikawa M, Okabe M, Nojima H (2007) Lats2 is an essential mitotic regulator required for the coordination of cell division. J Biol Chem 282:19259–19271

Youngren KK, Coveney D, Peng X, Bhattacharya C, Schmidt LS, Nickerson ML, Lamb BT, Deng JM, Behringer RR, Capel B, Rubin EM, Nadeau JH, Matin A (2005) The Ter mutation in the dead end gene causes germ cell loss and testicular germ cell tumours. Nature 435:360–364

Zafarana G, Grygalewicz B, Gillis AJ, Vissers LE, van de Vliet W, van Gurp RJ, Stoop H, Debiec-Rychter M, Oosterhuis JW, van Kessel AG, Schoenmakers EF, Looijenga LH, Veltman JA (2003) 12p-amplicon structure analysis in testicular germ cell tumors of adolescents and adults by array CGH. Oncogene 22:7695–7701

Zeeman AM, Stoop H, Boter M, Gillis AJ, Castrillon DH, Oosterhuis JW, Looijenga LH (2002) VASA is a specific marker for both normal and malignant human germ cells. Lab Invest 82:159–166

Part D
Inherited Susceptibility

Chapter 7
Identification of Genetic Risk Factors for Prostate Cancer: Analytic Approaches Using Hereditary Prostate Cancer Families

Ethan M. Lange

7.1 Introduction

In 2009, prostate cancer is the most commonly diagnosed nonskin cancer among men in the United States, with an estimated 192,280 new cases, and a leading cause of cancer-related mortality, with an estimated 27,360 related deaths (Jemal et al. 2008). Increasing age, positive family history, and African ancestry are established major risk factors for prostate cancer (Bostwick et al. 2004).

The clustering of prostate cancer cases among families has motivated the search for genetic risk factors for the disease. The identification of genetic factors that predispose men to prostate cancer will likely result in a better understanding of the disease etiology. It also has the potential to help identify at-risk individuals, to suggest new drug targets and therapies, and to assist in chemoprevention strategies. Characterization of prostate cancer susceptibility genes will open the way to a new level of inquiry in the genetic epidemiology of this disease, in which the joint effects of specific genetic variants and putative environmental risk factors can be examined more directly.

In this chapter, I describe analytic approaches for identifying genetic risk factors for prostate cancer using data collected from families that typically contain multiple men with the disease. Many of these past and current approaches are not unique to prostate cancer. In fact, these same approaches have been or are currently used to identify genetic risk factors for numerous other human diseases including type I and type II diabetes, psoriasis, asthma, cardiovascular diseases, psychiatric disorders, addiction disorders, and other cancers. The one obvious difference between prostate cancer (and other male cancers) and these other diseases is that females could be carriers of genetic susceptibility, but they would not demonstrate

E.M. Lange
Department of Genetics, University of North Carolina at Chapel Hill,
4300D Medical Biomolecular Research Building, CB #7264, 103 Mason Farm Road,
Chapel Hill, NC, 27599-7264, USA
e-mail: elange@med.unc.edu

W.D. Foulkes and K.A. Cooney (eds.), *Male Reproductive Cancers:*
Epidemiology, Pathology and Genetics, Cancer Genetics,
DOI 10.1007/978-1-4419-0449-2_7, © Springer Science+Business Media, LLC 2010

any clinical characteristics of the disease. This fact impacts study design and can make it more difficult to unravel the genetic mechanisms involved. Additional complications in identifying prostate cancer genetic risk factors that will be considered in the course of this discussion include the high prevalence, the typically late age of onset, and the highly variable presentation of the disease; the range of alternative methods to detect the disease (most notably the variable use of PSA screening); and a poor understanding of environmental (nongenetic) risk factors.

7.2 Establishing that Genetic Risk Factors Exist for Prostate Cancer

Before embarking on costly efforts to identify genetic variants that are associated (and ultimately causal) with prostate cancer or any other disease, it is critical to establish that such genetic risk factors exist and that they are sufficiently strong to be detected for the proposed study designs. The observation of positive family history as a significant risk factor for prostate cancer is a strong indicator of an underlying genetic mechanism in the etiology of the disease. One of the most common measures to evaluate to role of genetics in disease susceptibility is the calculation of the sibling recurrence risk ratio, λ_s (Risch 1990). This measure is defined as the risk of disease manifestation for a subject conditional on having a sibling with the disease divided by the overall population risk. The λ_s measure has been shown to be highly sensitive to ascertainment bias and cannot separate the role of shared environmental and genetic risk factors in siblings (Guo 1998). Obtaining a valid estimate of λ_s for prostate cancer is very difficult given the increased screening in men with positive family history, the late age of onset of the disease, the increasing risk of disease with increasing age (which likely approaches near certainty if a man were to live long enough), and the observed differences in disease prevalence in different populations. For these reasons, estimates of λ_s in prostate cancer are dubious. In any case, there remains strong evidence for a genetic influence in prostate cancer susceptibility.

The evidence for family history as a strong risk factor for prostate cancer comes from a variety of studies, including case-control, cohort, twin, and family-based studies. Results from these numerous different types of studies have been summarized succinctly by Schaid (2004). A large number of case-control studies have consistently supported that having at least one first-degree relative diagnosed with prostate cancer conveys an odds ratio (OR) of ~2.5 (Schaid 2004; Zeegers et al. 2003). Steinberg et al. partitioned the OR estimates by the number of first-degree relatives with prostate cancer (Steinberg et al. 1990). Their estimated ORs increased from 2.2 to 4.9 to 10.9 if there were one, two, or three or more first-degree relatives with prostate cancer. Several cohort studies have also supported a positive family history as a strong risk factor for prostate cancer. Using 690 consecutive prostate cancer cases undergoing radical prostatectomy, Isaacs et al. estimated a relative risk of 1.76 for first-degree relatives (Isaacs et al. 1995). Epidemiological studies have suggested that the relative risk attributed to a positive family history is similar between African-American and European-American families (Hayes et al. 1995; Whittemore et al. 1995).

The risk associated with family history can be partitioned into shared genetic and environmental risk factors. Twin studies are useful for assessing the genetic etiology of traits that are known to segregate in families. A large twin study by Lichtenstein et al. based on Swedish, Danish, and Finnish twin registries estimated the recurrence risk in a cotwin of a prostate cancer case to be 21.1% in monozygotic (MZ) twins and 6.4% in dizygotic (DZ) twins (Lichtenstein et al. 2000). Lichtenstein et al. estimated that 42% of the risk of prostate cancer in these populations could be explained by heritable factors, though it should be noted that this estimate is highly sensitive to the estimated prevalence of the disease. Page et al. presented similar results from a large twin study based on USA World War II veterans that estimated the recurrence risk in a cotwin of a prostate cancer case to be 27.1% for MZ twins and 7.1% for DZ twins (Page et al. 1997). Together with the previously described epidemiological studies, these results demonstrate the presence of strong genetic risk factors for prostate cancer.

It has been shown that early-onset prostate cancer is a marker for heritable forms of the disease. On average, hereditary prostate cancer is diagnosed 6–7 years earlier than sporadic prostate cancer, but does not otherwise differ in clinical presentation than the sporadic form of the disease (Bastacky et al. 1995; Keetch et al. 1996; Valeri et al. 2000; Bratt et al. 2002; Bratt 2002). In Sweden, where screening for prostate cancer is not generally recommended, the relative risk for developing prostate cancer for a man whose father has been diagnosed with prostate cancer at age 60 or older was estimated to be 1.5; this estimated relative risk increased to 2.5 if the father was diagnosed prior to 60 years of age. Similarly, if one brother was diagnosed with prostate cancer at age 60 or older then the relative risk (λ_s) for a man developing prostate cancer was estimated to be 2, whereas the relative risk was estimated to be 3 if one brother was diagnosed with prostate cancer prior to age 60 (Bratt 2002). These findings show that early-onset prostate cancer patients are more likely to be carriers of genetic susceptibility factors than older cases. These findings are also consistent with what has been found with breast cancer, where women diagnosed with early-onset breast cancer are far more likely to carry mutations at the *BRCA1* or *BRCA2* genes, particularly if there is also a strong family history of breast cancer.

7.2.1   Segregation Analysis

In most gene searches, the underlying genetic mechanism is initially a complete mystery. Historically, the first step in identifying the susceptibility genes involves performing segregation analysis. The purpose of segregation analysis is to identify, in broad terms, the genetic mechanisms that confer susceptibility to a trait or disease of interest. Segregation analysis is often performed to estimate a set of parameters to be used for parametric linkage analysis – specifically, to estimate the number of contributing susceptibility genes and, for each putative susceptibility gene (whose location and identity is unknown), to estimate the underlying genetic mode of inheritance (e.g., dominant, recessive, etc.), the penetrance for each possible genotype at the gene (where genotype confers the number of mutated gene copies a person carries – 0,1, or 2), and the frequency of mutated copies of the gene in the general population. The penetrance function reflects the probability that an individual would be affected given his or her genotype at the disease gene. For a given genotype, penetrance is sometimes estimated separately for specific age or gender groups. Segregation analysis is performed by assimilating phenotype data on a collection of families that have at least one affected individual. The parameters of interest are estimated by maximum likelihood calculations. In order to remove bias introduced through how the families were collected (usually through identification of a proband – a single individual who was identified by seeking medical attention, though in some cases families are ascertained based on having a minimum number of individuals with the trait or some other criteria), an ascertainment correction is included in these calculations to maintain valid parameter estimates. Segregation analyses for prostate cancer have suggested the presence of at least one strong dominant susceptibility gene in addition to one or more recessive and/or X-linked prostate cancer susceptibility genes. One report suggested that as many as 43% of early-onset prostate cancer cases (diagnosed prior to 55 years) could be explained by a rare, highly penetrant dominant risk allele (Carter et al. 1992).

7.3 Historical Approach for Identifying Susceptibility Genes

In the late 1980s and early 1990s, disease susceptibility genes for a number of monogenic (or single-gene) Mendelian disorders were identified, including genes for Huntington's disease, cystic fibrosis, Duchenne muscular dystrophy, sickle cell anemia, Tay Sachs disease, and ataxia–telangiectasia. Monogenic Mendelian disorders are disorders that are caused by an adverse copy or copies (an individual has two copies of each gene – one inherited from each parent) of a single gene. For many monogenic Mendelian disorders, if individuals inherit genetic susceptibility then they will develop disease with 100% certainty (termed full penetrance) and individuals who do not inherit genetic susceptibility will not develop disease (cases of disease not due to genetic susceptibility are termed phenocopies or sporadics). Huntington's disease, an autosomal dominantly inherited disorder, is caused by microsatellite expansion in a single copy of a single gene at chromosome 4p. Individuals who carry two gene copies with 35 or fewer polyglutamine $(CAG)_n$ repeats are not at risk for developing Huntington's disease. Individuals who carry at least one gene copy with 36–39 CAG repeats have intermediate risk, while individuals who carry at least one gene copy with 40 or more CAG repeats will develop Huntington's disease with near certainty (Langbehn et al. 2004). Many Mendelian disorders follow an autosomal (gene not on chromosomes X or Y) recessive mode of inheritance (e.g., cystic fibrosis, sickle cell anemia, Tay Sachs disease, ataxia–telangiectasia). Recessive means that two copies of the mutated gene are necessary to confer genetic susceptibility, one inherited from the mother, and one from the father. A person who has only one mutated copy of a recessive gene is said to be a carrier for the trait or disease, but they typically do not have any health problems from carrying one copy of the mutated gene.

Linkage analysis was a highly successful approach for identifying the chromosomal regions that harbored causative genes for a number of Mendelian disorders. For example, in 1988 the gene for ataxia–telangiectasia was firmly localized to chromosome 11q based on linkage results from one large Amish pedigree that segregated the disease (Gatti et al. 1988). The *ATM* (or ataxia–telangiectasia mutated) gene was localized to ~800 kb region on chromosome 11q22-23 based on linkage results from 176 families from an international linkage consortium in 1995 and subsequently cloned months later (Lange et al. 1995; Savitsky et al. 1995). The identification of the *ATM* gene was aided by the fact that all ataxia–telangiectasia patients could have their disease explained by mutations in the *ATM* gene.

The success in identifying causative genes for single-gene Mendelian disorders led investigators to conduct similar linkage-based study designs for detecting genes for more genetically complex diseases such as prostate cancer. The basic study design is to collect DNA and phenotypes from families that have multiple individuals with the disease under study and use these pedigrees to identify chromosomal regions that contain the susceptibility genes.

7.3.1   Parametric Linkage Analysis

Parametric linkage analyses was a basic and powerful tool used to identify chromosomal regions that harbored susceptibility genes for a number of Mendelian disorders and continues to be the method of choice for rare disorders that are suspected to be due to rare but highly penetrant mutations. Linkage analysis is used to evaluate the coinheritance within families of genetic markers with a trait. In parametric linkage analysis, we stipulate that there is a susceptibility gene that comes in two forms, a normal copy and a mutated copy. Typically we assume that all mutations in a putative gene have the same detrimental effect. The goal of linkage analysis is to place the putative gene locus (the gene is treated as a genetic marker) in a map of nonfunctional genetic markers of known location using maximum likelihood-based methods. Placing one genetic marker in a map containing other genetic markers in fixed locations is not typically difficult when observed genotype data are available on the entire set of genetic markers, including the genetic marker being placed. However, in the case of mapping a putative disease gene, we do not observe the genotype at the disease gene itself (the identity of the gene is unknown) but instead we rely on each individual's trait phenotype to tell us something about the genotype for that individual at the disease gene locus. Probabilities for each possible genotype at the putative disease locus for the individual pedigree members are calculated based on the assumed genetic model parameters obtained from segregation analyses and the observed data across all members in the pedigree – hence, it is critically important to accurately estimate these parameters. Genome-wide linkage analysis studies have been routinely performed using microsatellite genetic markers (genetic markers that take many different variant forms) with a typical marker spacing of one microsatellite every 5–10 cM (or approximately 5–10 million bases apart). Likelihood-based methods are then used to assess the relative likelihood of each possible location for the putative disease gene locus at each considered location in the genome. Specifically, for a given location, we calculate the ratio of the likelihood that the trait gene is at this specific location (linked) versus the likelihood that it is unlinked (on a different chromosome or far away on the same chromosome) to this location. The metric used to evaluate the strength of the evidence for linkage at a given location is the LOD score, which is defined on the log-based-10 scale. A LOD score of 3 at a given location implies that the putative gene locus is 1,000 times more likely to be linked at this location than to not be. We typically require a high LOD threshold (LOD > 3.3) in order to conclude the evidence of linkage is statistically significant. The high LOD threshold takes into account the low prior probability of linkage at any given location in the genome and the impact of multiple testing when evaluating linkage across the genome.

Parametric linkage analysis is robust against allelic heterogeneity but suffers considerable loss of power when there is genetic heterogeneity. That is, the power of linkage analysis is robust even if each family with disease segregates a unique causal mutation, provided the mutations are all in the same gene (allelic heterogeneity) or within a tight gene cluster. However, power of linkage analysis is severely impacted if there are multiple unlinked genes with mutations that can cause the same disease phenotype (genetic heterogeneity). A parametric linkage approach that assumes genetic heterogeneity has been developed to allow for a proportion of families to not be linked to a given location when linkage is being evaluated at that location (Cavalli-Sforza and King 1986). The resulting heterogeneity LOD score, or HLOD, has been shown to be more robust in the presence of genetic heterogeneity, but there still remains a substantial loss of statistical power to detect linkage when there is genetic heterogeneity.

7.3.2 Nonparametric Linkage Analysis

The etiology of prostate cancer is complex; there are likely many different genetic and nongenetic factors that contribute to the risk of disease. In addition, because of the late age of onset of the disease, many men currently without prostate cancer will develop the disease in the future. These complicating factors have made the specification of any single parametric disease model for linkage analysis problematic. Of particular concern is the robustness of parametric linkage analysis to misclassification of the genetic mode-of-inheritance model (e.g., specifying a disease gene acts in a dominant fashion when in fact it acts in a recessive fashion) and to misclassification of the disease phenotype within families – particularly unaffected men who may carry genetic susceptibility. These concerns, similar to other common diseases as well, have led to an alternative form of linkage analysis termed "nonparametric" or "mode-of-inheritance free" linkage analysis. Nonparametric linkage analysis uses only phenotype data from the affected family members in a pedigree to avoid the problem of phenotype misclassification among family members who have not yet overtly manifested the disease. Family members with unaffected or unknown phenotypes do not directly contribute to the linkage score statistics, but do contribute potentially valuable information regarding inheritance patterns in their affected family members, particularly when there are missing genotype data on the pedigree founders. Pedigree founders are the individuals in a family who establish who is related to whom in the family. For example, if two brothers are affected, then the parents (the pedigree founders) will also need to be included in the pedigree, as it is the siblings' shared inheritance of their parents DNA that establishes how they are genetically related. A pedigree with first cousins would have four founders: two of the founders would be their shared grandparents and the other pedigree founders would be each of their unrelated parents.

Conceptually, nonparametric linkage analysis is rather intuitive. When more than one related pedigree member has the same disease, then there is a good chance that these affected family members have inherited the same susceptibility allele from the same pedigree founder. Two alleles that are the same ancestral copy of a founder allele are said to be identical by descent (IBD). Nonparametic linkage analysis is used to identify chromosomal regions where there is an excess of sharing of IBD founder DNA among related affected individuals (that would occur due to the affected family members inheriting the same susceptibility allele). To evaluate the evidence for linkage to a particular chromosomal location, we construct a Z-statistic for each pedigree, combine the Z-statistics across pedigrees by calculating a weighted-sum, and evaluate the statistical significance of the resulting combined Z-statistic (termed NPL Z-score) using a standard Z-test. To construct the Z-statistics, we first must choose a statistic that will be used to measure the extent of IBD allele sharing among affected individuals in the same family. Numerous choices of allele-sharing statistics have been proposed, with the two most widely used allele-sharing statistics being the "pairs" and "all" statistics introduced by Whittemore and Halpern (1994).

The pairs' allele-sharing statistic is the easiest to describe. For a given pedigree, the pairs' statistic simply counts the number of alleles shared IBD between each possible pair of related affected individuals and then sums these counts across all possible pairs of affected individuals in the family. The Z-statistic is calculated by subtracting the expected value of the sharing statistic (under the null hypothesis of no linkage) from the observed value of the sharing statistic and then by dividing this difference by the standard deviation of the sharing statistic (also under the null hypothesis of no linkage). Z-statistics are subsequently summed across pedigrees, typically after down-weighting each pedigree's Z-score by a factor equal to the square root of the number of pedigrees analyzed, to obtain an overall NPL Z-score statistic. This NPL Z-score statistic asymptotically follows the standard normal distribution under the null hypothesis of no linkage assuming IBD can be determined unambiguously within families. When founder genotype data are missing or uninformative this assumption is not valid (due to overestimation of the variance of the score statistic) and the resulting Z-scores will follow an approximate normal distribution with mean 0 but with a variance <1, making the use of the standard normal distribution to evaluate the statistical significance of the NPL Z-score somewhat conservative. Given the loss in power in applying the standard normal distribution to the resulting NPL Z-score, statistical significance of NPL Z-scores are often computed either empirically (using "gene-dropping" approaches) or they are converted to LOD scores using a statistical parametric model, where the individual family Z-scores are fit into either a linear or exponential model (Kong and Cox 1997).

Debate still exists regarding use of classic parametric versus nonparametric linkage analysis for complex traits such as prostate cancer. While nonparametric linkage analysis offers considerable flexibility and robustness to model misspecification, parametric linkage analysis can be statistically more powerful should a reasonably correct parametric model be specified. In any case, both methods suffer considerable reduction in power when there are many genes (genetic heterogeneity) that influence genetic susceptibility. Both methods have been routinely employed in prostate cancer linkage studies and, unfortunately, the level of success using either approach has been underwhelming.

7.3.3   Genome-Wide Linkage Screens for Prostate Cancer

Approximately 20 genome-wide linkage screens for prostate cancer have been conducted in the past decade. Results from these scans have implicated few specific and consistent chromosomal regions for linkage. It is important to recognize, however, that these studies differ in many ways, including the populations studied, sample sizes, ascertainment criteria (sib-pairs versus extended pedigrees), methods of diagnosis, analytic methods, and definitions used for subset analyses. These differences, combined with the complex genetic etiology of prostate cancer (including genetic heterogeneity, high rates of sporadic disease, and heterogeneity of the phenotype itself), have major implications for the power to detect specific prostate cancer susceptibility genes via linkage analysis. Recognizing the need to analyze a large set of homogeneous pedigrees, the International Consortium for Prostate Cancer Genetics (ICPCG) was formed to conduct joint linkage analyses using uniform analytic strategies, methods of diagnosis, and definitions for subset analyses and stricter inclusion rules for pedigrees in general. In 2005, the ICPCG reported linkage results from a genome-wide scan on 1,233 pedigrees from ten different prostate cancer research groups, identifying five regions with suggestive linkage (parametric or nonparametric LOD $\geq$ 1.86): 5q12, 8p21, 15q11, 17q21, and 22q12 (Xu et al. 2005).

An approach that has been widely used in linkage studies of complex traits is to focus on subsets of pedigrees that are more likely to segregate highly penetrant susceptibility alleles. Specifically, the idea has been to focus on pedigrees with large numbers of cases or pedigrees with early mean age at diagnosis. This approach was successful in mapping and subsequently identifying, among others, the breast/ovarian cancer genes *BRCA1* and *BRCA2*, the colorectal cancer genes *MSH2* and *MLH1*, and the melanoma gene *CDKN2A*. Six regions were identified with suggestive linkage by the ICPCG when focusing on the 269 prostate cancer families with at least five confirmed familial prostate cancer cases (LOD ≥ 1.86): 1q25, 8q13, 13q14, 16p13, 17q21, and 22q12. In addition, four regions with suggestive linkage for prostate cancer were identified in 606 families with mean age at prostate cancer diagnosis ≤ 65: 3p24, 5q35, 11q22, and Xq12(Xu et al. 2005). Again however, no region had linkage evidence reaching the threshold of statistical significance.

The cumulative results from the large number of prostate cancer linkage studies cast doubt regarding the segregation analysis conclusions of Carter et al., which evaluated a very select number of extreme high-density prostate cancer pedigrees and suggested much of hereditary and early-onset prostate cancer could be explained by a single rare highly penetrant risk allele(s) (Carter et al. 1992). If such were the case, given the extensive linkage studies focused on high density and early-onset prostate cancer families, such a gene likely would have been localized by now. It should be noted that segregation analyses can be dubious for complex traits given drastic oversimplification of the alternative disease models in the presence of strong genetic heterogeneity, high rates of sporadic disease increasing with age, strongly shared environmental components, and difficulties in adequately correcting for family ascertainment criteria among many concerns.

7.3.4   Linkage Analysis and Clinically Aggressive Disease

One major potential complication in identifying prostate cancer susceptibility genes is the tremendous heterogeneity of the prostate cancer phenotype. Specifically, aggressiveness of tumors in the prostate varies considerably, even within families. This variability of tumor aggressiveness has led to two separate hypotheses that have guided additional linkage studies. The first hypothesis is that aggressive prostate cancer, being a more severe and homogeneous phenotype, is more likely to be caused by common genetic risk factors than less aggressive prostate cancer, and therefore greater power to detect prostate cancer genes can be achieved by focusing analyses on men with aggressive disease only. The second hypothesis is that there exist genes that modify the severity of prostate cancer tumors in men afflicted with prostate cancer.

7.3.5 Aggressive Prostate Cancer

Linkage analysis for aggressive prostate cancer is conducted in a similar fashion to prostate cancer, but involves reducing the number of men defined to have the disease phenotype (i.e., aggressive prostate cancer). Operationally, linkage analysis of aggressive prostate cancer involves reclassifying the phenotype of some men diagnosed with prostate cancer in prostate cancer pedigrees. Specifically, men without aggressive disease are recoded as being phenotype "unknown" rather than being coded as "affected" and, after these changes are made, the analysis is conducted as described before. By this convention, aggressive prostate cancer, like prostate cancer, is a dichotomous trait. The rationale of focusing on aggressive prostate cancer in linkage studies is twofold. First, the genes that specifically cause susceptibility to aggressive prostate cancer (if there are genes that specifically predispose men to aggressive prostate cancer) are clearly the genes of greatest clinical importance. Second, by focusing on a more homogeneous phenotype, we may improve our power to find genes for prostate cancer. The latter assumption is not necessarily true as there is a clear trade-off, in terms of statistical power, between evaluating a more homogeneous phenotype on a smaller number of prostate cancer cases in a smaller number of families and a less homogeneous phenotype on a larger number of prostate cancer cases in a larger number of families. Despite this uncertainty, it is clearly important to evaluate aggressive prostate cancer by itself given the possibility that such a focus would increase our probability of finding genes associated with the greatest mortality from the disease.

Several moderately-sized studies have performed genome-wide linkage studies for aggressive prostate cancer (see Chap. 10, Sect. 10.6). A study from the University of Michigan on 71 informative families with two or cases of aggressive prostate cancer found significant evidence for linkage (LOD = 3.5) to chromosome 15q12 (a region that overlapped 15q11, previously identified for suggestive prostate cancer linkage by the ICPCG)(Lange et al. 2006). No other study found any evidence for linkage to aggressive prostate cancer at this location. The definition of what constitutes aggressive prostate cancer was very similar across studies. The ICPCG conducted a combined genome-wide linkage study on aggressive prostate cancer on 166 families with three or more aggressive prostate cancer cases (which included a subset of 22 University of Michigan pedigrees in the above report that met the more stringent criteria of the ICPCG) (Schaid et al. 2006). In this study, men were defined to have aggressive prostate cancer if they had at least one of the following characteristics: regional or distant stage (stages T3, T4, N1, or M1, based on the radical prostatectomy specimen for patients treated with surgery; otherwise based on clinical stage); tumor Gleason grade at diagnosis ≥ 7 (or poorly differentiated grade if no Gleason grade was available); pretreatment PSA at diagnosis ≥ 20 ng/mL; death from metastatic prostate cancer before age 65 years (if deceased). The ICPCG study did not find any region to be significantly linked to aggressive prostate cancer. Several regions (6p22.3, LOD = 3.0; 11q14.1-14.3, LOD = 2.4; and 20p11.21-q11.21, LOD = 2.5) reached a suggestive level of linkage. For chromosome

Table 7.1 Summary of regions with suggestive evidence for linkage (LOD/HLOD > 1.86) obtained from 1,233 prostate cancer families from the ICPCG

Strata	Number of pedigrees	Chromosome	Distance from Pter cM	Analysis type	LOD/HLOD
All[a]	1,233	5q12	77	Nonparametric	2.28
		8p21	46	Dominant	1.97
		15q11	1	Recessive	2.10
		17q21	77	Dominant	1.99
		22q12	42	Dominant	1.95
Families with at least five affected relatives[a]	269	1q25	184	Nonparametric	2.62
		8q13	81	Recessive	2.41
		13q14	56	Recessive	2.27
		16p13	34	Nonparametric	1.88
		17q21	77	Dominant	2.04
		22q12	42	Dominant	3.57
Families with average age of diagnosis ≤65 years[a]	606	3p24	57	Dominant	2.37
		5q35	179	Dominant	2.05
		11q22	102	Recessive	2.20
		Xq12	80	Dominant	2.30
Aggressive prostate cancer (3 or more cases)[b]	166	6p22	42	Nonparametric	3.00
		11q14	89	Recessive	2.40
		20p11	54	Dominant	2.49

[a]As reported by Xu et al. (2005)
[b]As reported by Schaid et al. (2006)

11q14, stronger evidence for linkage (LOD = 3.3) was found among the subset of 73 pedigrees with an average age of diagnosis of 65 years or younger. These results suggest that several regions may contain genes that, when mutated, predispose men to develop aggressive prostate cancer. Given the relatively small number of pedigrees that met the strict inclusion criteria in these analyses, the inclusion of additional prostate cancer families with multiple cases of aggressive disease could be particularly valuable to help prioritize regions for further study. Results from the linkage study on 1,233 families from the ICPCG are summarized in Table 7.1 for all families and for subsets of families identified to have five or more affected families members, average age of diagnosis for all family prostate cancer cases less than age 66 years, or three or more cases of aggressive disease (and only aggressive disease cases defined as "affected").

7.3.6   Genetic Modifiers of Prostate Cancer Severity – Study of Gleason Grade

To test for genetic modifiers of prostate cancer aggressiveness, prostate cancer researchers used Gleason grade, an ordinal quantitative outcome measure, as a measure of disease severity (see also Chap. 10, Sect. 10.2). In families collected for linkage analysis for prostate cancer, Gleason grade often varies considerably among men diagnosed with prostate cancer in the same family. This phenomenon is at least in part due to the mechanism in which prostate cancer families are collected for linkage analysis studies. Specifically, probands with severe disease typically come to the attention of prostate cancer researchers. The identification of probands with disease would likely result in increased screening in other men in the same family (men who otherwise showed little or no indications of disease) which would in turn subsequently lead to an increased detection of men with mild forms of the disease. Families with multiple affected men with prostate cancer would then be candidates for inclusion in linkage studies. The typical collection of prostate cancer families used for most linkage studies is not ideal for measuring the heritability of Gleason grade (given the mentioned source of screening bias), but these families could be quite powerful for identifying genetic variants that modify disease severity (as measured by Gleason grade) among men with prostate cancer.

Analytically, the identification of chromosomal regions containing genetic modifiers through linkage analysis involves finding regions of the genome where IBD between pairs of related men with prostate cancer is associated with the difference in Gleason grades between the men. Specifically, we look to identify chromosomal regions where there is significant evidence that related men who have similar Gleason grade values share more alleles IBD than would be expected by chance and evidence that related men with prostate cancer who have dissimilar Gleason grade values share fewer alleles IBD than would be expected by chance. This type of linkage analysis is often referred to as quantitative trait linkage analysis. A number of studies have been performed searching for regions linked to Gleason grade. Of note, several studies have reported evidence for linkage to chromosome 19q (Witte et al. 2000; Slager et al. 2003; Neville et al. 2003; Schaid et al. 2007). A combined linkage scan by the ICPCG for regions linked to Gleason grade has yet to be performed, the delay in part due to the variability in Gleason grade scoring methodologies across the different ICPCG participating groups, and in some cases, different scoring methods applied to samples within the same group. Still, the consistency of the results from these smaller studies suggests the existence of important genetic modifiers of prostate cancer disease severity.

7.4   Genetic Association Studies

Genetic association studies are now the most popular method for identifying genetic susceptibility variants in the human genome. Linkage studies are powered to identify chromosomal regions that harbor rare, but highly penetrant, gene mutations that cause disease – especially when the underlying cause can be attributed to a single gene. Genetic association studies are better powered to detect individual genetic polymorphisms that are associated with disease when the underlying disease susceptibility is due to common modestly penetrant genetic variants (Risch 2000). As the scientific community expanded their quest from identifying the genes that cause rare but purely genetic diseases to diseases that can be explained only in part by genetic susceptibility, it quickly became clear to researchers that linkage analysis is not the optimal strategy for finding genes that are associated with common diseases with complex etiologies. In particular, the risk for developing prostate cancer is influenced by many common genetic variants (both in genes and, as we are now beginning to observe, in key regulatory regions outside of genes). Genetic association studies estimate the association between specific genetic variants and the phenotype of interest. For disease studies, genetic association studies simply involve comparing the frequency of variants between a sample of individuals with and without disease and determining whether any observed difference in these frequencies reaches a level of statistical significance. For quantitative traits such as blood pressure or PSA levels, we test whether the mean of the quantitative measures significantly differs by genotype. These tests are often performed separately for each individual genetic marker, but sometimes can be based on haplotypes containing several tightly linked genetic markers simultaneously.

7.4.1   Association Studies for Prostate Cancer in Regions Identified by Linkage Analysis

Several prostate cancer candidate genes have been identified under suggestive linkage peaks; these include *RNASEL* at 1q, *MSR1* at 8p, *BRCA1* at 17q and *ELAC* at 17p (Carpten et al. 2002; Xu et al. 2003; Zuhlke et al. 2004; Tavtigian et al. 2001). Germline mutations were detected within all of these genes; however, it was found that the frequency spectrum of rare nonsense or missense mutations within these candidate genes varied significantly across studies and ethnicities. Confirmation studies have failed to consistently replicate the association between variants in these genes and prostate cancer, suggesting that these genes likely account for only a small fraction of the observed genetic predisposition to prostate cancer.

A genome-wide linkage scan on 323 prostate cancer families from Iceland identified a suggestive linkage signal (LOD = 2.11) on chromosome 8q24(Amundadottir et al. 2006). Investigators from deCODE genetics then genotyped an additional 358 microsatellite and indel markers spanning the 18.6 cM region on chromosome 8q24 from 125 to 135 Mb, based on NCBI build 24, in 869 unrelated men with prostate cancer and 569 population controls and found a strong association between the microsatellite DG8S737 and prostate cancer ($p = 3.0 \times 10^{-6}$; OR = 1.8). These findings were strongly replicated in four additional case-control samples from different populations: a second population from Iceland ($p = 1.8 \times 10^{-3}$; OR = 1.7), a population from Sweden ($p = 4.5 \times 10^{-3}$; OR = 1.4), a European American population from Illinois ($p = 2.9 \times 10^{-3}$; OR = 2.1), and an African American population from Michigan, ($p = 2.2 \times 10^{-3}$; OR = 1.6). Specifically, the DG8S737 −8 allele was found to be more prevalent in subjects diagnosed with prostate cancer than population controls in all five case-control samples.

7.4.2   Candidate Gene-Based Association Studies
for Prostate Cancer

BRCA1 and *BRCA2* have been studied extensively with respect to risk of prostate
cancer, particularly in families with a history of early-onset breast cancer. Men from
families with germline mutations in *BRCA1* or *BRCA2* are at increased risk for developing prostate cancer (Rosen et al. 2001). The relative risk for mutation carriers compared to noncarriers has been estimated to be between 2 and 5, with a higher risk for
BRCA2 carriers than *BRCA1*(Ford et al. 1994; The Breast Cancer Linkage Consortium
1999; Johannsson et al. 1999). Sequence analysis of *BRCA1* in University of Michigan
prostate cancer probands resulted in no evidence for deleterious mutations segregating
with prostate cancer in high-density prostate cancer pedigrees that linked to 17q;
however, a recent study on University of Michigan prostate cancer families found
some evidence for a common Gln(356)Arg substitution in exon 11 of *BRCA1* being
associated with prostate cancer (Zuhlke et al. 2004; Douglas et al. 2007). Evidence
that *BRCA2* mutations increase the risk for early-onset prostate cancer is presented in
chapter 8, section 8.5. However in total, given the very low frequency of *BRCA1* and
BRCA2 deleterious mutations, together *BRCA1* and *BRCA2* likely explain very little
of the genetic susceptibility to prostate cancer (Sinclair et al. 2000).

Association studies have also been conducted for other genes thought to play
important biological roles in the development of prostate cancer. Candidate gene-
based association studies have been controversial in the history of complex trait
genetics. In a review of 166 putative associations (for any complex trait) that have
been studied three or more times, Hirschhorn and colleagues identified only six that
have been replicated consistently (Hirschhorn et al. 2002). These findings are consistent with results from candidate gene studies in prostate cancer, where genes
such as *AR*, *CYP3A4*, *CYP17*, *SRD5A2,* and *IGF1* have been extensively studied
with mixed results. Some failures to replicate could be due to true differences
between study populations, others are limited by power and design problems, and
many other results are likely false positives subject to publication bias and inadequate control of the overall type I error (failure to account for the number of candidate genes previously studied). Many candidate gene studies rely on assumptions
of gene function and proposed role in development of prostate cancer. As our
understanding of molecular genetic pathways is incomplete, many genes likely to
be associated with prostate cancer have yet to be identified. In addition, empirical
evidence now suggests that many important SNPs associated with complex traits
are not in known genes but are rather in key regulatory regions of the genome.

7.5   Changing Focus

The field of genetics is evolving at an amazing rate. Technological advances in
laboratory science, the increasing availability of low-cost powerful computing, and
the results from the considerable public and private investments in the Human

Genome Project over the past decade have changed the way we search for genetic risk factors for human disease and have significantly improved our ability to find such risk factors.

The Human Genome Project was a 13-year, multibillion-dollar project completed in 2003 that was primarily funded by the U.S. Dept of Energy, U.S. National Institutes of Health (NIH), and the Wellcome Trust (UK)(Lander et al. 2001). Additional contributions were made from the governments of Japan, China, France, Germany, and other nations. Celera, a private company, also completed sequencing the human genome at approximately the same time as the completion of the Human Genome Project. The primary motivation of the Human Genome Project was to provide scientists with powerful new tools to help them understand the molecular etiology of common devastating diseases. The stated goals (see genomics.energy. gov) of the human genome project were to: (1) Identify all the approximately 20,000–25,000 genes in human DNA, (2) Determine the sequences of the 3 billion chemical base pairs that make up human DNA, (3) Store the information in databases, (4) Improve tools for data analysis, (5) Transfer-related technologies to the private sector and (6) Address the ethical, legal, and social issues that result from the project.

The Human Genome Project has identified the location and sequence of genes throughout the human genome but was not designed to catalog the differences in the DNA sequence that make us all unique. The Human Genome Project's sequencing efforts were based on a small number of individuals, and consequently the project was not designed to accurately measure the variability in DNA sequence between humans.

Millions of genetic variants called single nucleotide polymorphisms (SNPs) have been identified in the human genome. SNPs almost always have just two alleles (two different bases from A, C, G, or T) and identify the variability at a single specific base location in the genome in a population. As of August 2008, the dbSNP database (www.ncbi.nlm.nih.gov/SNP) contains 14.7 million SNPs, with 6.6 million of those validated (build 129). Methods to genotype SNPs have improved dramatically in the past several years. Techniques have been developed that allow many SNPs to be genotyped in the same reaction, or multiplexed. Multiplexing has substantially reduced genotyping costs for individually selected SNPs. Importantly, this increased throughput has been accompanied by increased genotype accuracy and completion rates.

While a genomic region may contain many SNPs, often only a relatively few are needed to capture the majority of the genetic variability (for a given population) across the defined region. The reason only a small number of SNPs are necessary to capture the variability in a genomic region is due to linkage disequilibrium (LD), which often occurs between physically close SNPs. Two SNPs are in LD if their genotypes are not independent. The International HapMap project (www.hapmap. org) was established to characterize common genetic variability and linkage disequilibrium patterns, reducing the number of SNPs required to efficiently examine a genomic region (or the entire genome) for association with a trait. The HapMap database contains high-density genotype data for 90 European individuals

(30 parent–parent–child trios from the U.S.A. with northern and western European ancestry) 90 Yoruban individuals (30 trios from Ibadan, Nigeria), 45 unrelated individuals from Tokyo, Japan, and 45 unrelated individuals from Beijing, China. The average SNP density throughout the genome is now more than one SNP every kilobase.

7.6   Genome-Wide Association Studies

Genome-wide association (GWA) studies are a genetic study design in which a sample of cases and controls, or a collection of families, is genotyped for a large number of genetic markers spanning the human genome – usually SNPs due to their relative ease of multiplexing. Unlike the genetic association studies of the past few decades which focused only on specific genes identified by linkage analysis or biological function, the aim of the GWA study design is to capture all common variation across the genome and to relate this variation to disease risk or quantitative measures of interest. It is debatable just how many SNPs are needed to capture the vast majority of variability in the genome (and this number varies across different ethnic populations), but it is conceivable that in the near future all common SNPs will be included on genome-wide SNP panels. Today, commercially available platforms containing 1,000,000 SNPs are commonplace.

GWA studies were made feasible by technological advances yielded by most notably the Human Genome Project (http://genome.ucsc.edu) and the International HapMap Project (http://www.hapmap.org) (Lander et al. 2001; International HapMap Consortium 2005). Using commercial genotyping platforms, the cost per genotype has dropped orders of magnitude in the past decade. Moreover, the principal genotyping products that are currently available provide excellent coverage for most of the human genome, are highly accurate, and are continually improving.

A GWA study is explicitly designed to detect common variants associated with common diseases. When a phenotype, usually Mendelian in nature, is driven by rare highly penetrant mutations then linkage analysis and sequencing are still the preferred approach. GWA studies, initially treated with some skepticism primarily due to cost and power concerns, have proved to be very successful in identifying promising genetic regions associated with disease. Among other successes, GWA scans have identified SNPs associated with traits such as age-related macular degeneration, inflammatory bowel disease, type 1 diabetes, Crohn's disease, bipolar disorder, rheumatoid arthritis, coronary artery diseases, type 2 diabetes, episodic memory, obesity, breast cancer, colorectal cancer, and prostate cancer (Klein et al. 2005; Duerr et al. 2006; Wellcome Trust Case Control Consortium 2007; Sladek et al. 2007; Papassotiropoulos et al. 2006; Herbert et al. 2006; Easton et al. 2007; Hunter et al. 2007; Tomlinson et al. 2007; Zanke et al. 2007; Yeager et al. 2007; Gudmundsson et al. 2007a; Gudmundsson et al. 2007b; Eeles et al. 2008). In almost all instances to date, the SNPs identified and their associated genes/genomic regions were not previously thought to play a role in the phenotype under study.

GWA studies are complex but have the enormous potential to add considerably more insight into the genetic etiology of complex traits than candidate gene association studies. GWA studies provide a relatively unbiased screening of the human genome in terms of location and can lead to the discovery of new hypotheses about previously unsuspected genetic variants whose frequencies substantially differ between those with and without the phenotype under study. GWA studies are predicated upon the idea that our hypotheses about the etiology of medical disorders are relatively incomplete and that susceptibility may be due to genomic regions not previously considered. The scale of GWA studies is massive and they are still relatively costly compared to small candidate gene association studies. Consideration must be given whether it is more appropriate to follow up existing GWA study results or to conduct a new GWA studies. Should one decide to conduct a GWA study, considerable care must be taken to ensure an appropriate study design, maintain strict quality control, and utilize a sound analytic strategy.

GWA studies for prostate cancer, while only conducted in earnest recently, have enjoyed excellent success in identifying common genetic variants that are associated with the disease. These results, summarized in another chapter in this book (Chap. 8, Sect. 8.4), represent an exciting development for prostate cancer research. I will spend the remainder of this chapter briefly describing a few alternative genetic association study designs, paying particular attention to the utility of prostate cancer cases identified and collected from hereditary prostate cancer families.

7.7 Sample Selection Strategies for Genetic Association Studies

Two fundamentally different study designs are used in genetic association studies for qualitative trails: designs that use unrelated individuals (case-control, cohort, and case-cohort studies) and those that use families. Both study designs have their strengths and weaknesses.

7.7.1 Case-Control and Cohort Designs

Most genetic association studies are case-control or cohort studies of unrelated individuals. Cohort studies typically involve following up a large sample of unrelated individuals, without disease at baseline, for a long period of time. In order to have sufficient statistical power, cohort studies typically must follow an identified set of individuals for a long period of time. Because tracking large numbers of individuals for a long period of time can be expensive, cohort studies are often initiated in older populations containing individuals that are at greatest risk for the disease of interest.

Case-control studies are often more economically palatable than cohort studies. Case-control selection strategies vary considerably across studies. Prostate cancer association studies have been performed using a variety of case populations including population-based cases, family-based cases, cases with early-onset disease, and cases with aggressive disease. A wide range of controls have also been used including unscreened controls, PSA screened controls, and elderly controls. Several theoretical and simulation studies have demonstrated that greater power can be achieved in genetic case-control association studies by selecting cases from families with multiple cases over selecting unrelated cases with no family history of the disease (Risch and Teng 1998; Risch 2001; Fingerlin et al. 2004; Li et al. 2006). Empirical results from prostate cancer genetic association studies support these conclusions. Specifically, stronger evidence for prostate cancer association with 8q24 variants was observed when using cases from high-density hereditary prostate cancer families than when using unrelated prostate cancer cases collected independent of family history in a study from John Hopkins University (Sun et al. 2008). A recently completed GWA study for prostate cancer using early-onset disease cases diagnosed prior to age 61 or cases with a family history of disease was tremendously successful in not only strongly replicating the results from previous GWA studies (namely, variants associated with prostate cancer on 8q and 17q) but also in identifying a number of new regions that harbor genetic variants significantly associated with the disease (Eeles et al. 2008). These studies demonstrate the considerable power that can be gained by studying cases, such as those collected through linkage studies, which are enriched for carrying genetic susceptibility variants.

7.7.2 Controlling False-Positive Results Due to Population Stratification

Population stratification is a phenomenon in genetic association studies where differences in allele or genotype frequencies at a particular polymorphism between a sample of cases and controls are due to systematic differences in ethnic origins between the two samples, rather than a real effect of the variation at the polymorphism on disease risk. Allele frequencies for SNPs in the human genome vary considerably across different ethnic populations. Risk for some diseases such as prostate cancer varies considerably across different ethnic groups. Analytical methods and study designs that address subtle and complex population stratification are necessary to address the problems in genetic association studies caused by this phenomenon.

Several methods have been described to account for population stratification in genetic association studies. These methods include genomic control, structured association, and principal components' analysis (Devlin and Roeder 1999; Pritchard and Rosenberg 1999; Pritchard et al. 2000; Price et al. 2006). Genomic control corrects for population stratification by adjusting association test statistics at each marker by a uniform inflation factor determined by evaluating the distribution of test statistics across all markers. Structured association uses a Bayesian clustering algorithm to assign individuals to subpopulations and then performs association analyses conditional on the inferred assignments. Principal components analysis is a data reduction method designed to capture most of the variability across all SNPs using a relatively small number of independent continuous variables. Critical to the validity of case-control genetic association study results is the ability of analytic methods to account for population stratification, particularly for SNPs in regions of selection. Results from numerous association studies that have used analytic methods to control for population stratification have demonstrated good control of systematic type I errors. However, it is important to note that if the causal polymorphisms are highly associated with underlying population structure (e.g., because of natural selection), it will be difficult to distinguish between true and false positives statistically, and any attempt to remove the population structure will reduce the power to detect truly associated markers.

7.7.3   Family-Based Association Studies

The recognition of population stratification as a concern in genetic association studies led to an alternative study design, based on family data, for genetic association studies. Family-based association methods evaluate whether particular alleles are transmitted from parents down to affected offspring in a proportion that is different than expectation under the null hypothesis of no association between marker and disease. Because these methods utilize nontransmitted alleles from the same parents as the control sample, these methods are not susceptible to population stratification. Family-based association methods were originally proposed for a parent–parent-affected offspring design, but have been extended to include siblings discordant for the disease under study and general family-designs (Spielman et al. 1993; Spielman and Ewens 1998; Lake et al. 2000). Since many of the diseases of interest typically have a late age of onset, the consequential unavailability of parents has made these more general forms of the transmission disequilibrium test popular.

While family-based study designs offer protection from false positives due to population stratification, they have not been the design of choice for genetic association studies due to the higher costs associated with collecting family-based samples. In addition, case-control studies have greater statistical power than family-based studies when comparing samples of the same size. Many family-based samples have already been collected through linkage studies; thus, the additional cost of collecting these family-based samples is often not a major concern. However, the additional costs associated with having to genotype a significantly larger number of samples to achieve equivalent power still likely renders performing large-scale genetic association studies using family-based association methods (even on previously collected samples) inefficient. Given the continuing concerns of population stratification, family-based association methods still have value for validating specific association results from case-control association studies.

7.8   Conclusions

Family-based samples have played an important role in understanding the genetic etiology of prostate cancer. Initially, these samples were used to gain a basic understanding of the overall genetic risk of diseases such as prostate cancer through twin and segregation-analysis studies. Family-based samples were subsequently collected for linkage studies to identify chromosomal regions that harbor rare but highly penetrant genetic variants or mutations that dramatically increase risk for disease. The search for highly penetrant prostate cancer genes through linkage analysis has been somewhat disappointing. Simply put, we have not yet identified any genes that can compare to the impact of *BRCA1* and *BRCA2* in breast cancer through our linkage study efforts, and it is looking increasingly unlikely that any such major impact genes exists for prostate cancer. Still, there are a number of promising regions that have been identified by linkage studies. Fine-mapping efforts for finding these genes may be aided by the addition of new prostate cancer families. One of the biggest obstacles for identifying relatively rare but highly penetrant prostate cancer genes in candidate regions identified by linkage analysis is the prohibitive cost of large-scale sequence analysis. The expense of sequence analysis is expected to come down dramatically in the next decade, and this decrease in cost could reinvigorate efforts to find high penetrant genes for diseases such as prostate cancer. In the meantime, genetic association studies for common, but less penetrant, genetic variants are the current study design of choice for diseases like prostate cancer. Contrary to linkage analysis, excellent success has been achieved in identifying these common variants.

A number of genetic variants have been found to be associated with prostate cancer across multiple studies. While this success will provide some insights into the genetic etiology of prostate cancer, it is unclear how useful these identified variants will be from a clinical perspective given their very modest impact on disease risk. It will be particularly important to evaluate the role of these common susceptibility markers, identified primarily using nonfamilial cases, in hereditary prostate cancer. Individuals with a strong family history of a disease are the individuals that are most likely to seek genetic counseling and subsequent genotyping for genetic risk factors for that disease. Evaluating the role of common variants in hereditary prostate cancer families will be critical in determining whether an accumulation of common risk variants is responsible for hereditary prostate cancer or whether there exist a number of yet to be identified rare, but high penetrant, mutations that explains the significant clustering of the disease within families.

References

Amundadottir LT, Sulem P, Gudmundsson J, Helgason A, Baker A, Agnarsson BA, Sigurdsson A, Benediktsdottir KR, Cazier JB, Sainz J, Jakobsdottir M, Kostic J, Magnusdottir DN, Ghosh S, Agnarsson K, Birgisdottir B, Le RL, Olafsdottir A, Blondal T, Andresdottir M, Gretarsdottir

OS, Bergthorsson JT, Gudbjartsson D, Gylfason A, Thorleifsson G, Manolescu A, Kristjansson K, Geirsson G, Isaksson H, Douglas J, Johansson JE, Balter K, Wiklund F, Montie JE, Yu X, Suarez BK, Ober C, Cooney KA, Gronberg H, Catalona WJ, Einarsson GV, Barkardottir RB, Gulcher JR, Kong A, Thorsteinsdottir U, Stefansson K (2006) A common variant associated with prostate cancer in European and African populations. Nat Genet 38(6):652–658

Bastacky SI, Wojno KJ, Walsh PC, Carmichael MJ, Epstein JI (1995) Pathological features of hereditary prostate cancer. J Urol 153:987–992

Bostwick DG, Burke HB, Djakiew D, Euling S, Ho SM, Landolph J, Morrison H, Sonawane B, Shifflett T, Waters DJ, Timms B (2004) Human prostate cancer risk factors. Cancer 101:2371–2490

Bratt O (2002) Hereditary prostate cancer: clinical aspects. J Urol 168:906–913

Bratt O, Damber JE, Emanuelsson M, Gronberg H (2002) Hereditary prostate cancer: clinical characteristics and survival. J Urol 167:2423–2426

Carpten J, Nupponen N, Isaacs S, Sood R, Robbins C, Xu J, Faruque M, Moses T, Ewing C, Gillanders E, Hu P, Bujnovszky P, Makalowska I, Baffoe-Bonnie A, Faith D, Smith J, Stephan D, Wiley K, Brownstein M, Gildea D, Kelly B, Jenkins R, Hostetter G, Matikainen M, Schleutker J, Klinger K, Connors T, Xiang Y, Wang Z, De MA, Papadopoulos N, Kallioniemi OP, Burk R, Meyers D, Gronberg H, Meltzer P, Silverman R, Bailey-Wilson J, Walsh P, Isaacs W, Trent J (2002) Germline mutations in the ribonuclease L gene in families showing linkage with HPC1. Nat Genet 30:181–184

Carter BS, Beaty TH, Steinberg GD, Childs B, Walsh PC (1992) Mendelian inheritance of familial prostate cancer. Proc Natl Acad Sci U S A 89:3367–3371

Cavalli-Sforza LL, King MC (1986) Detecting linkage for genetically heterogeneous diseases and detecting heterogeneity with linkage data. Am J Hum Genet 38:599–616

Devlin B, Roeder K (1999) Genomic control for association studies. Biometrics 55:997–1004

Douglas JA, Levin AM, Zuhlke KA, Ray AM, Johnson GR, Lange EM, Wood DP, Cooney KA (2007) Common variation in the BRCA1 gene and prostate cancer risk. Cancer Epidemiol Biomarkers Prev 16:1510–1516

Duerr RH, Taylor KD, Brant SR, Rioux JD, Silverberg MS, Daly MJ, Steinhart AH, Abraham C, Regueiro M, Griffiths A, Dassopoulos T, Bitton A, Yang H, Targan S, Datta LW, Kistner EO, Schumm LP, Lee AT, Gregersen PK, Barmada MM, Rotter JI, Nicolae DL, Cho JH (2006) A genome-wide association study identifies IL23R as an inflammatory bowel disease gene. Science 314:1461–1463

Easton DF, Pooley KA, Dunning AM, Pharoah PD, Thompson D, Ballinger DG, Struewing JP, Morrison J, Field H, Luben R, Wareham N, Ahmed S, Healey CS, Bowman R, Meyer KB, Haiman CA, Kolonel LK, Henderson BE, Le ML, Brennan P, Sangrajrang S, Gaborieau V, Odefrey F, Shen CY, Wu PE, Wang HC, Eccles D, Evans DG, Peto J, Fletcher O, Johnson N, Seal S, Stratton MR, Rahman N, Chenevix-Trench G, Bojesen SE, Nordestgaard BG, Axelsson CK, Garcia-Closas M, Brinton L, Chanock S, Lissowska J, Peplonska B, Nevanlinna H, Fagerholm R, Eerola H, Kang D, Yoo KY, Noh DY, Ahn SH, Hunter DJ, Hankinson SE, Cox DG, Hall P, Wedren S, Liu J, Low YL, Bogdanova N, Schurmann P, Dork T, Tollenaar RA, Jacobi CE, Devilee P, Klijn JG, Sigurdson AJ, Doody MM, Alexander BH, Zhang J, Cox A, Brock IW, MacPherson G, Reed MW, Couch FJ, Goode EL, Olson JE, Meijers-Heijboer H, van den OA, Uitterlinden A, Rivadeneira F, Milne RL, Ribas G, Gonzalez-Neira A, Benitez J, Hopper JL, McCredie M, Southey M, Giles GG, Schroen C, Justenhoven C, Brauch H, Hamann U, Ko YD, Spurdle AB, Beesley J, Chen X, Mannermaa A, Kosma VM, Kataja V, Hartikainen J, Day NE, Cox DR, Ponder BA (2007) Genome-wide association study identifies novel breast cancer susceptibility loci. Nature 447:1087–1093

Eeles RA, Kote-Jarai Z, Giles GG, Olama AA, Guy M, Jugurnauth SK, Mulholland S, Leongamornlert DA, Edwards SM, Morrison J, Field HI, Southey MC, Severi G, Donovan JL, Hamdy FC, Dearnaley DP, Muir KR, Smith C, Bagnato M, rdern-Jones AT, Hall AL, O'Brien LT, Gehr-Swain BN, Wilkinson RA, Cox A, Lewis S, Brown PM, Jhavar SG, Tymrakiewicz M, Lophatananon A, Bryant SL, Horwich A, Huddart RA, Khoo VS, Parker CC, Woodhouse CJ, Thompson A, Christmas T, Ogden C, Fisher C, Jamieson C, Cooper CS, English DR,

Hopper JL, Neal DE, Easton DF (2008) Multiple newly identified loci associated with prostate cancer susceptibility. Nat Genet 40:316–321

Fingerlin TE, Boehnke M, Abecasis GR (2004) Increasing the power and efficiency of disease-marker case-control association studies through use of allele-sharing information. Am J Hum Genet 74:432–443

Ford D, Easton DF, Bishop DT, Narod SA, Goldgar DE (1994) Risks of cancer in BRCA1-mutation carriers. Breast Cancer Linkage Consortium. Lancet 343:692–695

Gatti RA, Berkel I, Boder E, Braedt G, Charmley P, Concannon P, Ersoy F, Foroud T, Jaspers NG, Lange K et al (1988) Localization of an ataxia–telangiectasia gene to chromosome 11q22-23. Nature 336:577–580

Gudmundsson J, Sulem P, Manolescu A, Amundadottir LT, Gudbjartsson D, Helgason A, Rafnar T, Bergthorsson JT, Agnarsson BA, Baker A, Sigurdsson A, Benediktsdottir KR, Jakobsdottir M, Xu J, Blondal T, Kostic J, Sun J, Ghosh S, Stacey SN, Mouy M, Saemundsdottir J, Backman VM, Kristjansson K, Tres A, Partin AW, bers-Akkers MT, Godino-Ivan MJ, Walsh PC, Swinkels DW, Navarrete S, Isaacs SD, Aben KK, Graif T, Cashy J, Ruiz-Echarri M, Wiley KE, Suarez BK, Witjes JA, Frigge M, Ober C, Jonsson E, Einarsson GV, Mayordomo JI, Kiemeney LA, Isaacs WB, Catalona WJ, Barkardottir RB, Gulcher JR, Thorsteinsdottir U, Kong A, Stefansson K (2007a) Genome-wide association study identifies a second prostate cancer susceptibility variant at 8q24. Nat Genet 39:631–637

Gudmundsson J, Sulem P, Steinthorsdottir V, Bergthorsson JT, Thorleifsson G, Manolescu A, Rafnar T, Gudbjartsson D, Agnarsson BA, Baker A, Sigurdsson A, Benediktsdottir KR, Jakobsdottir M, Blondal T, Stacey SN, Helgason A, Gunnarsdottir S, Olafsdottir A, Kristinsson KT, Birgisdottir B, Ghosh S, Thorlacius S, Magnusdottir D, Stefansdottir G, Kristjansson K, Bagger Y, Wilensky RL, Reilly MP, Morris AD, Kimber CH, Adeyemo A, Chen Y, Zhou J, So WY, Tong PC, Ng MC, Hansen T, Andersen G, Borch-Johnsen K, Jorgensen T, Tres A, Fuertes F, Ruiz-Echarri M, Asin L, Saez B, Van BE, Klaver S, Swinkels DW, Aben KK, Graif T, Cashy J, Suarez BK, van Vierssen TO, Frigge ML, Ober C, Hofker MH, Wijmenga C, Christiansen C, Rader DJ, Palmer CN, Rotimi C, Chan JC, Pedersen O, Sigurdsson G, Benediktsson R, Jonsson E, Einarsson GV, Mayordomo JI, Catalona WJ, Kiemeney LA, Barkardottir RB, Gulcher JR, Thorsteinsdottir U, Kong A, Stefansson K (2007b) Two variants on chromosome 17 confer prostate cancer risk, and the one in TCF2 protects against type 2 diabetes. Nat Genet 39:977–983

Guo SW (1998) Inflation of sibling recurrence-risk ratio, due to ascertainment bias and/or over-reporting. Am J Hum Genet 63:252–258

Hayes RB, Liff JM, Pottern LM, Greenberg RS, Schoenberg JB, Schwartz AG, Swanson GM, Silverman DT, Brown LM, Hoover RN (1995) Prostate cancer risk in U.S. blacks and whites with a family history of cancer. Int J Cancer 60:361–364

Herbert A, Gerry NP, McQueen MB, Heid IM, Pfeufer A, Illig T, Wichmann HE, Meitinger T, Hunter D, Hu FB, Colditz G, Hinney A, Hebebrand J, Koberwitz K, Zhu X, Cooper R, Ardlie K, Lyon H, Hirschhorn JN, Laird NM, Lenburg ME, Lange C, Christman MF (2006) A common genetic variant is associated with adult and childhood obesity. Science 312:279–283

Hirschhorn JN, Lohmueller K, Byrne E, Hirschhorn K (2002) A comprehensive review of genetic association studies. Genet Med 4:45–61

Hunter DJ, Kraft P, Jacobs KB, Cox DG, Yeager M, Hankinson SE, Wacholder S, Wang Z, Welch R, Hutchinson A, Wang J, Yu K, Chatterjee N, Orr N, Willett WC, Colditz GA, Ziegler RG, Berg CD, Buys SS, McCarty CA, Feigelson HS, Calle EE, Thun MJ, Hayes RB, Tucker M, Gerhard DS, Fraumeni JF Jr, Hoover RN, Thomas G, Chanock SJ (2007) A genome-wide association study identifies alleles in FGFR2 associated with risk of sporadic postmenopausal breast cancer. Nat Genet 39:870–874

International HapMap Consortium (2005) A haplotype map of the human genome. Nature 437:1299–1320

Isaacs SD, Kiemeney LA, Baffoe-Bonnie A, Beaty TH, Walsh PC (1995) Risk of cancer in relatives of prostate cancer probands. J Natl Cancer Inst 87:991–996

Jemal A, Siegel R, Ward E, Hao Y, Xu J, Murray T, Thun MJ (2008) Cancer statistics, 2008. CA Cancer J Clin 58:71–96

Johannsson O, Loman N, Moller T, Kristoffersson U, Borg A, Olsson H (1999) Incidence of malignant tumours in relatives of BRCA1 and BRCA2 germline mutation carriers. Eur J Cancer 35:1248–1257

Keetch DW, Humphrey PA, Smith DS, Stahl D, Catalona WJ (1996) Clinical and pathological features of hereditary prostate cancer. J Urol 155:1841–1843

Klein R, Klein BE, Knudtson MD (2005) Frailty and age-related macular degeneration: the Beaver Dam Eye Study. Am J Ophthalmol 140:129–131

Kong A, Cox NJ (1997) Allele-sharing models: LOD scores and accurate linkage tests. Am J Hum Genet 61:1179–1188

Lake SL, Blacker D, Laird NM (2000) Family-based tests of association in the presence of linkage. Am J Hum Genet 67:1515–1525

Lander ES, Linton LM, Birren B, Nusbaum C, Zody MC, Baldwin J, Devon K, Dewar K, Doyle M, FitzHugh W, Funke R, Gage D, Harris K, Heaford A, Howland J, Kann L, Lehoczky J, LeVine R, McEwan P, McKernan K, Meldrim J, Mesirov JP, Miranda C, Morris W, Naylor J, Raymond C, Rosetti M, Santos R, Sheridan A, Sougnez C, Stange-Thomann N, Stojanovic N, Subramanian A, Wyman D, Rogers J, Sulston J, Ainscough R, Beck S, Bentley D, Burton J, Clee C, Carter N, Coulson A, Deadman R, Deloukas P, Dunham A, Dunham I, Durbin R, French L, Grafham D, Gregory S, Hubbard T, Humphray S, Hunt A, Jones M, Lloyd C, McMurray A, Matthews L, Mercer S, Milne S, Mullikin JC, Mungall A, Plumb R, Ross M, Shownkeen R, Sims S, Waterston RH, Wilson RK, Hillier LW, McPherson JD, Marra MA, Mardis ER, Fulton LA, Chinwalla AT, Pepin KH, Gish WR, Chissoe SL, Wendl MC, Delehaunty KD, Miner TL, Delehaunty A, Kramer JB, Cook LL, Fulton RS, Johnson DL, Minx PJ, Clifton SW, Hawkins T, Branscomb E, Predki P, Richardson P, Wenning S, Slezak T, Doggett N, Cheng JF, Olsen A, Lucas S, Elkin C, Uberbacher E, Frazier M, Gibbs RA, Muzny DM, Scherer SE, Bouck JB, Sodergren EJ, Worley KC, Rives CM, Gorrell JH, Metzker ML, Naylor SL, Kucherlapati RS, Nelson DL, Weinstock GM, Sakaki Y, Fujiyama A, Hattori M, Yada T, Toyoda A, Itoh T, Kawagoe C, Watanabe H, Totoki Y, Taylor T, Weissenbach J, Heilig R, Saurin W, Artiguenave F, Brottier P, Bruls T, Pelletier E, Robert C, Wincker P, Smith DR, Doucette-Stamm L, Rubenfield M, Weinstock K, Lee HM, Dubois J, Rosenthal A, Platzer M, Nyakatura G, Taudien S, Rump A, Yang H, Yu J, Wang J, Huang G, Gu J, Hood L, Rowen L, Madan A, Qin S, Davis RW, Federspiel NA, Abola AP, Proctor MJ, Myers RM, Schmutz J, Dickson M, Grimwood J, Cox DR, Olson MV, Kaul R, Raymond C, Shimizu N, Kawasaki K, Minoshima S, Evans GA, Athanasiou M, Schultz R, Roe BA, Chen F, Pan H, Ramser J, Lehrach H, Reinhardt R, McCombie WR, Dela BM, Dedhia N, Blocker H, Hornischer K, Nordsiek G, Agarwala R, Aravind L, Bailey JA, Bateman A, Batzoglou S, Birney E, Bork P, Brown DG, Burge CB, Cerutti L, Chen HC, Church D, Clamp M, Copley RR, Doerks T, Eddy SR, Eichler EE, Furey TS, Galagan J, Gilbert JG, Harmon C, Hayashizaki Y, Haussler D, Hermjakob H, Hokamp K, Jang W, Johnson LS, Jones TA, Kasif S, Kaspryzk A, Kennedy S, Kent WJ, Kitts P, Koonin EV, Korf I, Kulp D, Lancet D, Lowe TM, McLysaght A, Mikkelsen T, Moran JV, Mulder N, Pollara VJ, Ponting CP, Schuler G, Schultz J, Slater G, Smit AF, Stupka E, Szustakowski J, Thierry-Mieg D, Thierry-Mieg J, Wagner L, Wallis J, Wheeler R, Williams A, Wolf YI, Wolfe KH, Yang SP, Yeh RF, Collins F, Guyer MS, Peterson J, Felsenfeld A, Wetterstrand KA, Patrinos A, Morgan MJ, De JP, Catanese JJ, Osoegawa K, Shizuya H, Choi S, Chen YJ (2001) Initial sequencing and analysis of the human genome. Nature 409:860–921

Langbehn DR, Brinkman RR, Falush D, Paulsen JS, Hayden MR (2004) A new model for prediction of the age of onset and penetrance for Huntington's disease based on CAG length. Clin Genet 65:267–277

Lange E, Borresen AL, Chen X, Chessa L, Chiplunkar S, Concannon P, Dandekar S, Gerken S, Lange K, Liang T et al (1995) Localization of an ataxia–telangiectasia gene to an approximately 500-kb interval on chromosome 11q23.1: linkage analysis of 176 families by an international consortium. Am J Hum Genet 57:112–119

Lange EM, Ho LA, Beebe-Dimmer JL, Wang Y, Gillanders EM, Trent JM, Lange LA, Wood DP, Cooney KA (2006) Genome-wide linkage scan for prostate cancer susceptibility genes in men with aggressive disease: significant evidence for linkage at chromosome 15q12. Hum Genet 119:400–407

Li M, Boehnke M, Abecasis GR (2006) Efficient study designs for test of genetic association using sibship data and unrelated cases and controls. Am J Hum Genet 78:778–792

Lichtenstein P, Holm NV, Verkasalo PK, Iliadou A, Kaprio J, Koskenvuo M, Pukkala E, Skytthe A, Hemminki K (2000) Environmental and heritable factors in the causation of cancer–analyses of cohorts of twins from Sweden, Denmark, and Finland. N Engl J Med 343:78–85

Neville PJ, Conti DV, Krumroy LM, Catalona WJ, Suarez BK, Witte JS, Casey G (2003) Prostate cancer aggressiveness locus on chromosome segment 19q12-q13.1 identified by linkage and allelic imbalance studies. Genes Chromosomes Cancer 36:332–339

Page WF, Braun MM, Partin AW, Caporaso N, Walsh P (1997) Heredity and prostate cancer: a study of World War II veteran twins. Prostate 33:240–245

Papassotiropoulos A, Stephan DA, Huentelman MJ, Hoerndli FJ, Craig DW, Pearson JV, Huynh KD, Brunner F, Corneveaux J, Osborne D, Wollmer MA, Aerni A, Coluccia D, Hanggi J, Mondadori CR, Buchmann A, Reiman EM, Caselli RJ, Henke K, de Quervain DJ (2006) Common Kibra alleles are associated with human memory performance. Science 314:475–478

Price AL, Patterson NJ, Plenge RM, Weinblatt ME, Shadick NA, Reich D (2006) Principal components analysis corrects for stratification in genome-wide association studies. Nat Genet 38:904–909

Pritchard JK, Rosenberg NA (1999) Use of unlinked genetic markers to detect population stratification in association studies. Am J Hum Genet 65:220–228

Pritchard JK, Stephens M, Donnelly P (2000) Inference of population structure using multilocus genotype data. Genetics 155:945–959

Risch N (1990) Linkage strategies for genetically complex traits II. The power of affected relative pairs. Am J Hum Genet 46:229–241

Risch NJ (2000) Searching for genetic determinants in the new millennium. Nature 405:847–856

Risch N (2001) Implications of multilocus inheritance for gene-disease association studies. Theor Popul Biol 60:215–220

Risch N, Teng J (1998) The relative power of family-based and case-control designs for linkage disequilibrium studies of complex human diseases I DNA pooling. Genome Res 8:1273–1288

Rosen EM, Fan S, Goldberg ID (2001) BRCA1 and prostate cancer. Cancer Invest 19:396–412

Savitsky K, Bar-Shira A, Gilad S, Rotman G, Ziv Y, Vanagaite L, Tagle DA, Smith S, Uziel T, Sfez S, Ashkenazi M, Pecker I, Frydman M, Harnik R, Patanjali SR, Simmons A, Clines GA, Sartiel A, Gatti RA, Chessa L, Sanal O, Lavin MF, Jaspers NG, Taylor AM, Arlett CF, Miki T, Weissman SM, Lovett M, Collins FS, Shiloh Y (1995) A single ataxia telangiectasia gene with a product similar to PI-3 kinase. Science 268:1749–1753

Schaid DJ (2004) The complex genetic epidemiology of prostate cancer. Hum Mol Genet 13(Spec No 1):R103–R121

Schaid DJ, McDonnell SK, Zarfas KE, Cunningham JM, Hebbring S, Thibodeau SN, Eeles RA, Easton DF, Foulkes WD, Simard J, Giles GG, Hopper JL, Mahle L, Moller P, Badzioch M, Bishop DT, Evans C, Edwards S, Meitz J, Bullock S, Hope Q, Guy M, Hsieh CL, Halpern J, Balise RR, Oakley-Girvan I, Whittemore AS, Xu J, Dimitrov L, Chang BL, Adams TS, Turner AR, Meyers DA, Friedrichsen DM, Deutsch K, Kolb S, Janer M, Hood L, Ostrander EA, Stanford JL, Ewing CM, Gielzak M, Isaacs SD, Walsh PC, Wiley KE, Isaacs WB, Lange EM, Ho LA, Beebe-Dimmer JL, Wood DP, Cooney KA, Seminara D, Ikonen T, Baffoe-Bonnie A, Fredriksson H, Matikainen MP, Tammela TL, Bailey-Wilson J, Schleutker J, Maier C, Herkommer K, Hoegel JJ, Vogel W, Paiss T, Wiklund F, Emanuelsson M, Stenman E, Jonsson BA, Gronberg H, Camp NJ, Farnham J, Cannon-Albright LA, Catalona WJ, Suarez BK, Roehl KA (2006) Pooled genome linkage scan of aggressive prostate cancer: results from the International Consortium for Prostate Cancer Genetics. Hum Genet 120:471–485

Schaid DJ, Stanford JL, McDonnell SK, Suuriniemi M, McIntosh L, Karyadi DM, Carlson EE, Deutsch K, Janer M, Hood L, Ostrander EA (2007) Genome-wide linkage scan of prostate cancer Gleason score and confirmation of chromosome 19q. Hum Genet 121:729–735

Sinclair CS, Berry R, Schaid D, Thibodeau SN, Couch FJ (2000) BRCA1 and BRCA2 have a limited role in familial prostate cancer. Cancer Res 60:1371–1375

Sladek R, Rocheleau G, Rung J, Dina C, Shen L, Serre D, Boutin P, Vincent D, Belisle A, Hadjadj S, Balkau B, Heude B, Charpentier G, Hudson TJ, Montpetit A, Pshezhetsky AV, Prentki M, Posner BI, Balding DJ, Meyre D, Polychronakos C, Froguel P (2007) A genome-wide association study identifies novel risk loci for type 2 diabetes. Nature 445:881–885

Slager SL, Schaid DJ, Cunningham JM, McDonnell SK, Marks AF, Peterson BJ, Hebbring SJ, Anderson S, French AJ, Thibodeau SN (2003) Confirmation of linkage of prostate cancer aggressiveness with chromosome 19q. Am J Hum Genet 72:759–762

Spielman RS, Ewens WJ (1998) A sibship test for linkage in the presence of association: the sib transmission/disequilibrium test. Am J Hum Genet 62:450–458

Spielman RS, McGinnis RE, Ewens WJ (1993) Transmission test for linkage disequilibrium: the insulin gene region and insulin-dependent diabetes mellitus (IDDM). Am J Hum Genet 52:506–516

Steinberg GD, Carter BS, Beaty TH, Childs B, Walsh PC (1990) Family history and the risk of prostate cancer. Prostate 17:337–347

Sun J, Lange EM, Isaacs SD, Liu W, Wiley KE, Lange L, Gronberg H, Duggan D, Carpten JD, Walsh PC, Xu J, Chang BL, Isaacs WB, Zheng SL (2008) Chromosome 8q24 risk variants in hereditary and non-hereditary prostate cancer patients. Prostate 68:489–497

Tavtigian SV, Simard J, Teng DH, Abtin V, Baumgard M, Beck A, Camp NJ, Carillo AR, Chen Y, Dayananth P, Desrochers M, Dumont M, Farnham JM, Frank D, Frye C, Ghaffari S, Gupte JS, Hu R, Iliev D, Janecki T, Kort EN, Laity KE, Leavitt A, Leblanc G, rthur-Morrison J, Pederson A, Penn B, Peterson KT, Reid JE, Richards S, Schroeder M, Smith R, Snyder SC, Swedlund B, Swensen J, Thomas A, Tranchant M, Woodland AM, Labrie F, Skolnick MH, Neuhausen S, Rommens J, Cannon-Albright LA (2001) A candidate prostate cancer susceptibility gene at chromosome 17p. Nat Genet 27:172–180

The Breast Cancer Linkage Consortium (1999) Cancer risks in BRCA2 mutation carriers. The Breast Cancer Linkage Consortium. J Natl Cancer Inst 91:1310–1316

Tomlinson I, Webb E, Carvajal-Carmona L, Broderick P, Kemp Z, Spain S, Penegar S, Chandler I, Gorman M, Wood W, Barclay E, Lubbe S, Martin L, Sellick G, Jaeger E, Hubner R, Wild R, Rowan A, Fielding S, Howarth K, Silver A, Atkin W, Muir K, Logan R, Kerr D, Johnstone E, Sieber O, Gray R, Thomas H, Peto J, Cazier JB, Houlston R (2007) A genome-wide association scan of tag SNPs identifies a susceptibility variant for colorectal cancer at 8q24.21. Nat Genet 39:984–988

Valeri A, Azzouzi R, Drelon E, Delannoy A, Mangin P, Fournier G, Berthon P, Cussenot O (2000) Early-onset hereditary prostate cancer is not associated with specific clinical and biological features. Prostate 45:66–71

Wellcome Trust Case Control Consortium (2007) Genome-wide association study of 14,000 cases of seven common diseases and 3,000 shared controls. Nature 447:661–678

Whittemore AS, Halpern J (1994) A class of tests for linkage using affected pedigree members. Biometrics 50:118–127

Whittemore AS, Wu AH, Kolonel LN, John EM, Gallagher RP, Howe GR, West DW, Teh CZ, Stamey T (1995) Family history and prostate cancer risk in black, white, and Asian men in the United States and Canada. Am J Epidemiol 141:732–740

Witte JS, Goddard KA, Conti DV, Elston RC, Lin J, Suarez BK, Broman KW, Burmester JK, Weber JL, Catalona WJ (2000) Genomewide scan for prostate cancer-aggressiveness loci. Am J Hum Genet 67:92–99

Xu J, Zheng SL, Komiya A, Mychaleckyj JC, Isaacs SD, Chang B, Turner AR, Ewing CM, Wiley KE, Hawkins GA, Bleecker ER, Walsh PC, Meyers DA, Isaacs WB (2003) Common sequence variants of the macrophage scavenger receptor 1 gene are associated with prostate cancer risk. Am J Hum Genet 72:208–212

Xu J, Dimitrov L, Chang BL, Adams TS, Turner AR, Meyers DA, Eeles RA, Easton DF, Foulkes WD, Simard J, Giles GG, Hopper JL, Mahle L, Moller P, Bishop T, Evans C, Edwards S, Meitz J, Bullock S, Hope Q, Hsieh CL, Halpern J, Balise RN, Oakley-Girvan I, Whittemore AS, Ewing CM, Gielzak M, Isaacs SD, Walsh PC, Wiley KE, Isaacs WB, Thibodeau SN, McDonnell SK, Cunningham JM, Zarfas KE, Hebbring S, Schaid DJ, Friedrichsen DM, Deutsch K, Kolb S, Badzioch M, Jarvik GP, Janer M, Hood L, Ostrander EA, Stanford JL, Lange EM, Beebe-Dimmer JL, Mohai CE, Cooney KA, Ikonen T, Baffoe-Bonnie A, Fredriksson H, Matikainen MP, Tammela TL, Bailey-Wilson J, Schleutker J, Maier C, Herkommer K, Hoegel JJ, Vogel W, Paiss T, Wiklund F, Emanuelsson M, Stenman E, Jonsson BA, Gronberg H, Camp NJ, Farnham J, Cannon-Albright LA, Seminara D (2005) A combined genomewide linkage scan of 1, 233 families for prostate cancer-susceptibility genes conducted by the international consortium for prostate cancer genetics. Am J Hum Genet 77:219–229

Yeager M, Orr N, Hayes RB, Jacobs KB, Kraft P, Wacholder S, Minichiello MJ, Fearnhead P, Yu K, Chatterjee N, Wang Z, Welch R, Staats BJ, Calle EE, Feigelson HS, Thun MJ, Rodriguez C, Albanes D, Virtamo J, Weinstein S, Schumacher FR, Giovannucci E, Willett WC, Cancel-Tassin G, Cussenot O, Valeri A, Andriole GL, Gelmann EP, Tucker M, Gerhard DS, Fraumeni JF Jr, Hoover R, Hunter DJ, Chanock SJ, Thomas G (2007) Genome-wide association study of prostate cancer identifies a second risk locus at 8q24. Nat Genet 39:645–649

Zanke BW, Greenwood CM, Rangrej J, Kustra R, Tenesa A, Farrington SM, Prendergast J, Olschwang S, Chiang T, Crowdy E, Ferretti V, Laflamme P, Sundararajan S, Roumy S, Olivier JF, Robidoux F, Sladek R, Montpetit A, Campbell P, Bezieau S, O'Shea AM, Zogopoulos G, Cotterchio M, Newcomb P, McLaughlin J, Younghusband B, Green R, Green J, Porteous ME, Campbell H, Blanche H, Sahbatou M, Tubacher E, Bonaiti-Pellie C, Buecher B, Riboli E, Kury S, Chanock SJ, Potter J, Thomas G, Gallinger S, Hudson TJ, Dunlop MG (2007) Genome-wide association scan identifies a colorectal cancer susceptibility locus on chromosome 8q24. Nat Genet 39:989–994

Zeegers MP, Jellema A, Ostrer H (2003) Empiric risk of prostate carcinoma for relatives of patients with prostate carcinoma: a meta-analysis. Cancer 97:1894–1903

Zuhlke KA, Madeoy JJ, Beebe-Dimmer J, White KA, Griffin A, Lange EM, Gruber SB, Ostrander EA, Cooney KA (2004) Truncating BRCA1 mutations are uncommon in a cohort of hereditary prostate cancer families with evidence of linkage to 17q markers. Clin. Cancer Res. 10:5975–5980

Chapter 8
The Identification of Rare and Common Variants Which Predispose to Prostate Cancer

Rosalind A. Eeles, Zsofia Kote-Jarai, Michelle Guy, and Douglas Easton

8.1 Introduction and Evidence for a Genetic Predisposition

Prostate cancer is now the commonest cancer in men in the Western world, with over 34,000 new cases per annum and a lifetime risk of 1 in 11 in the UK (Cancer Research UK Factsheets 2008). However, its aetiology remains very poorly understood. There is substantial worldwide variation in disease incidence, with the disease being much commoner in the Western countries than in the developing world and the Far East (Marugame and Katanoda 2006). These observations, together with studies of incidence rates in migrant populations (Lee et al. 2007), suggest strongly that lifestyle risk factors are important determinants of prostate cancer risk. To date, however, no definite lifestyle risk factors have been identified.

Aside from demographic factors, the only long-established risk factor for prostate cancer is a family history of the disease. The risk of the disease in first-degree relatives of cases, estimated consistently from multiple studies, is approximately twice that in the general population (Goldgar et al. 1994; Edwards and Eeles 2004). This familial risk is greater amongst young cases, being more than fourfold for cases below age 60. Analyses based on the Nordic twin registries have found higher risks in monozygotic than dizygotic twins, supporting the hypothesis that much of this familial aggregation is due to genetic rather than shared lifestyle factors (Hemminki and Vaittinen 1998; Lichtenstein et al. 2000). The higher incidence of prostate cancer in African Americans (and lower rate in Americans of Asian ancestry) suggests that genetic factors may also be important determinants of the variation in disease risk at a population level (Zeigler-Johnson et al. 2008) (for more detail, see Chapter by Lange, Section 7.2).

R.A. Eeles (✉), Z. Kote-Jarai, and M. Guy
Translational Cancer Genetics Team, The Institute of Cancer Research,
15 Cotswold Road, Sutton, Surrey, UK
e-mail: rosalind.eeles@icr.ac.uk

D. Easton
Cancer Research UK Genetic Epidemiology Unit, Department of Public Health and Primary Care, University of Cambridge, Strangeways Laboratory, Worts Causeway, Cambridge, UK

W.D. Foulkes and K.A. Cooney (eds.), *Male Reproductive Cancers:*
Epidemiology, Pathology and Genetics, Cancer Genetics,
DOI 10.1007/978-1-4419-0449-2_8, © Springer Science+Business Media, LLC 2010

8.2   Models of Susceptibility to Prostate Cancer

In general, genetic variation in the risk of a disease may result from rare highly penetrant genetic mutations, from genetic variants conferring more moderate risks, and from a combination of both. Until the mid-2000s most research focused on the identification of high-risk susceptibility loci, since they were more tractable to the existing technologies and had more obvious clinical application. Several segregation analyses, based on systematic series of pedigrees of prostate cancer patients, have suggested that prostate cancer susceptibility has a major gene component (Carter et al. 1992; Grönberg et al. 1997; Schaid et al. 1998; Gong et al. 2002). Although segregation analyses have rather poor power to discriminate between different genetic models, these studies have provided an impetus to search for high-risk genes. Such genes are amenable to mapping through genetic linkage studies in multiple case families, and several groups have used this approach. This is described in more detail elsewhere in this book (see chapter by Lange, Section 7.3.3). These studies have identified loci with reasonable evidence for linkage, including loci on chromosomes 1, 3, 5, 8, 11, 17, 19, 20, 22 and X (Smith et al. 1996; Gibbs et al. 1999; Berthon et al. 1998; Xu et al. 1998; Badzioch et al. 2000; Berry et al. 2000a; Schleutker et al. 2000; Xu 2000; Tavtigian et al. 2001; Xu et al. 2001; Zheng et al. 2001; Xu et al. 2003; Wiklund et al. 2003; Schleutker et al. 2003). However, these linkage peaks have not been consistently replicated in other studies (McIndoe et al. 1997; Eeles et al. 1998; Singh et al. 2000; Berry et al. 2000b; Hsieh et al. 2001; Cancel-Tansin et al. 2001; Edwards et al. 2003a; Cunningham et al. 2003; Easton et al. 2003; Janer et al. 2003; Schaid et al. 2005; Slager et al. 2006). A recent analysis by the International Consortium for Prostate Cancer Genetics (ICPCG) combined data on 1,233 families from 10 groups (Xu et al. 2005). In this analysis, no loci with LOD scores in excess of 3 were identified in the total set of families, and only one LOD score over 3 was identified in subgroup analyses (on 22q, in families with over 5 cases and early onset disease). Linkage studies have led to identification of three putative prostate cancer genes (*RNASEL*, *MSR1* and *ELAC2*) by virtue of their position under linkage peaks, and the identification of potential disease-associated mutations in these genes in prostate cancer families. In each case, however, these associations could not be replicated consistently (e.g., Meitz et al. 2002; Hope et al. 2005; Wiklund et al. 2004; Maier et al. 2005), and their status as susceptibility genes remains in doubt.

The failure of linkage studies to identify prostate cancer loci suggests strongly that prostate cancer is genetically complex, with many genes involved. It remains possible that some of these genes confer a high risk, but that such loci only explain a small fraction of the familial risk. An alternative model, however, is that susceptibility is mediated through a combination of loci conferring more moderate risks of the disease.

8.3   Association Studies

Linkage mapping, which is based on segregation of genetic markers through families, lacks the power to detect loci in which the susceptibility variants confer only a moderate risk of the disease. Genetic association studies provide a much more powerful strategy (see also chapter by Lange, Sections 7.5 and 7.6). In these studies, susceptibility variants are identified by finding a difference in genotype frequency between cases and controls. These studies can either be based on typing presumed functional variants, or on typing a set of variants (usually single nucleotide polymorphisms or SNPs) that are associated with a neighbouring functional variant indirectly, through linkage disequilibrium. Given a sufficiently large case-control sample, these studies are able to identify reliably variants that confer quite moderate risks (as low as 1.1-fold or less), far below that detectable by linkage. Although these approaches are very powerful, they are relatively expensive. Until recently, therefore, such studies have concentrated on a few genes that were thought to be strong candidate susceptibility genes. Such studies have been conducted in prostate cancer by several groups. As with the linkage studies, this approach has not yet yielded a definite susceptibility gene.

Over the past 2–3 years, new genotyping platforms have become available that allow association studies to be conducted on a genome-wide basis (that enable hundreds of thousands of SNPs to be assayed, so called Genome-Wide Association Studies, or GWAS). These platforms provide the ability to assay simultaneously almost all common SNPs in the genome, without prior selection of loci on the basis of position or function. It is estimated that there are approximately 11 million SNPs in the genome with a minor allele frequency of 1% or greater, of which ~7 million have a frequency of >5% (Kruglyak and Nickerson 2001; Livingston et al. 2004). In principle, it would be possible to assess whether each of them was associated with prostate cancer by determining their genotype frequencies in a sufficiently large number of cases and controls, but this would be prohibitively expensive and, in any event, not all SNPs have been identified. Fortunately, this is not necessary because many neighbouring SNPs are highly correlated (are in strong linkage disequilibrium), so that one SNP can often report on many others (so called tagSNPs). As a result, associations with any common SNP should be detectable by typing a more limited number of 'tagging SNPs'. The required size of this set in European populations has been variously estimated to be in the range of 200,000 to 500,000 SNPs (larger sets are required to cover the genome in African populations). Suitable SNP sets are available on commercially available genotyping arrays and are now in widespread use.

8.4   Results of GWAS in Prostate Cancer

At least 20 prostate cancer susceptibility loci have been identified to date through association studies. The first and most important region to be identified was 8q24. This region was first suggested by a linkage study conducted by the deCODE group in Iceland. Subsequent association analysis of markers in the region identified a SNP, rs1447295, associated with a 1.6-fold risk of prostate cancer (Amundadottir et al. 2006). An admixture scan conducted in African–Americans also identified 8q24 as a susceptibility region (Freedman et al. 2006). Subsequent association analyses identified two further regions on 8q24 as harbouring susceptibility loci (Fig. 8.1, Yeager et al. 2007; Gudmundsson et al. 2007a). All of these loci have been confirmed in subsequent GWAS (Eeles et al. 2008a; Thomas et al. 2008). Analyses by Haiman et al. 2007 identified at least seven independent risk alleles in these blocks, and Salinas et al. 2008 suggest that there may be further susceptibility alleles which extend the region of association, though fine mapping will be required to determine the true number of independent 'causal' loci. Intriguingly, the susceptibility alleles at the three major 8q24 loci are commoner in Yoruban (North African) and African–Americans, and thus may explain at least in part the higher frequency of the disease in African populations. The three loci are all distinct from a breast cancer locus that has been identified in the same region (Easton et al. 2007), which falls in a separate LD block (Fig. 8.1; Ghoussaini et al. 2008). However, in one of the three loci (region 3 in Fig. 8.1) the SNP mostly strongly associated with prostate cancer (rs6983267) is also associated with colorectal cancer with a similar odds ratio. This SNP has also been shown to be associated with ovarian cancer (Ghoussaini et al. 2008). Recent resequencing results indicate that SNP rs6983267 is only highly correlated with one other SNP; this, together with a high degree of conservation, suggests that this SNP may be causal but this remains to be proven (Yeager et al. 2008). All of these loci fall in a 1.2-Mb region that contains no known genes. The closest distal gene is the oncogene *c-MYC*, leading to suggestions that the susceptibility results from long-range control of myc expression, and this has recently been shown to be the case in colon cancer (Pomerantz et al., 2009).

Subsequent analyses of GWAS data by the deCODE group, based on a scan of 1,500 men with prostate cancer and the Illumina 317-k array, identified two further loci on 17q. One of these maps to the *HNF1B* (*TCF2*) gene. Coding mutations in *HNF1B* cause maturity-onset diabetes in the young (MODY). Gudmundsson et al. (2007b) found that the susceptibility prostate cancer allele at this locus was inversely associated with diabetes. Some studies have suggested that prostate cancer

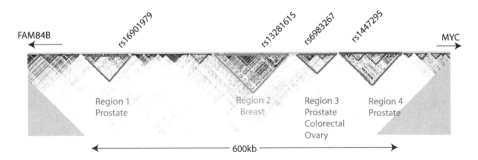

Fig. 8.1 Schematic of the 8q24 region (adapted from Ghoussaini et al. 2008)

is less common in patients with diabetes, raising the possibility that other susceptibility loci may be associated with both diseases (Calton et al. 2007). A second,
independent association at *HNF1B* 26 kb telomeric to the first has recently been
found (Sun et al. 2008).

In the largest study to date, (Eeles et al. 2008b) conducted, a GWAS using 1854
prostate cancer cases diagnosed at <60 years or with a family history of the disease, and 1894 controls selected for low prostate-specific antigen (PSA) (<0.5 ng/
ml), based on the Illumina 550-k array (Eeles et al 2008 a,b). The selection of cases
was designed to enrich for genetic variants by virtue of their young age or familial
clustering. The controls were selected for low PSA since such individuals have a
lower risk of prostate cancer than the general population, thus increasing the likely
difference in genotype frequency between cases and controls. Regions significant
at $p < 10^{-6}$ were followed up in an additional 3268 cases and 3366 controls from the
UK and Australia. Using this strategy they identified seven novel loci on chromosomes 3, 6, 7, 10, 11, 19 and *X* (Table 8.1; Fig. 8.2). These loci were validated in a
further analysis by the PRACTICAL association consortium, that included 7370
cases and 5742 controls from 13 studies (Kote-Jarai et al. 2008). Evidence for association was found for all loci, and the odds ratios were very similar to those estimated by Eeles et al.

The seven novel susceptibility regions contain several strong plausible candidate
genes. rs10993994 and rs7920517 lie within an LD block of ~ 100 kb on chromosome 10, containing the microseminoprotein beta gene, *MSMB*. The most strongly
associated SNP, rs10993994, lies 2 bp upstream of the transcription start site of
MSMB. Its location and the strength of the association raises the possibility that this
SNP may be causally related to disease risk, and resequencing and molecular studies
have shown that the SNP does have a functional efferct (Lou et al., 2009).

rs2735839 lies between *KLK2* (Kallikrein-related peptidase 2; *hK2*) and *KLK3*.
The kallikreins are a subgroup of serine proteases. *KLK2* and *KLK3* are 2 of 15
kallikrein subfamily members located in a cluster on chromosome 19. PSA, which
is the protein product of the *KLK3* gene, is a serine protease which liquefies semen
and as a serum marker is used in screening and disease monitoring; there is also
evidence that hK2 may also be useful for screening and prognosis (Steuber et al.
2006, 2007). Multiple SNPs in the *KLK3* promoter region have been associated
with PSA levels (Cramer et al. 2003) and some have been suggested to be associated with prostate cancer risk (Lai et al. 2007). rs27358389 lies 3' of *KLK3* and
shows a much stronger association with PSA levels than those previously reported,
suggesting a novel functional effect. rs27358389 is also strongly associated with
PSA level, leading to the argument proposed that the identification of this susceptibility allele may have been confounded by the use of low PSA in controls (Ahn
et al. 2008). However the effect was still seen in both the second stage of the
GWAS (Eeles et al. 2008a, b) and in the PRACTICAL analysis, in which control
groups were not selected for low PSA (Kote-Jarai et al. 2008).

rs6465657 lies on chromosome 7 in intron 9 of *LMTK2* (*cprk; BREK;* Brain-
Enriched Kinase) (Kawa et al. 2004). It encodes a neuronal kinase, cyclin-dependent
kinase 5 (cdk5)/p35-regulated kinase (cprk). Somatic mutations in *LMTK2* have

234   R.A. Eeles et al.

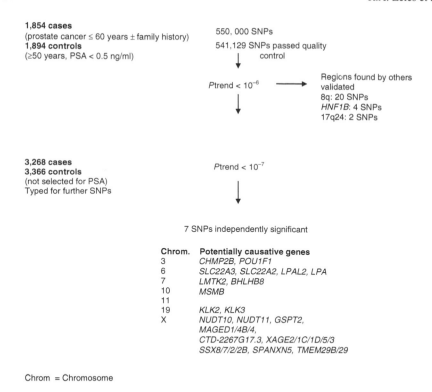

Fig. 8.2 Outline of the GWAS conducted by Eeles et al. (Eeles et al. 2008 a,b)

been found in a small proportion of cancers at other sites, but prostate cancer has not been analysed (Greenman et al. 2007). rs6465657 also lies upstream of basic helix-loop-helix *BHLHB8* which is a transcription factor expressed at high levels in the adult seminal vesicle and during seminal gland differentiation.

rs9364554 lies in intron 5 of the gene *SLC22A3* which is one of the solute carrier family 22 (organic cation transporter; OCT) genes. Polyspecific OCTs are critical for elimination of some drugs and environmental toxins. This gene is one of three similar cation transporter genes located in a cluster on chromosome 6. Two of these, *SLC22A3* and *SLC22A2*, are both in the LD block containing rs9364554. *SLC22A2* is part of the PI3 kinase and cyclic AMP-dependent protein kinase A catalytic subunit pathway (Cetinkaya et al. 2003).

rs5945619 is in an LD block of approximately 2 MB on Xp. It lies between *NUDT10* and *NUDT11* [nudix (nucleoside diphosphate-linked moiety X)-type motif 11], about 2 kb upstream of the latter. These genes encode isoforms of diphosphoinositol polyphosphate phosphohydrolase which determine the rate of phosphorylation in DNA repair, stress responses and apoptosis (Hidaka et al. 2002). Also in the LD block are *GSPT2* (a GTP binding protein)*; MAGEDs 1, 4B, 4* (melanoma antigen genes expressed in the testes)*; CTD-2267G17.3; XAGEs 2, 1C, 1D, 5, 3* (encoding a family of cancer/testis-associated antigens)*; SSXs 8, 7, 2,* 2B (a

Table 8.1 Prostate cancer susceptibility loci reaching genome-wide significance as identified through GWAS

Locus	Chrom	SNP(s)	Risk allele frequency[a]	Per allele OR[b]	p-value[c]	References[d]
2p15	2	rs721048	0.19	1.15	8×10^{-9}	Gudmundsson et al. (2008)
3p12	3	rs2660753	0.11	1.18	3×10^{-8}	Eeles et al. (2008a, b)
6q25	6	rs9364554	0.29	1.17	6×10^{-10}	Eeles et al. (2008a, b)
LMTK2	7	rs6465657	0.46	1.12	10^{-9}	Eeles et al. (2008a, b)
JAZF1	7	rs10486567	0.77	1.12	10^{-7}	Eeles et al. (2008a, b)
8q24	8	rs1447295, DG8S737	0.10	1.62	3×10^{-11}	Amundadottir et al. (2006)
8q24	8	rs6983267	0.50	1.26	9×10^{-13}	Yeager et al. (2007)
8q24	8	rs16901979, hapC	0.03	2.1	3×10^{-15}	Gudmundsson et al. (2007a)
HNF1B	17	rs4430796	0.49	1.24	10^{-11}	Gudmundsson et al. (2007b)
HNF1B	17	rs11649743	0.80	1.28	2×10^{-9}	Sun et al. (2008)
17q24	17	rs1859962	0.46	1.25	3×10^{-10}	Gudmundsson et al. (2007b)
MSMB	10	rs10993994	0.40	1.25	9×10^{-29}	Eeles et al. (2008a, b); Thomas et al. (2008)
CTBP2	10	rs4962416	0.27	1.17	3×10^{-8}	Thomas et al. (2008)
11q13	11	rs7931342	0.51	1.19	2×10^{-12}	Eeles et al. (2008a, b); Thomas et al. (2008)
KLK2/KLK3	19	rs2735839	0.85	1.20	2×10^{-18}	Eeles et al. (2008a, b)
Xp11	X	rs5945572	0.35	1.24	4×10^{-13}	Gudmundsson et al. (2008); Eeles et al. (2008a, b)

[a] Reported risk allele frequency in Europeans
[b] Estimated per allele odds ratio from the largest available study
[c] *p* for trend, rounded up to the nearest whole number value, from the most significant study reporting the association (not necessarily the current combined evidence)
[d] Studies first reporting the association at this locus. The SNP with the most significant association is listed. Other SNPs at these loci have also been associated with prostate cancer

family of synovial sarcoma *X* breakpoint proteins which may function as transcriptional repressors); *SPANXN5* and *TMEMs 29B* and *29*.

rs2660753 is in a gene-poor region on chromosome 3. It is 170 kb upstream of *CHMP2B* (chromatin-modifying protein 2B), which encodes a component of the endosomal ESCRTIII complex. The LD block also contains *POU1F1* (*PIT1*) which is a pituitary-specific transcription factor. Finally, rs7931342 lies in an LD block of 70 kb on chromosome 11 that contains no recognised genes.

A second GWAS of 527, 869 SNPs was conducted by the CGEMS group based on 1,172 cases and 1157 controls selected from the Prostate, Lung, Colorectal and Ovarian screening (PLCO) trial, using the Illumina 550-k array. 26,958 SNPs showing associations in this study were followed up in a further 3941 cases and 3964 controls from 4 independent studies (Thomas et al. 2008). After these two stages, they identified four loci associated with prostate cancer risk at or near genome-wide significance. These included same SNP, rs10993994, on chromosome 10 identified by Eeles et al. and an association on 11q with an SNP closely linked to that found by Eeles et al. (Eeles et al. 2008a). In addition, they identified associations with SNPs in *JAZF1*, a transcriptional repressor of NR2C2, and another locus on chromosome 10 containing the *CTBP2* gene (Thomas et al. 2008). In a further analysis of the deCODE study, Gudmundsson et al. also found an association with an SNP at Xp11.22, 3 kb downstream of *NUDT10* in the same LD block as that identified by Eeles et al. together with an additional locus on 2p.

The identification of these susceptibility loci marks a huge step forward in the characterization of the genetic basis of prostate cancer (Fig. 8.3). The understanding of the biology underlying these associations is still, however, in its infancy. A critical first step is the identification of the variant (or variants) that are causally related to the disease. Moving from the associated variant to the causal variant is problematic because variants within LD blocks are often strongly correlated. Resequencing of these regions, followed by large association studies in multiple populations, will be required to narrow down the set of possible causal variants, but epidemiological studies alone are unlikely to be sufficient to identify the causal variant unambiguously and additional functional studies will be required. The limited fine-scale mapping and resequencing that has been conducted to date (and similar evidence from loci identified for other common cancers) suggests that the associations are unlikely to reflect changes in the coding sequences of genes. Of the 23 susceptibility variants identified to date, some evidence of causality has been obtained for only two of these - the 8q24 SNP rs6983267 and rs10993994 upstream of *MSMB*. For only four of the loci is the relevant gene (*MSMB, HNF1B, KLK2* or *KLK3, LMTK2*) reasonably certain. Several of the regions contain multiple genes but others are in gene deserts, notably 8q24, and also 11q. The mechanisms underlying these associations are obscure. They may reflect promoter or enhancer elements leading to control of gene expression in genes located elsewhere, but other mechanisms, for example involving structural rearrangements, micro-RNAs, or changes in DNA structure, may be important.

Meta analyses of GWAS, further analysis of SNPs identified (at $p > 10^{-6}$) from the GWAS described above and new GWAS in further sample sets and samples from different ethnic origins are very likely to find further prostate cancer susceptiblity loci.

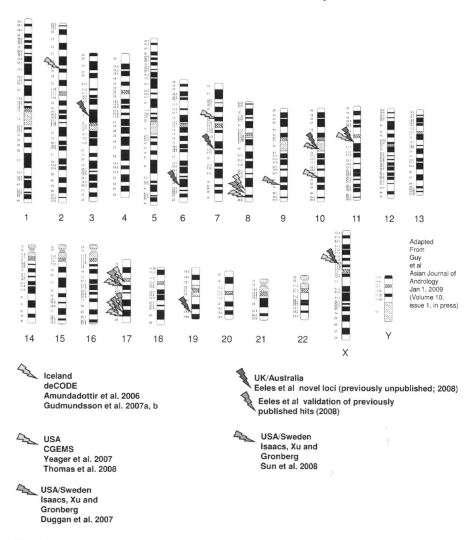

Fig. 8.3 Summary of loci associated with prostate cancer risk identified by the various GWAS study groups

8.5 Rare Variants

The current generation of GWAS provides excellent power to identify common variants associated with prostate cancer with frequencies of 5% or more. However, they lack power to detect rarer susceptibility alleles, which are not well tagged by the arrays. The identification of these alleles is much more problematic, requiring direct testing of the much larger number of uncommon alleles, or resequencing of cases and controls. It is likely that this will become possible on a genome-wide basis, but this is not currently feasible and such studies have therefore focused on candidate genes.

One gene for which there is clear evidence of rare variants predisposing to prostate cancer is *BRCA2*. Studies by the Breast Cancer Linkage Consortium (BCLC) showed that germline *BRCA2* mutations segregating in breast-ovarian cancer families confer a prostate cancer risk of approximately fivefold, increasing to more than sevenfold below age 65 years (The Breast Cancer Linkage Consortium 1999, Thompson et al. 2001). This association has been confirmed in multiple studies. Edwards et al. (2003b) reported a 2% germline mutation rate in *BRCA2* in prostate cancer cases diagnosed at <55 years unselected for family history. There is some evidence of a genotype–phenotype correlation with mutations in the ovarian cancer cluster region (OCCR) in the centre of the gene associated with a lower risk than those outside, particularly those downstream of this region. Several groups have shown that prostate cancer in *BRCA2* mutation carriers is more aggressive and has a poorer prognosis (Tryggvadóttir et al. 2007; Mitra et al. 2008; Narod et al. 2008). This finding has important clinical implications as discussed below.

Several other DNA repair genes have been analysed for mutations in prostate cancer cases, including the *CHEK2*, *PALB2* and *NBS1* genes. Truncating mutations in *CHEK2* and *PALB2* are associated with a moderate risk of breast cancer, while *NBS1* mutations are the cause of Nijmegen Breakage Syndrome. In each case, some evidence of an association has been found with prostate cancer cases in some populations, but not others, so the evidence is not conclusive (Cybulski et al. 2004; Cybulski et al. 2006; Thompson et al. 2006; Erkko et al. 2007; Tischkowitz et al. 2008). An association with the *NBS1* founder mutation, common only in Slavic populations was reported in a Polish study, but this was not replicated in a US study (Hebbring et al. 2006). An association between the Finnish *PALB2* founder mutation and prostate cancer has been reported (Erkko et al. 2007). This association was not replicated by Montreal group, although the study was small and based on a different population (Tischkowitz et al. 2008).

8.6   Conclusions

The substantial risk of prostate cancer in *BRCA2* mutation carriers raises particular clinical issues. Such mutations are usually identified through genetic testing of breast-ovarian cancer families, and as such testing is becoming more straightforward, the number of male carriers that is identified is growing ever larger. The fact that *BRCA2* mutations predispose to an aggressive disease with poor prognosis poses particular issues. The appropriate management strategy for such carriers is unclear; an international study to evaluate screening of this group (IMPACT) is currently ongoing. The development of targeted drugs (PARP inhibitors) for tumours harbouring *BRCA* mutations has resulted in promising response rates in other tumour sites (Farmer et al. 2005; Fong et al. 2008), and this provides a new therapeutic option for this disease. If efficacy with such agents could be demonstrated in prostate cancer due to *BRCA2* mutations, this would raise the possibility of the clinical use of more widespread testing for *BRCA2* mutations in prostate

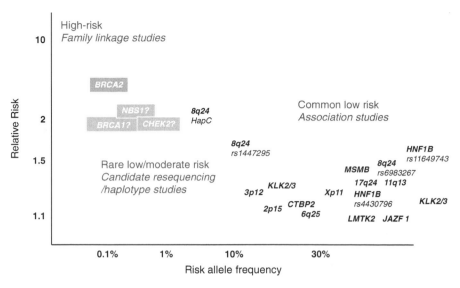

Fig. 8.4 The pattern of genetic predisposition to prostate cancer

cancer patients. The RR of prostate cancer in young *BRCA1* mutation carriers is more contentious and needs further studies.

The value of more general genetic testing for risk profiling has been hotly debated. As described earlier, prostate cancer is genetically complex, involving a combination of many loci and both rare and common variants (Fig. 8.4). The current set of variants explain about 15% of the genetic variance of the disease, indicating that any test based on current knowledge will be provisional and likely to change substantially over the next few years. Nevertheless, such tests are being developed. These latter genetic variants are easy to identify using saliva or blood DNA testing, and at least three commercial tests based on some of the known variants are available. The question then is how useful such tests will be, either for individual risk prediction or for population screening. The risks conferred by the common susceptibility SNP alleles are low, generally 1.3-fold or less (Table 8.1); however, these alleles are common. The combined effects may, however, be sufficiently large to be useful for risk prediction, and targeted screening and prevention. The top 1% of the risk distribution using the currently known SNPs has 3 times the risk of the average of the population (Eeles et al., 2008). Zheng et al. (2008) have shown the risks associated with the SNPs can be combined with family history to improve risk assessment. Identification of this higher-risk group may be useful, but this depends critically on the efficacy of any intervention.

A serious disadvantage with prostate cancer screening is that uncovers a large incidence of indolent disease that would never have progressed to metastatic disease, thus diagnosing the disease unnecessarily in the majority of men. Genetic risk profiling could be much more useful if it could be linked to clinical outcome (as in the case of *BRCA2*). Early analyses suggest that at least some of the genetic profiles may be associated with aggressive disease (Helfand et al. 2008; Cussenot et al. 2008; Cheng et al. 2008; Tan et al. 2008), but this is contradicted by others (Xu et al. 2008). If genetic profiling could determine when men should have a prostate biopsy, and did detect clinically significant disease, such genetic profiling would have a greater public health benefit as it would target prostate cancer screening to those most likely to benefit and may reduce the diagnosis of indolent cancers which do not need detection.

References

Ahn J, Berndt SI, Wacholder S, Kraft P, Kibel AS, Yeager M, Albanes D, Giovannucci E, Stampfer MJ, Virtamo J, Thun MJ, Feigelson HS, Cancel-Tassin G, Cussenot O, Thomas G, Hunter DJ, Fraumeni JF Jr, Hoover RN, Chanock SJ, Hayes RB (2008) Variation in KLK genes, prostate specific antigen and risk of prostate cancer. Nat Genet 40(9):1032–1034

Amundadottir LT, Sulem P, Gudmundsson J, Helgason A, Baker A, Agnarsson BA, Sigurdsson A, Benediktsdottir KR, Cazier JB, Sainz J, Jakobsdottir M, Kostic J, Magnusdottir DN, Ghosh S, Agnarsson K, Birgisdottir B, Le Roux L, Olafsdottir A, Blondal T, Andresdottir M, Gretarsdottir OS, Bergthorsson JT, Gudbjartsson D, Gylfason A, Thorleifsson G, Manolescu A, Kristjansson K, Geirsson G, Isaksson H, Douglas J, Johansson JE, Bälter K, Wiklund F, Montie JE, Yu X, Suarez BK, Ober C, Cooney KA, Gronberg H, Catalona WJ, Einarsson GV, Barkardottir RB, Gulcher JR, Kong A, Thorsteinsdottir U, Stefansson K (2006) A common variant associated with prostate cancer in European and African populations. Nat Genet 38:652–658

Badzioch M, Eeles R, Leblanc G, Foulkes WD, Giles G, Edwards S, Goldgar D, Hopper JL, Bishop DT, Moller P, Heimdahl K, Easton D, The CRC/BPG Familial Prostate Cancer Study Coordinators and Collaborators, The EU Biomed Collaborators, Simard J (2000) Suggestive evidence for a site specific prostate cancer gene on 1p36. J Med Genet 37:947–948

Berry R, Schroeder J, French A, McDonnell S, Peterson B, Cunningham J, Thibodeau S, Schaid D (2000a) Evidence for a prostate cancer-susceptibility locus on chromosome 20. Am J Hum Genet 7:82–91

Berry R, Schaid DJ, Smith JR, French AJ, Schroeder JJ, McDonnell SK, Peterson BJ, Wang ZY, Carpten JD, Roberts SG, Tester DJ, Blute ML, Trent JM, Thibodeau SN (2000b) Linkage analyses at the chromosome 1 loci 1q24-25 (HPRCA1), 1q42.2-43 (PRCAAP), and 1p36 (CAPB) in families with hereditary prostate cancer. Am J Hum Genet 66:539–546

Berthon P, Valeri A, Cohen-Akenine A, Drelon E, Paiss T, Wohr G, Latil A, Millasseau P, Mellah I, Cohen N, Blanche H, Bellane-Chantelot C, Demenais F, Teillac P, Le Duc A, de Petriconi R, Hautmann R, Chumakov I, Bachner L, Maitland NJ, Lindereeau R, Vogel W, Fournier G, Mangin P, Cussenot O (1998) Predisposing gene for early-onset prostate cancer, localized on chromosome 1q42.2-43. Am J Hum Genet 62:1416–1424

Calton BA, Chang SC, Wright ME, Kipnis V, Lawson K, Thompson FE, Subar AF, Mouw T, Campbell DS, Hurwitz P, Hollenbeck A, Schatzkin A, Leitzmann MF (2007) History of diabetes mellitus and subsequent prostate cancer risk in the NIH-AARP Diet and Health Study. Cancer Causes Control 18(5):93–503

Cancel-Tansin G, Latil A, Valeri A, Guillaume E, Mangin P, Fournier G, Berthon P, Cussenot O (2001) No evidence of linkage to HPRCA20 on chromosome 20q13 in hereditary prostate cancer. Int J Cancer 93:455–456

Carter BS, Beaty TH, Steinberg GD, Childs B, Walsh P (1992) Mendelian inheritance of familial prostate cancer. Proc Natl Acad Sci USA 89:3367–3371

Cetinkaya I, Ciarimboli G, Yalçinkaya G, Mehrens T, Velic A, Hirsch JR, Gorboulev V, Koepsell H, Schlatter E (2003) Regulation of human organic cation transporter hOCT2 by PKA, PI3K, and calmodulin-dependent kinases. Am J Physiol-Renal Physiol 284:F293–F302

Cheng I, Plummer SJ, Jorgenson E, Liu X, Rybicki BA, Casey G, Witte JS (2008) 8q24 and prostate cancer: Association with advanced disease and meta-analysis. Eur J Hum Genet
16:496–505

Cramer SD, Rao A, Hawkins GA, Zheng SL, Wade WN, Cooke RT, Thomas LN, Bleecker ER,
Catalona WJ, Sterling DA, Meyers DA, Ohar J, Xu J (2003) Association between genetic
polymorphisms in the prostate-specific antigen gene promoter and serum prostate-specific
antigen levels. J Natl Cancer Inst 95:1044–1053

Cunningham JM, McDonnell SK, Marks A, Hebbring S, Anderson SA, Peterson BJ, Slager S,
French A, Blute ML, Schaid DJ, Thibodeau SN (2003) Genome linkage screen for prostate
cancer susceptibility loci: Results from the Mayo Clinic Familial Prostate Cancer Study.
Prostate 57:335–346

Cussenot O, Azzouzi A-R, Bantsimba-Malanda G, Gaffory C, Mangin P, Cormier L, Fournier G,
Valeri A, Jouffe L, Roupret M, Fromont G, Sibony M, Comperat E, Cancel-Tassin G (2008)
Effect of genetic variability within 8q24 on aggressiveness patterns at diagnosis and familial
status of prostate cancer. Clin Cancer Res 14(17):5635–5639

Cybulski C, Górski B, Debniak T, Gliniewicz B, Mierzejewski M, Masoj B, Jakubowska A,
Matyjasik J, Złowocka E, Sikorski A, Narod SA, Lubi ski J (2004) NBS1 is a prostate cancer
susceptibility gene. Cancer Res 64(4):1215–9

Cybulski C, Wokołorczyk D, Huzarski T, Byrski T, Gronwald J, Górski B, Debniak T, Masoj B,
Jakubowska A, Gliniewicz B, Sikorski A, Stawicka M, Godlewski D, Kwias Z, Antczak A,
Krajka K, Lauer W, Sosnowski M, Sikorska-Radek P, Bar K, Klijer R, Zdrojowy R, Małkiewicz
B, Borkowski A, Borkowski T, Szwiec M, Narod SA, Lubi ski JA (2006) Large germline dele-
tion in the Chek2 kinase gene is associated with an increased risk of prostate cancer. J Med
Genet 43(11):863–6

Donovan J, Hamdy F, Neal D, Peters T, Oliver S, Brindle L, Jewell D, Powell P, Gillatt D, Dedman
D, Mills N, Smith M, Noble S, Lane A, ProtecT Study Group (2003) Prostate Testing for
Cancer and Treatment (ProtecT) feasibility study. Health Technol Assess 7(14):1–88

Duggan D, Zheng SL, Knowlton M, Benitez D, Dimitrov L, Wiklund F, Robbins C, Isaacs SD,
Cheng Y, Li G, Sun J, Chang BL, Marovich L, Wiley KE, Bälter K, Stattin P, Adami HO,
Gielzak M, Yan G, Sauvageot J, Liu W, Kim JW, Bleecker ER, Meyers DA, Trock BJ, Partin
AW, Walsh PC, Isaacs WB, Grönberg H, Xu J, Carpten JD (2007) Two genome-wide associa-
tion studies of aggressive prostate cancer implicate putative prostate tumor suppressor gene
DAB2IP. J Natl Cancer Inst 99(24):1836–1844

Easton DF, Schaid DJ, Whittemore AS, Isaacs WJ, International Consortium for Prostate Cancer
Genetics (2003) Where are the prostate cancer genes? – A summary of eight genome wide
searches. Prostate 57(4):261–269

Easton DF, Pooley KA, Dunning AM, Pharoah PD, Thompson D, Ballinger DG, Struewing JP,
Morrison J, Field H, Luben R, Wareham N, Ahmed S, Healey CS, Bowman R, SEARCH col-
laborators, Meyer KB, Haiman CA, Kolonel LK, Henderson BE, Le Marchand L, Brennan P,
Sangrajrang S, Gaborieau V, Odefrey F, Shen CY, Wu PE, Wang HC, Eccles D, Evans DG,
Peto J, Fletcher O, Johnson N, Seal S, Stratton MR, Rahman N, Chenevix-Trench G, Bojesen
SE, Nordestgaard BG, Axelsson CK, Garcia-Closas M, Brinton L, Chanock S, Lissowska J,
Peplonska B, Nevanlinna H, Fagerholm R, Eerola H, Kang D, Yoo KY, Noh DY, Ahn SH,
Hunter DJ, Hankinson SE, Cox DG, Hall P, Wedren S, Liu J, Low YL, Bogdanova N,
Schürmann P, Dörk T, Tollenaar RA, Jacobi CE, Devilee P, Klijn JG, Sigurdson AJ, Doody
MM, Alexander BH, Zhang J, Cox A, Brock IW, MacPherson G, Reed MW, Couch FJ, Goode
EL, Olson JE, Meijers-Heijboer H, van den Ouweland A, Uitterlinden A, Rivadeneira F, Milne
RL, Ribas G, Gonzalez-Neira A, Benitez J, Hopper JL, McCredie M, Southey M, Giles GG,
Schroen C, Justenhoven C, Brauch H, Hamann U, Ko YD, Spurdle AB, Beesley J, Chen X,
kConFab; AOCS Management Group, Mannermaa A, Kosma VM, Kataja V, Hartikainen J,
Day NE, Cox DR, Ponder BA (2007) Genome-wide association study identifies novel breast
cancer susceptibility loci. Nature 447(7148):1087–1093

Edwards SM, Eeles RA (2004) Unravelling the genetics of prostate cancer. Am J Med Genetics
129C:65–73

Edwards S, Meitz J, Evans C, Easton D, Hopper GG, Foulkes WD, Narod S, Simard J, Badzoich M, Maehle L, PI Eeles R (2003a) Results of a genome-wide linkage analysis in prostate cancer families ascertained through the ACTANE consortium. The international ACTANE consortium. Prostate 57(4):270–279

Edwards SM, Kote-Jarai Z, Meitz J, Hamoudi R, Hope Q, Osin P, Jackson R, Southgate C, Singh R, Falconer A, Dearnaley DP, Ardern-Jones A, Murkin A, Dowe A, Kelly J, Williams S, Oram R, Stevens M, Teare DM, Ponder BA, Gayther SA, Easton DF, Eeles RA, Cancer Research UK/Bristish Prostate Group UK Familial Prostate Cancer Study Collaborators and British Association of Urological Surgeons Section of Oncology (2003b) Two percent of men with early onset prostate cancer harbour germline mutations in the BRCA2 gene. Am J Hum Genet 72:1–12

Eeles RA, Durocher F, Edwards S, Teare D, Badzioch M, Hamoudi R, Gill S, Biggs P, Dearnaley D, Ardern-Jones A, Dowe A, Shearer R, McLennan DL, Norman RW, Ghadirian P, Aprikian A, Ford D, Amos C, King TM, The CRC/BPG UK Familial Prostate Cancer Study Collaborators, Labrie F, Simard J, Narod S, Easton D, Foulkes W (1998) Linkage analysis of chromosome 1q markers in 136 prostate cancer families. Am J Hum Genet 62:653–658

Eeles RA, Kote-Jarai Z, Giles GG, Olama AA, Guy M, Jugurnauth SK, Mulholland S, Leongamornlert DA, Edwards SM, Morrison J, Field HI, Southey MC, Severi G, Donovan JL, Hamdy FC, Dearnaley DP, Muir KR, Smith C, Bagnato M, Ardern-Jones AT, Hall AL, O'Brien LT, Gehr-Swain BN, Wilkinson RA, Cox A, Lewis S, Brown PM, Jhavar SG, Tymrakiewicz M, Lophatananon A, Bryant SL, UK Genetic Prostate Cancer Study Collaborators; British Association of Urological Surgeons' Section of Oncology; UK ProtecT Study Collaborators, Horwich A, Huddart RA, Khoo VS, Parker CC, Woodhouse CJ, Thompson A, Christmas T, Ogden C, Fisher C, Jamieson C, Cooper CS, English DR, Hopper JL, Neal DE, Easton DF (2008a) Identification of multiple novel prostate cancer susceptibility loci by a genome-wide association study. Nat Genet 40:316–321

Eeles R, Giles G, Neal D, Hamdy F, Donovan J, Muir K, Easton DF, for the PRACTICAL Consortium (2008b) Reply to Variation in KLK genes, prostate specific antigen and risk of prostate cancer. Nat Genet 40(9):1035

Erkko H, Xia B, Nikkilä J, Schleutker J, Syrjäkoski K, Mannermaa A, Kallioniemi A, Pylkäs K, Karppinen SM, Rapakko K, Miron A, Sheng Q, Li G, Mattila H, Bell DW, Haber DA, Grip M, Reiman M, Jukkola-Vuorinen A, Mustonen A, Kere J, Aaltonen LA, Kosma VM, Kataja V, Soini Y, Drapkin RI, Livingston DM, Winqvist R (2007) A recurrent mutation in PALB2 in Finnish cancer families. Nature 446:316–319

Farmer H, McCabe N, Lord CJ, Tutt AN, Johnson DA, Richardson TB, Santarosa M, Dillon KJ, Hickson I, Knights C, Martin NM, Jackson SP, Smith GC, Ashworth A (2005) Targeting the DNA repair defect in BRCA mutant cells as a therapeutic strategy. Nature 434(7035):917–921

Fong PC, Boss DS, Carden M et al (2008) AZD2281 (KU-0059436), a PARP inhibitor with single agent anticancer activity in patients with BRCA deficient ovarian cancer. ASCO presentation Abstract 5510 ASCO meeting proceedings

Freedman ML, Haiman CA, Patterson N, McDonald GJ, Tandon A, Waliszewska A, Penney K, Steen RG, Ardlie K, John EM, Oakley-Girvan I, Whittemore AS, Cooney KA, Ingles SA, Altshuler D, Henderson BE, Reich D (2006) Admixture mapping identifies 8q24 as a prostate cancer risk locus in African–American men. Proc Natl Acad Sci USA 103:14068–14073

Ghoussaini M, Song H, Koessler T, Al Olama AA, Kote-Jarai Z, Driver KE, Pooley KA, Ramus SJ, Kjaer SK, Hogdall E, DiCioccio RA, Whittemore AS, Gayther SA, Giles GG, Guy M, Edwards SM, Morrison J, Donovan JL, Hamdy FC, Dearnaley DP, Ardern-Jones AT, Hall AL, O'Brien LT, Gehr-Swain BN, Wilkinson RA, Brown PM, Hopper JL, Neal DE, Pharoah PD, Ponder BA, Eeles RA, Easton DF, Dunning AM, The UK Genetic Prostate Cancer Study Collaborators/British Association of Urological Surgeons' Section of Oncology; UK ProtecT Study Collaborators (2008) Multiple loci with different cancer specificities within the 8q24 gene desert. J Natl Cancer Inst 100:962–966

Gibbs M, Stanford JL, McIndoe RA, Jarvik GP, Kolb S, Goode EL, Chakrabarti L, Schuster EF,
   Buckley VA, Miller EL, Brandzel S, Li S, Hood L, Ostrander EA (1999) Evidence for a rare
   prostate cancer-susceptibility locus at chromosome 1p36. Am J Hum Genet 64:776–787
Goldgar DE, Easton DF, Cannon-Albright LA, Skolnick MH (1994) Systematic population-based
   assessment of cancer risk in first-degree relatives of cancer probands. J Natl Cancer Inst
   86:1600–1608
Gong G, Oakley-Girvan I, Wu AH, Kolonel LN, John EM, West DW, Felberg A, Gallagher RP,
   Whittemore AS (2002) Segregation analysis of prostate cancer in 1, 719 white, African–
   American and Asian–American families in the United States and Canada. Cancer Causes
   Control 13(5):471–82
Greenman C, Stephens P, Smith R, Dalgliesh GL, Hunter C, Bignell G, Davies H, Teague J, Butler
   A, Stevens C, Edkins S, O'Meara S, Vastrik I, Schmidt EE, Avis T, Barthorpe S, Bhamra G,
   Buck G, Choudhury B, Clements J, Cole J, Dicks E, Forbes S, Gray K, Halliday K, Harrison
   R, Hills K, Hinton J, Jenkinson A, Jones D, Menzies A, Mironenko T, Perry J, Raine K,
   Richardson D, Shepherd R, Small A, Tofts C, Varian J, Webb T, West S, Widaa S, Yates A,
   Cahill DP, Louis DN, Goldstraw P, Nicholson AG, Brasseur F, Looijenga L, Weber BL, Chiew
   YE, DeFazio A, Greaves MF, Green AR, Campbell P, Birney E, Easton DF, Chenevix-Trench
   G, Tan MH, Khoo SK, Teh BT, Yuen ST, Leung SY, Wooster R, Futreal PA, Stratton MR
   (2007) Patterns of somatic mutation in human cancer genomes. Nature 446:153–158
Grönberg H, Damber L, Damber JE, Iselius L (1997) Segregation analysis of prostate cancer in
   Sweden: Support for dominant inheritance. Am J Epidemiol 146(7):552–557
Gudmundsson J, Sulem P, Manolescu A, Amundadottir LT, Gudbjartsson D, Helgason A, Rafnar
   T, Bergthorsson JT, Agnarsson BA, Baker A, Sigurdsson A, Benediktsdottir KR, Jakobsdottir
   M, Xu J, Blondal T, Kostic J, Sun J, Ghosh S, Stacey SN, Mouy M, Saemundsdottir J,
   Backman VM, Kristjansson K, Tres A, Partin AW, Albers-Akkers MT, Godino-Ivan Marcos J,
   Walsh PC, Swinkels DW, Navarrete S, Isaacs SD, Aben KK, Graif T, Cashy J, Ruiz-Echarri
   M, Wiley KE, Suarez BK, Witjes JA, Frigge M, Ober C, Jonsson E, Einarsson GV, Mayordomo
   JI, Kiemeney LA, Isaacs WB, Catalona WJ, Barkardottir RB, Gulcher JR, Thorsteinsdottir U,
   Kong A, Stefansson K (2007a) Genome-wide association study identifies a second prostate
   cancer susceptibility variant at 8q24. Nat Genet 39:631–637
Gudmundsson J, Sulem P, Steinthorsdottir V, Bergthorsson JT, Thorleifsson G, Manolescu A,
   Rafnar T, Gudbjartsson D, Agnarsson BA, Baker A, Sigurdsson A, Benediktsdottir KR,
   Jakobsdottir M, Blondal T, Stacey SN, Helgason A, Gunnarsdottir S, Olafsdottir A, Kristinsson
   KT, Birgisdottir B, Ghosh S, Thorlacius S, Magnusdottir D, Stefansdottir G, Kristjansson K,
   Bagger Y, Wilensky RL, Reilly MP, Morris AD, Kimber CH, Adeyemo A, Chen Y, Zhou J, So
   WY, Tong PC, Ng MC, Hansen T, Andersen G, Borch-Johnsen K, Jorgensen T, Tres A, Fuertes
   F, Ruiz-Echarri M, Asin L, Saez B, van Boven E, Klaver S, Swinkels DW, Aben KK, Graif T,
   Cashy J, Suarez BK, van Vierssen Trip O, Frigge ML, Ober C, Hofker MH, Wijmenga C,
   Christiansen C, Rader DJ, Palmer CN, Rotimi C, Chan JC, Pedersen O, Sigurdsson G,
   Benediktsson R, Jonsson E, Einarsson GV, Mayordomo JI, Catalona WJ, Kiemeney LA,
   Barkardottir RB, Gulcher JR, Thorsteinsdottir U, Kong A, Stefansson K (2007b) Two variants
   on chromosome 17 confer prostate cancer risk, and the one in TCF2 protects against type 2
   diabetes. Nat Genet 39:977–983
Gudmundsson J, Sulem P, Rafnar T, Bergthorsson JT, Manolescu A, Gudbjartsson D, Agnarsson
   BA, Sigurdsson A, Benediktsdottir KR, Blondal T, Jakobsdottir M, Stacey SN, Kostic J,
   Kristinsson KT, Birgisdottir B, Ghosh S, Magnusdottir DN, Thorlacius S, Thorleifsson G,
   Zheng SL, Sun J, Chang BL, Elmore JB, Breyer JP, McReynolds KM, Bradley KM, Yaspan
   BL, Wiklund F, Stattin P, Lindström S, Adami HO, McDonnell SK, Schaid DJ, Cunningham
   JM, Wang L, Cerhan JR, St Sauver JL, Isaacs SD, Wiley KE, Partin AW, Walsh PC, Polo S,
   Ruiz-Echarri M, Navarrete S, Fuertes F, Saez B, Godino J, Weijerman PC, Swinkels DW, Aben
   KK, Witjes JA, Suarez BK, Helfand BT, Frigge ML, Kristjansson K, Ober C, Jonsson E,
   Einarsson GV, Xu J, Gronberg H, Smith JR, Thibodeau SN, Isaacs WB, Catalona WJ,
   Mayordomo JI, Kiemeney LA, Barkardottir RB, Gulcher JR, Thorsteinsdottir U, Kong A,

Stefansson K (2008) Common sequence variants on 2p15 and Xp11.22 confer susceptibility to prostate cancer. Nat Genet 40:281–283

Guy M, Kote-Jarai Z, Giles GG, Al Olama AA, jugurnauth SK, Mulholland S, Leongamornlert DA, Edwards SM, Morrison J, Field HI, Southey MC, Severi G, Donovan JL, Hamdy FC, Dearnaley DP, Muir KR, Smith C, Bagnato M, Ardern-jones AT, Hall al, O;Brien LT, Gehr-Swain BN, Wilkinson RA, Cox A, Lewis S, Brown PM, Jhavar SG, Tymrakiewicz M, Lophatananon A, Bryant SL; UK Genetic prostate Cancer Study Collaborators; British Association of Urological Surgeons' Section of Oncology; UK protecT Study Collaborators, Horwich A, Huddart RA, Khoo VS, Parker CC, Woodhouse CJ, Thompson A, Christmas T, Ogden C, Fisher C, Jameson C, Cooper CS, English DR, Hopper JL, Neal DE, Easton DF, Eeles RA. Asian J Androl. 2009 Jan; 11(1):49–55

Haiman CA, Patterson N, Freedman ML, Myers SR, Pike MC, Waliszewska A, Neubauer J, Tandon A, Schirmer C, McDonald GJ, Greenway SC, Stram DO, Le Marchand L, Kolonel LN, Frasco M, Wong D, Pooler LC, Ardlie K, Oakley-Girvan I, Whittemore AS, Cooney KA, John EM, Ingles SA, Altshuler D, Henderson BE, Reich D (2007) Multiple regions within 8q24 independently affect risk for prostate cancer. Nat Genet 39:638–644

Hebbring SJ, Fredriksson H, White KA, Maier C, Ewing C, McDonnell SK, Jacobsen SJ, Cerhan J, Schaid DJ, Ikonen T, Autio V, Tammela TL, Herkommer K, Paiss T, Vogel W, Gielzak M, Sauvageot J, Schleutker J, Cooney KA, Isaacs W, Thibodeau SN (2006) Role of the Nijmegen breakage syndrome 1 gene in familial and sporadic prostate cancer. Cancer Epidemiol Biomarkers Prev 15(5):935–938

Helfand BT, Loeb S, Cashy J, Meeks JJ, Thaxton CS, Han M, Catalona WJ (2008) Tumor characteristics of carriers and noncarriers of the deCODE 8q24 prostate cancer susceptibility alleles. J Urol 179:2197–2202

Hemminki K, Vaittinen P (1998) Familial breast cancer in the family-cancer database. Int J Cancer 77:386–391

Hidaka K, Caffrey JJ, Hua L, Zhang T, Falck JR, Nickel GC, Carrel L, Barnes LD, Shears SB (2002) An adjacent pair of human NUDT genes on chromosome X are preferentially expressed in testis and encode two new isoforms of diphosphoinositol polyphosphate phosphohydrolase. J Biol Chem 277:32730–32738

Hope Q, Bullock S, Evans C, Meitz J, Hamel N, Edwards SM, Severi G, Dearnaley D, Jhavar S, Southgate C, Falconer A, Dowe A, Muir K, Houlston RS, Engert JC, Roquis D, Sinnett D, Simard J, Heimdal K, Moller P, Maehle L, Badzioch M, Eeles RA, Easton DF, English DR, Southey MC, Hopper JL, Foulkes WD, Giles GG (2005) Macrophage scavenger receptor 1 999C>T (R293X) mutation and risk of prostate cancer. Cancer Epidemiol Biomarkers Prev 14(2):397–402

Hsieh C-L, Oakley-Girvan I, Balise RR, Halpern J, Gallagher RP, Wu AH, Kolonel LN, O'Brien LE, Lin IG, Van Den Berg DJ, Teh CZ, West DW, Whittemore AS (2001) A genome screen of families with multiple cases of prostate cancer: Evidence of genetic heterogeneity. Am J Hum Genet 69:148–158

Janer M, Friedrichsen DM, Stanford JL, Badzioch MD, Kolb S, Deutsch K, Peters MA, Goode EL, Welti R, DeFrance HB, Iwasaki L, Li S, Hood L, Ostrander EA, Jarvik GP (2003) Genomic scan of 254 hereditary prostate cancer families. Prostate 57:309–319

Kawa S, Fujimoto J, Tezuka T, Nakazawa T, Yamamoto T (2004) Involvement of BREK, a serine/threonine kinase enriched in brain, in NGF signalling. Genes Cells 9:219–232

Kote-Jarai Z, Easton DF, Stanford JL, Ostrander EA, Schleutker J, Ingles SA, Schaid D, Thibodeau S, Dörk T, Neal D, Hamdy F, Donovan J, Cox A, Maier C, Vogel W, Guy M, Muir K, Lophatananon A, Kedda MA, Spurdle A, Steginga S, John EM, Giles G, Hopper J, Chappuis PO, Hutter P, Foulkes WD, Hamel N, Salinas CA, Koopmeiners JS, Karyadi DM, Johanneson B, Wahlfors T, Tammela TL, Stern MC, Corral R, McDonnell SK, Schürmann P, Meyer A, Kuefer R, Leongamornlert DA, Tymrakiewicz M, Liu JF, O'Mara T, Gardiner RA, Aitken J, Joshi AD, Severi G, English DR, Southey M, Edwards SM, Al Olama AA, PRACTICAL Consortium, Eeles RA (2008) Multiple novel prostate cancer predispostion loci confirmed by an international study: The PRACTICAL Consortium. Cancer Epidemiol Biomarkers Prev 17(8):2052–2061

Kruglyak L, Nickerson DA (2001) Variation is the spice of life. Nat Genet 27:234

Lai J, Kedda MA, Hinze K, Smith RL, Yaxley J, Spurdle AB, Morris CP, Harris J, Clements JA (2007) PSA/KLK3 AREI promoter polymorphism alters androgen receptor binding and is associated with prostate cancer susceptibility. Carcinogenesis 28:1032–1039

Lamerato LE, Marcus PM, Jacobsen G, Johnson CC (2008) Recruitment in the prostate, lung, colorectal, and ovarian (PLCO) cancer screening trial: The first phase of recruitment at Henry Ford Health System. Cancer Epidemiol Biomarkers Prev 17(4):827–33

Lee J, Demissie K, Lu SE, Rhoads GG (2007) Cancer incidence among Korean–American immigrants in the United States and native Koreans in South Korea. Cancer Control 14(1):78–85

Lichtenstein P, Holm NV, Verkasalo PK, Iliadou A, Kaprio J, Koskenvuo M, Pukkala E, Skytthe A, Hemminki K (2000) Environmental and heritable factors in the causation of cancer – Analyses of cohorts of twins from Sweden, Denmark, and Finland. N Engl J Med 343:78–85

Livingston RJ, von Niederhausern A, Jegga AG, Crawford DC, Carlson CS, Rieder MJ, Gowrisankar S, Aronow BJ, Weiss RB, Nickerson DA (2004) Pattern of sequence variation across 213 environmental response genes. Genome Res 14:1821–1831

Lou H, Yeager M, Li H, Bosquet JG, Hayes RB, Orr N, Yu K, Hutchinson A, Jacobs KB, Kraft P, Wacholder S, Chatterjee N, Feigelson HS, Thun MJ, Diver WR, Albanes D, Virtamo J, Weinstein S, Ma J, Gaziano JM, Stampfer M, Schummacher FR, Giovannucci E, Cancel-Tassin G,Cussenot O, Valeri A, Andriole GL, Crawford ED, Anderson SK, Tucker M, Hoover RN, Fraumeni JF Jr, Thomas G, Hunter DJ, Dean M, Chanock SJ. Proc Natl Acad Sci USA. 2009 May 12; 106(19):7933–7938

Maier C, Haeusler J, Herkommer K, Vesovic Z, Hoegel J, Vogel W, Paiss T (2005) Mutation screening and association study of RNASEL as a prostate cancer susceptibility gene. Br J Cancer 92:1159–1164

Marugame T, Katanoda K (2006) International comparisons of cumulative risk of breast and prostate cancer, from cancer incidence in five continents IARC Press, Lyon, France Vol. VIII. Jpn J Clin Oncol 36(6):399–400

McIndoe RA, Stanford JL, Gibbs M, Jarvik GP, Brandzel S, Neal CL, Li S, Gammack JT, Gay AA, Goode EL, Hood L, Ostrander EA (1997) Linkage analysis of 49 high-risk families does not support a common familial prostate cancer-susceptibility gene at 1q24-25. Am J Hum Genet 61:347–353

Meitz J, Edwards S, Easton D, Murkin A, Ardern-Jones A, Jackson R, Williams S, Dearnaley D, Stratton M, Houlston R, The CRC/BPGUK Familial Prostate Cancer Study Collaborators, Eeles RA (2002) HPC2/ELAC2 polymorphisms and prostate cancer risk: Analysis by age of onset of disease. Br J Cancer 87:905–908

Mitra A, Fisher C, Foster CS, Jameson C, Barbachanno Y, Bartlett J, Bancroft E, Doherty R, Kote-Jarai Z, Peock S, Easton D, IMPACT and EMBRACE Collaborators, Eeles R (2008) Prostate cancer in male BRCA1 and BRCA2 mutation carriers has a more aggressive phenotype. Br J Cancer 98((2):502–507

Narod SA, Neuhausen S, Vichodez G, Armel S, Lynch HT, Ghadirian P, Cummings S, Olopade O, Stoppa-Lyonnet D, Couch F, Wagner T, Warner E, Foulkes WD, Saal H, Weitzel J, Tulman A, Poll A, Nam R, Sun P; Hereditary Breast Cancer Study Group, Danquah J, Domchek S, Tung N, Ainsworth P, Horsman D, Kim-Sing C, Maugard C, Eisen A, Daly M, McKinnon W, Wood M, Isaacs C, Gilchrist D, Karlan B, Nedelcu R, Meschino W, Garber J, Pasini B, Manoukian S, Bellati C (2008) Rapid progression of prostate cancer in men with a BRCA2 mutation. Br J Cancer 99(2):371–374

Pomerantz MM, Ahmadiyeh N, Jia L, Herman P, Verzi MP, Doddapaneni H, Beckwith CA, Chan JA, Hills A, Davis M, Yao K, Kehoe SM, Lenz HJ, Haiman CA, Yan C, Henderson BE, Frenkel B, Barretina J, Bass A, Tabernero J, Baselga J, Regan MM, Manak JR, Shivdasani R, Coetzee GA, Freedman ML. Nat Genet. 2009 Aug; 41(8):882–884

Salinas CA, Kwon E, Carlson CS, Koopmeiners JS, Feng Z, Karyadi DM, Ostrander EA, Stanford JL (2008) Multiple independent genetic variants in the 8q24 region are associated with prostate cancer risk. Cancer Epidemiol Biomarkers Prev 17(5):1203–1213

Schaid DJ, McDonnell SK, Blute ML, Thibodeau SN (1998) Evidence for autosomal dominant inheritance of prostate cancer. Am J Hum Genet 62(6):1425–1438

Schaid DJ, Chang BL, The International Consortium For Prostate Cancer Genetics (2005) Description of the International Consortium for Prostate Cancer Genetics, and failure to replicate linkage of hereditary prostate cancer to 20q13. Prostate 63(3):276–290

Schleutker J, Matikainen M, Smith J, Koivisto P, Baffoe-Bonnie A, Kainu T, Gillanders E, Sankila R, Pukkala E, Carpten J, Stephan D, Tammela T, Brownstein M, Bailey-Wilson J, Trent J, Kallioniemi OP (2000) A genetic epidemiological study of hereditary prostate cancer (HPC) in Finland: Frequent HPCX linkage in families with late-onset disease. Clin Cancer Res 6:4810–4815

Schleutker J, Baffoe-Bonnie AB, Gillanders E, Kainu T, Jones MP, Freas-Lutz D, Markey C, Gildea D, Riedesel E, Albertus J, Gibbs KD Jr, Matikainen M, Koivisto PA, Tammela T, Bailey-Wilson JE, Trent JM, Kallioniemi OP (2003) Genome-wide scan for linkage in finish hereditary prostate cancer (HPC) families identifies novel susceptibility loci at 11q14 and 3p25-26. Prostate 57(4):280–289

Schröder FH (2008) Screening for prostate cancer (PC) – an update on recent findings of the European Randomized Study of Screening for Prostate Cancer (ERSPC). Urol Oncol 26(5):533–541

Singh R, The ACTANE Consortium, Eeles RA (2000) No evidence of linkage to chromosome 1q42.2-43 in 131 prostate cancer families from the ACTANE consortium. Br J Cancer 83:1654–1658

Slager SL, Zarfas KE, Brown WM, Lange EM, McDonnell SK, Wojno KJ, Cooney KA (2006) Genome-wide linkage scan for prostate cancer aggressiveness loci using families from the University of Michigan Prostate Cancer Genetics Project. Prostate 66(2):173–9

Smith JR, Freije D, Carpten JD, Grönberg H, Xu J, Isaacs SD, Brownstein MJ, Bova GS, Guo H, Bujinovszky P, Nusskern DR, Damber JE, Bergh A, Emanuelsson M, Kallioniemi OP, Walker-Daniels J, Bailey-Wilson JE, Beaty TH, Meyers DA, Walsh PRCA, Collins FS, Trent JM, Isaacs WB (1996) Major susceptibility locus for prostate cancer on chromosome 1 suggested by a genome-wide search. Science 274:1371–1374

Steuber T, Vickers AJ, Haese A, Becker C, Pettersson K, Chun FK, Kattan MW, Eastham JA, Scardino PT, Huland H, Lilja H (2006) Risk assessment for biochemical recurrence prior to radical prostatectomy: Significant enhancement contributed by human glandular kallikrein 2 (hk2) and free prostate specific antigen (PSA) in men with moderate PSA-elevation in serum. Int J Cancer 118:1234–1240

Steuber T, Helo P, Lilja H (2007) Circulating biomarkers for prostate cancer. World J Urol 25:111–119

Sun J, Zheng SL, Wiklund F, Isaacs SD, Purcell LD, Gao Z, Hsu FC, Kim ST, Liu W, Zhu Y, Stattin P, Adami HO, Wiley KE, Dimitrov L, Sun J, Li T, Turner AR, Adams TS, Adolfsson J, Johansson JE, Lowey J, Trock BJ, Partin AW, Walsh PC, Trent JM, Duggan D, Carpten J, Chang BL, Grönberg H, Isaacs WB, Xu J (2008) Evidence for two independent prostate cancer risk-associated loci in the HNF1B gene at 17q12. Nat Genet 40(10):1153–1155

Tan Y-C, Zeigler-Johnson C, Mittal RD, Mandhani A, Mital B, Rebbeck TR, Rennert H (2008) Common 8q24 sequence variations are associated with Asian Indian advanced prostate cancer risk. Cancer Epidemiol Biomarkers Prev 17(9):2431–2435

Tavtigian SV, Simard J, Teng DH, Abtin V, Baumgard M, Beck A, Camp NJ, Carillo AR, Chen Y, Dayananth P, Desrochers M, Dumont M, Farnham JM, Frank D, Frye C, Ghaffari S, Gupte JS, Hu R, Iliev D, Janecki T, Kort EN, Laity KE, Leavitt A, Leblanc G, McArthur-Morrison J, Pederson A, Penn B, Peterson KT, Reid JE, Richards S, Schroeder M, Smith R, Snyder SC, Swedlund B, Swensen J, Thomas A, Tranchant M, Woodland AM, Labrie F, Skolnick MH, Neuhausen S, Rommens J, Cannon-Albright LA (2001) A strong candidate prostate cancer susceptibility gene at chromosome 17p. Nat Genet 27:172–180

The Breast Cancer Linkage Consortium (1999) Cancer risks in BRCA2 mutation carriers. J Natl Cancer Inst 91:1310–1316

Thomas G, Jacobs KB, Yeager M, Kraft P, Wacholder S, Orr N, Yu K, Chatterjee N, Welch R, Hutchinson A, Crenshaw A, Cancel-Tassin G, Staats BJ, Wang Z, Gonzalez-Bosquet J, Fang J, Deng X, Berndt SI, Calle EE, Feigelson HS, Thun MJ, Rodriguez C, Albanes D, Virtamo J, Weinstein S, Schumacher FR, Giovannucci E, Willett WC, Cussenot O, Valeri A, Andriole GL, Crawford ED, Tucker M, Gerhard DS, Fraumeni JF Jr, Hoover R, Hayes RB, Hunter DJ, Chanock SJ (2008) Multiple loci identified in a genome-wide association study of prostate cancer. Nat Genet 40:310–315

Thompson D, Easton D, The Breast Cancer Linkage Consortium (2001) Variation in cancer risks, by mutation position, in BRCA2 mutation carriers. Am J Hum Genet 68(2):410–419

Thompson D, Seal S, Schutte M, McGuffog L, Barfoot R, Renwick A, Eeles R, Sodha N, Houlston R, Shanley S, Klijn J, Wasielewski M, Chang-Claude J, Futreal PA, Weber BL, Nathanson KL, Stratton M, Meijers-Heijboer H, Rahman N, Easton DF (2006) A multicenter study of cancer incidence in CHEK2 1100delC mutation carriers. Cancer Epidemiol Biomarkers Prev 15(12):2542–2545

Tischkowitz M, Sabbaghian N, Ray AM, Lange EM, Foulkes WD, Cooney KA (2008) Analysis of the gene coding for the BRCA2-interacting protein PALB2 in hereditary prostate cancer. Prostate 68(6):675–678

Tryggvadóttir L, Vidarsdóttir L, Thorgeirsson T, Jonasson JG, Olafsdóttir EJ, Olafsdóttir GH, Rafnar T, Thorlacius S, Jonsson E, Eyfjord JE, Tulinius H (2007) Prostate cancer progression and survival in BRCA2 mutation carriers. J Natl Cancer Inst 99(12):929–35

Wiklund F, Gillanders EM, Albertus JA, Bergh A, Damber JE, Emanuelsson M, Freas-Lutz DL, Gildea DE, Goransson I, Jones MS, Jonsson BA, Lindmark F, Markey CJ, Riedesel EL, Stenman E, Trent JM, Grönberg H (2003) Genome-wide scan of Swedish families with hereditary prostate cancer: Suggestive evidence of linkage at 5q11.2 and 19p13.3. Prostate 57:290–297

Wiklund F, Jonsson BA, Brookes AJ, Stromqvist L, Adolfsson J, Emanuelsson M, Adami HO, Augustsson-Balter K, Gronberg H (2004) Genetic analysis of the RNASEL gene in hereditary, familial, and sporadic prostate cancer. Clin Cancer Res 10(21):7150–7156

Xu J (2000) Combined analysis of hereditary prostate cancer linkage to 1q24-25: Results from 772 hereditary prostate cancer families from the International Consortium for Prostate Cancer Genetics. Am J Hum Genet 66:945–957

Xu J, Meyers D, Freije D, Isaacs S, Wiley K, Nusskern D, Ewing C, Wilkens E, Bujnovszky P, Bova GS, Walsh P, Isaacs W, Schleutker J, Matikainen M, Tammela T, Visakorpi T, Kallioniemi OP, Berry R, Schaid D, French A, McDonnell S, Schroeder J, Blute M, Thibodeau S, Gronberg H, Emanuelsson M, Damber JE, Bergh A, Jonsson BA, Smith J, Bailey-Wilson J, Carpten J, Stephan D, Gillanders E, Amundson I, Kainu T, Freas-Lutz D, Baffoe-Bonnie A, Van Aucken A, Sood R, Collins F, Brownstein M, Trent J (1998) Evidence for a prostate cancer susceptibility locus on the X chromosome. Nat Genet 20:175–179

Xu J, Zheng SL, Hawkins GA, Faith DA, Kelly B, Isaacs SD, Wiley KE, Chang B, Ewing CM, Bujinovszky P, Carpten JD, Bleecker ER, Walsh PRCA, Trent JM, Meyers DA, Isaacs WB (2001) Linkage and association studies of prostate cancer susceptibility: Evidence for linkage at 8p22-23. Am J Hum Genet 69:341–350

Xu J, Gillanders EM, Isaacs SD, Chang BL, Wiley KE, Zheng SL, Jones M, Gildea D, Riedesel E, Albertus J, Freas-Lutz D, Markey C, Meyers DA, Walsh PRCA, Trent JM, Isaacs WB (2003) Genome-wide scan for prostate cancer susceptibility genes in the Johns Hopkins hereditary prostate cancer families. Prostate 57:320–325

Xu J, Dimitrov L, Chang B-L, Adams TS, Turner AR, Meyers DA, Eeles R, Easton DF, Foulkes WD, Simard J, Giles G G, Hopper JL, Mahle L, Moller P, Bishop T, Evans C, Edwards S, Meitz J, Bullock S, Hope Q, Hsieh CL, Halpern J, Balise RN, Oakley-Girvan I, Whittemore AS, Ewing CM, Gielzak M, Isaacs SD, Walsh PC, Wiley KE, Isaacs WB, Thibodeau SN, McDonnell SK, Cunningham JM, Zarfas KE, Hebbring S, Schaid DJ, Friedrichsen DM, Deutsch K, Kolb S, Badzioch M, Jarvik GP, Janer M, Hood L, Ostrander EA, Stanford JL,

Lange EM, Beebe-Dimmer JL, Mohai CE, Conney KA, Ikonen T, Baffoe-Bonnie A, Fredriksson H, Matikainen MP, Tammela TL, Bailey-Wilson J, Schleutker J, Maier C, Herkommer K, Hoegal JJ, Vogel W, Paiss T, Siklund F, Emanuelsson M, Stenman E, Jonsson BA, Gronberg H, Camp NJ, Farnham J, Cannon-Albright LA, Seminara D, and The ACTANE Consortium (2005) A combined genome-wide linkage scan for prostate cancer susceptibility genes in 1,233 families conducted by the ICPCG. Am J Hum Genet 77(2):219–229, 11

Xu J, Isaacs SD, Sun J, Li G, Wiley KE, Zhu Y, Hsu FC, Wiklund F, Turner AR, Adams TS, Liu W, Trock BJ, Partin AW, Chang B, Walsh PC, Grönberg H, Isaacs W, Zheng S (2008) Association of prostate cancer risk variants with clinicopathologic characteristics of disease. Clin Cancer Res 14(18):5819–5824

Yeager M, Orr N, Hayes RB, Jacobs KB, Kraft P, Wacholder S, Minichiello MJ, Fearnhead P, Yu K, Chatterjee N, Wang Z, Welch R, Staats BJ, Calle EE, Feigelson HS, Thun MJ, Rodriguez C, Albanes D, Virtamo J, Weinstein S, Schumacher FR, Giovannucci E, Willett WC, Cancel-Tassin G, Cussenot O, Valeri A, Andriole GL, Gelmann EP, Tucker M, Gerhard DS, Fraumeni JF Jr, Hoover R, Hunter DJ, Chanock SJ, Thomas G (2007) Genome-wide association study of prostate cancer identifies a second risk locus at 8q24. Nat Genet 39:645–649

Yeager M, Xiao N, Hayes RB, Bouffard P, Desany B, Burdett L, Orr N, Matthews C, Qi L, Crenshaw A, Markovic Z, Fredrikson KM, Jacobs KB, Amundadottir L, Jarvie TP, Hunter DJ, Hoover R, Thomas G, Harkins TT, Chanock SJ (2008) Comprehensive resequence analysis of a 136 kb region of human chromosome 8q24 associated with prostate and colon cancers. Hum Genet 124:161–170

Zeigler-Johnson CM, Spangler E, Jalloh M, Gueye SM, Rennert H, Rebbeck TR (2008) Genetic susceptibility to prostate cancer in men of African descent: Implications for global disparities in incidence and outcomes. Can J Urol 15(1):3872–3882

Zheng SL, Xu J, Isaacs SD, Wiley K, Chang B, Bleecker ER, Walsh PRCA, Trent JM, Meyers DA, Isaacs WB (2001) Evidence for a prostate cancer linkage to chromosome 20 in 159 hereditary prostate cancer families. Hum Genet 108:430–435

Zheng SL, Sun J, Wiklund F, Smith S, Stattin P, Li G, Adami HO, Hsu FC, Zhu Y, Bälter K, Kader AK, Turner AR, Liu W, Bleecker ER, Meyers DA, Duggan D, Carpten JD, Chang BL, Isaacs WB, Xu J, Grönberg H (2008) Cumulative association of five genetic variants with prostate cancer. N Engl J Med 358:910–919

Chapter 9
Prostate Cancer in Special Populations

William D. Foulkes

Risk factors for prostate cancer have been discussed in detail in a previous chapter by Graham Giles (Chapter 1). As noted by Giles, in addition to the important effect of family history, it is notable that the incidence of prostate cancer varies substantially by ethnicity and nationality. This chapter explores these two factors in more detail, and focuses on special populations in which prostate cancer genetics has been explored in some detail including Icelanders, Poles, Ashkenazi Jews and African-Americans.

Icelanders are an example of a geographical isolate. The population of Iceland is approximately 300,000 individuals, and immigration is uncommon. In addition, there have been several important sudden declines in population, the most notable of which was the arrival of smallpox in 1707 which killed more than one quarter of Iceland's inhabitants. As a consequence of Iceland's isolation, genetic heterogeneity may be less pronounced in Iceland compared to other European countries. As discussed by Julius Gudmundsson and Kári Stefánsson, several important low to moderate penetrance prostate cancer alleles were first discovered in this population, and these findings have been subsequently confirmed in many other populations. Founder effects in several disease genes have been demonstrated in Iceland. Perhaps the most well-known cancer-associated mutation is the 999del5 mutation in *BRCA2*, which is associated with a substantially increased risk for breast cancer and accounts for the vast majority of hereditary breast cancer cases in Iceland. Importantly, as discussed in the chapter by Eeles and colleagues (Chapter 8), this mutation has been shown to be associated with aggressive prostate cancer. The presence of a founder mutation enabled these studies to be conducted, as systematically identifying all *BRCA2*-postive prostate cancer cases at low cost in an outbred population is not technically feasible at the current time.

W.D. Foulkes
Program in Cancer Genetics, Departments of Oncology and Human Genetics,
McGill University, 546 Pine Avenue West Montreal, QC, Canada H2W 1S6,
e-mail: william.foulkes@mcgill.ca

W.D. Foulkes and K.A. Cooney (eds.), *Male Reproductive Cancers:*
Epidemiology, Pathology and Genetics, Cancer Genetics,
DOI 10.1007/978-1-4419-0449-2_9, © Springer Science+Business Media, LLC 2010

Ashkenazi Jews are a genetic isolate for different reasons. Here, the isolation is mainly cultural and religious, rather than strictly geographical or linguistic. The worldwide Ashkenazi Jewish population is about 12 million, with the United States and Israel having the largest Ashkenazi Jewish populations. Founder mutations in BRCA1 and BRCA2 are important causes of breast cancer in this population, and in the chapter by William Foulkes and Sabrina Notte, the contribution of these and other alleles to prostate cancer risk in Ashkenazi Jewish men is discussed.

Recent studies have shown that, perhaps surprisingly, hereditary breast cancer in Poland can be attributed to a rather restricted number of alleles of BRCA1. Interestingly, one of these alleles, usually referred to as BRCA1: 5382insC (more properly c.5266dupC), is an important contributor to hereditary breast cancer in the Jewish population. In the contribution by Cezary Cybulski and Jan Lubiński, the role of BRCA1 alleles, as well as variants in NBS1, CHEK2 and other genes are discussed, further emphasizing the importance of population isolates in conducting prostate cancer research.

African-American men have the highest incidence of prostate cancer in the world. These men also suffer excess mortality from prostate cancer. A significant amount of research has been conducted in the last two decades to begin to address this health disparity. While the true explanation will likely be multifactorial and include issues regarding diet, environmental exposures as well as access to health care, genetic contributions will certainly be important. One genetic factor that seems to be particularly significant is the chromosome 8q24 region that is strongly associated with prostate cancer. Some of the risk alleles at this locus are much more frequent in the black Americans than in the white Americans. In the final sub-chapter by Baffoe-Bonnie and Powell, the main focus is on the African-American Hereditary Prostate Cancer Study, which has been one of the major groups working on the genetics of prostate cancer in blacks, with a particular focus on linkage approaches.

9.1 Genetics of Prostate Cancer in Iceland

Julius Gudmundsson and Kári Stefánsson

9.1.1 Introduction

In Iceland, like in most other Western countries, prostate cancer incidence has risen dramatically over the past four decades. According to the Icelandic Cancer Registry (ICR; www.http://www.krabbameinsskra.is) which contains data going back to 1955 about all Icelanders diagnosed with cancer the annual age-standardized incidence has increased close to sixfold. It has gone from about 16 individuals annually per 100,000 individuals during the years 1955–1960, to the current rate of over 90 individuals per 100,000. Prostate cancer is by far the most common cancer in Icelandic males, accounting for about 30% of all cancers (lung- and colon cancer come next accounting for about 10% and 8%, respectively). Despite the rapid rise in prostate cancer incidence over the past 40 years, the death rate has remained more or less stable over the same time period. Yet, prostate cancer is the second leading cause of death due to cancer, causing about 19% of all cancer-related deaths in males, only exceeded by lung cancer. Currently, there are more than 1,400 individuals alive with the disease in Iceland and over the past 5 years about 185 individuals were diagnosed annually with prostate cancer having an average age at diagnosis of 72 years.

9.1.2 Risk Variants and Familial Factors in Prostate Cancer

Of the various risk factors associated with prostate cancer, age, ethnicity, and positive family history are the ones most firmly established. In Iceland, the relative risk (RR) among first-degree male relatives of prostate cancer patients

J. Gudmundsson
deCODE genetics, Sturlugata 8, 101, Reykjavik, Iceland
julius.gudmundsson@decode.is

K. Stefánsson (✉)
deCODE genetics, Sturlugata 8, 101, Reykjavik, Iceland
kari.stefansson@decode.is

has been estimated to be about 1.7–1.9 (Eldon et al. 2003; Amundadottir et al. 2004). Furthermore, by making use of the extensive genealogic data existing in Iceland and data from the ICR, it has been shown that RR risk greater than one extends well beyond the nuclear family. Second- and third-degree relatives were found to have an RR of 1.36 and 1.19, respectively, whereas fourth- and fifth-degree relatives have an RR of 1.10 (Amundadottir et al. 2004). The familial coaggregation of prostate cancer and other cancer types, of which breast cancer is the most prevalent, has also been reported (Tulinius et al. 1992; Amundadottir et al. 2004).

9.1.3   Candidate Loci in Prostate Cancer

Several variants in the sequence of the human genome have been implicated in the aetiology of prostate cancer (reviewed in Simard et al. 2003; Schaid 2004; Dong 2006). Some variants have yielded conflicting results and the ones better established, like *BRCA1* and *BRCA2*, are only believed to explain a small proportion of the prostate cancer susceptibility. Of the candidate loci/genes studied so far in Iceland, *RNASEL (HPC1)*, *HPCX*, and *PCAP* produced negative LOD scores when studied in prostate cancer families (Bergthorsson et al. 2000). Hence, it is unlikely that these genes account for any substantial fraction of the familial contribution to prostate cancer susceptibility in Iceland. The breast cancer susceptibility gene *BRCA2* has been investigated extensively in Iceland where a single founder mutation, 999del5, is accountable for all *BRCA2*-related cancer cases (Gudmundsson et al. 1996; Thorlacius et al. 1996). This mutation has not only been detected in individuals with breast cancer belonging to high-risk cancer families, but also been detected in individuals diagnosed with several other cancer types, including prostate cancer (Thorlacius et al. 1996; Johannesdottir et al. 1996). Carriers of the 999del5 mutation among prostate cancer patients have a significantly worse prognosis than non-carriers (Tryggvadottir et al. 2007), and although it has been shown that the 999del5 mutation accounts for majority of the excess risk of prostate cancer in relatives of breast cancer patients (Tulinius et al. 2002), some residual risk remains unaccounted for (Baffoe-Bonnie et al. 2002). The frequency of 999del5 has only been shown to be elevated in Icelandic prostate cancer cases that either have young age at diagnosis (<65 years), or are relatives of breast cancer patients (Johannesdottir et al. 1996; Sigurdsson et al. 1997). On the contrary, when the frequency of the Icelandic *BRCA2* mutation was estimated in an unselected case series recruited over a period of six years (2000–2006) and consisting of about 1,600 prostate cancer cases, there was no statistically significant excess in the cases compared with the 2,000 controls used (deCODE, unpublished data). Therefore it is evident that *BRCA2* contributes only very little to the overall disease burden of prostate cancer in Iceland.

9.1.4   Chromosome 8q24

Recently, variants on chromosome 8q24 were shown to confer risk of prostate cancer (Amundadottir et al. 2006). The 8q24 region was originally discovered by applying classical methods of positional cloning where a suggestive linkage signal was detected after performing a genome-wide linkage scan on 871 Icelandic men grouped into 323 extended families. Fine-mapping with microsatellite markers of a 10 Mb region yielded the strongest association to prostate cancer for allele −8 of marker DG8S737, with an odds ratio (OR) of 1.79 ($P = 3.0 \times 10^{-6}$). A further refinement of the association signal resulted in allele A of SNP rs1447295 with an OR of 1.72 ($P = 1.7 \times 10^{-9}$). These two markers were genotyped in case-control samples of European descent from Sweden and the United States which resulted in a combined OR of 1.62 for allele −8 of DG8S737 and 1.51 for allele A of rs1447295 (both with $P < 3.0 \times 10^{-11}$). When the association on 8q24 was examined in cases and controls of African descent from the United States, only the −8 allele of the microsatellite marker DG8S737 yielded a replication. The observed OR was lower in this study group but the frequency of the allele was twice as high as in samples descended from Europeans (Amundadottir et al. 2006). This observation is of interest since SNPs are generally thought to be more stable and, therefore, more likely to replicate across populations and ethnic groups. In this region, however, the micro-satellite is capturing better the underlying risk variant than the SNP, even though the SNP, based on its frequency distribution, is apparently also of an African origin. The prostate cancer risk conferred by the variants on 8q24 has since been confirmed by several independent groups (Freedman et al. 2006; Schumacher et al. 2007; Severi et al. 2007; Suuriniemi et al. 2007; Wang et al. 2007; Haiman et al. 2007; Yeager et al. 2007).

   In order to study further the genetic risk of prostate cancer in Iceland, a genome-wide SNP association (GWA) study was conducted, involving 1,500 cases and over 3,000 controls (Gudmundsson et al. 2007a). In that study, the previously identified allele A of SNP rs1447295 showed the strongest result with an OR of 1.71 ($P = 1.7 \times 10^{-14}$) and was the only SNP exceeding a genome-wide significance level (~1.5 × 10^{-7}). However, a further elaboration of the data by using haplotypes defined in such a way that each spans only a single linkage disequilibrium (LD) block, resulted in the discovery of a new variant located in an LD-block 300 kb centromeric of the original 8q24 signal (region 1) and only very weakly correlated with it ($r^2 = 0.01$, $D' = 0.2$). This haplotype, designated HapC and defined by 14 SNPs, had an OR of 2.08 ($P = 1.4 \times 10^{-10}$) but the frequency was considerably lower than that of the SNP rs1447295 in region 1, or 3% in Icelandic controls compared to 10.4%, respec-tively. By examining the HapMap data and later by further genotyping in the Icelandic study group, allele A of rs16901979 was shown to be strongly correlated with HapC as well as associated to prostate cancer (OR = 1.80; $P = 9.9 \times 10^{-9}$). The combined population attributable risk (PAR) of the two variants on 8q24 is about 16.5% in Iceland. Both the results for HapC and the correlated SNP were replicated in case-control samples of European descent from Spain, the Netherlands, and the United States. The combined OR of allele A of rs16901979 in the three populations was about 1.8 ($P = 2.4 \times 10^{-5}$). When the SNP was genotyped in African-American samples it was found to be significantly associated to prostate cancer with an OR of 1.34 ($P = 5 \times 10^{-5}$) and similarly to the results for the variants in region 1, the frequency was found to be considerably higher (>10 times) than in the European descended samples (Gudmundsson et al. 2007a). When a closer look was taken at the impact of the 8q24 variants from the two regions on a more aggressive form of the disease, as reflected by high Gleason scores, the at-risk alleles of the two markers in region 1 had a greater frequency in individuals with high (7–10) compared with low (2–6) Gleason scores (Amundadottir et al. 2006). For the HapC region on the contrary, no evidence was found of a stronger association to the disease in individuals with a higher Gleason score. However, for each copy of allele A of rs16901979, carriers were diagnosed with prostate cancer 1.4 years younger than the non-carriers; HapC gave very similar results (Gudmundsson et al. 2007a). Based on this observation and the fact that familial cancer cases tend to have younger age at diagnosis, it is not surprising that the frequency of allele A of rs16901979 is greater in individuals who have at least one first- or second-degree relative with prostate cancer than in cases who have no closely related relative diagnosed with prostate cancer (OR of 1.6 and $P = 0.002$) (deCODE; unpublished results).

Based on the results discussed above, it is clear that the sequence variants on 8q24 play an important role in conferring genetic risk of prostate cancer in Iceland as well as in other parts of the world. However, despite being the only variants generating genome-wide significant results in the association analysis, the 8q24 variants are not the only sequence variants having significant impact on prostate cancer risk in Iceland.

9.1.5 Chromosome 17q

On the basis of the above-mentioned GWA-study, two common variants, having an allelic frequency between 45% and 50% in two distinct regions on the long arm of chromosome 17 were shown to confer risk of prostate cancer. The RR was estimated to be about 1.45 for the homozygous carriers and their frequency was between 20% and 25% in a combined analysis of four study populations, all of European descent (Gudmundsson et al. 2007b). One locus was on 17q12 (rs7501939 and rs4430796) encompassing the 5′ end of the *TCF2* (*HNF1β*) gene. The second locus is in a gene poor area on 17q24.3 (rs1859962). The two loci are separated by approximately 33 Mb and no correlation was observed between them. Chromosome 17q has been previously implicated in prostate cancer by linkage analysis (Lange et al. 2003; Xu et al. 2005) and the two loci reside within a region having LOD scores ranging from 1 to 2 but outside a proposed 10-cM candidate gene region reported in a recent linkage analysis (Lange et al. 2007). Based on the combined results from the four study populations, the two variants on 17q have an estimated PAR of 20% each, and a PAR of about 36% combined. The large PAR is a consequence of the high frequencies of these variants. However, as their relative risks, as estimated by the ORs, are not high, the sibling risk ratio accounted for by them is only approximately 1.009 each, and 1.018 jointly. As a consequence, they can only explain a small fraction of the familial clustering of the disease and can therefore only generate modest linkage scores.

The *TCF2* gene on 17q12 has been reported to be mutated in individuals diagnosed with renal cysts, pancreatic atrophy, genital tract abnormalities, and maturity-onset diabetes of the young, type 5 (MODY5) (Bellanne-Chantelot et al. 2005; Edghill et al. 2006). Interestingly, several epidemiological studies have demonstrated an inverse relationship between type 2 diabetes (T2D) and the risk of prostate cancer (Kasper and Giovannucci 2006 and references therein). When the effect of the two SNPs in *TCF2* showing association to prostate cancer were studied in an Icelandic T2D case-control group as well as in seven additional T2D case-control groups of African-, Asian-, and European descent, both SNPs on 17q12 showed a protection against the disease (i.e., OR < 1.0). The combined results from all groups including Iceland gave an OR of 0.91 ($P = 9.2 \times 10^{-7}$) for allele C of rs7501939, and an OR of 0.91 ($P = 2.7 \times 10^{-7}$) for allele A of rs4430796. The discovery of variants in TCF2 that confer risk of prostate cancer but protect against T2D explains at least partly the inverse relationship previously described between the two diseases. A more detailed study of the function of TCF2 may lead to the identification of mutual pathway(s) that could provide better diagnostic and/or therapeutic options for both diseases.

9.1.6   Conclusion

Four new sequence variants having significant impact on the risk of prostate cancer in Iceland and in other parts of the world have been discovered. Three of them are common (>5% freq.) and they all confer low to moderate risk. The 8q24 region is the first prostate cancer locus consistently replicated across populations and ethnic groups.

Based on combined results from several European populations, the four variants on 8q24 and 17q have an estimated joint PAR of about 44%, which is substantial from a public health point of view. On the contrary, the risk associated with each variant is relatively small. Therefore it is unlikely that any single variant will be of diagnostic importance alone. However, further studies on the combined effect of these and other prostate cancer risk factors may provide a sufficiently high predictive value to become clinically important.

Three of the four loci do not have an obvious candidate gene as a target for functional studies. Whether this makes it possible to further refine the association signal and thereby uncover greater risk conferred by new variants remains to be determined.

The fourth locus contains a gene that has no prior relevance to prostate cancer but at least partly accounts for the inverse correlation between prostate cancer and T2D.

Based on results from a genome-wide association analysis done in population-based case-control samples, it is clear that low to moderate risk variants contribute significantly to the overall prostate cancer susceptibility in Iceland. However, these variants do not contribute extensively to the familial clustering of prostate cancer. Hence, additional susceptibility variants remain to be identified.

Note Added in Proof

Further loci associated with an increased risk of prostate cancer on chromosomes Xp11.2 and 2p15 have been identified using icelandic cases and controls (Gudmundsson J et al, Nature Genetics, 40 (3), 281-283, 2008)

References

Amundadottir LT, Thorvaldsson S, Gudbjartsson DF, Sulem P, Kristjansson K, Arnason S, Gulcher JR, Bjornsson J, Kong A, Thorsteinsdottir U, Stefansson, K (2004) Cancer as a complex phenotype: Pattern of cancer distribution within and beyond the nuclear family. PLoS Med 1(3):e65 Epub 2004 Dec 28

Amundadottir LT, Sulem P, Gudmundsson J, Helgason A, Baker A, Agnarsson BA, Sigurdsson A, Benediktsdottir KR, Cazier JB, Sainz J, Jakobsdottir M, Kostic J, Magnusdottir DN, Ghosh S, Agnarsson K, Birgisdottir B, Le Roux L, Olafsdottir A, Blondal T, Andresdottir M, Gretarsdottir OS, Bergthorsson JT, Gudbjartsson D, Gylfason A, Thorleifsson G, Manolescu A, Kristjansson K, Geirsson G, Isaksson H, Douglas J, Johansson JE, Balter K, Wiklund F, Montie JE, Yu X, Suarez BK, Ober C, Cooney KA, Gronberg H, Catalona WJ, Einarsson GV, Barkardottir RB, Gulcher JR, Kong A, Thorsteinsdottir U, Stefansson K (2006) A common variant associated with prostate cancer in European and African populations. Nat Genet 38(6):652–658

Baffoe-Bonnie AB, Kiemeney LA, Beaty TH, Bailey-Wilson JE, Schnell AH, Sigvaldason H, Olafsdottir G, Tryggvadottir L, Tulinius H (2002) Segregation analysis of 389 Icelandic pedigrees with Breast and prostate cancer. Genet Epidemiol 23(4):349–363

Bellanne-Chantelot C, Clauin S, Chauveau D, Collin P, Daumont M, Douillard C, Dubois-Laforgue D, Dusselier L, Gautier JF, Jadoul M, Laloi-Michelin M, Jacquesson L, Larger E, Louis J, Nicolino M, Subra JF, Wilhem JM, Young J, Velho G, Timsit J (2005) Large genomic rearrangements in the hepatocyte nuclear factor-1beta (TCF2) gene are the most frequent cause of maturity-onset diabetes of the young type 5. Diabetes 54(11):3126–3132

Bergthorsson JT, Johannesdottir G, Arason A, Benediktsdottir KR, Agnarsson BA, Bailey-Wilson JE, Gillanders E, Smith J, Trent J, Barkardottir RB (2000) Analysis of HPC1, HPCX, and PCaP in Icelandic hereditary prostate cancer. Hum Genet 107(4):372–375

Dong JT. (2006) Prevalent mutations in prostate cancer. J Cell Biochem 97(3):433–447

Edghill EL, Bingham C, Ellard S, Hattersley AT (2006) Mutations in hepatocyte nuclear factor-1beta and their related phenotypes. J Med Genet 43(1):84–90

Eldon BJ, Jonsson E, Tomasson J, Tryggvadottir L, Tulinius H (2003) Familial risk of prostate cancer in Iceland. BJU Int 92(9):915–919

Freedman ML, Haiman CA, Patterson N, McDonald GJ, Tandon A, Waliszewska A, Penney K, Steen RG, Ardlie K, John EM, Oakley-Girvan I, Whittemore AS, Cooney KA, Ingles SA, Altshuler D, Henderson BE, Reich D (2006) Admixture mapping identifies 8q24 as a prostate cancer risk locus in African-American men. Proc Natl Acad Sci U S A 103(38):14068–14073

Gudmundsson J, Johannesdottir G, Arason A, Bergthorsson JT, Ingvarsson S, Egilsson V, Barkardottir RB (1996) Frequent occurrence of BRCA2 linkage in Icelandic breast cancer families and segregation of a common BRCA2 haplotype. Am J Hum Genet 58(4):749–756

Gudmundsson J, Sulem P, Manolescu A, Amundadottir LT, Gudbjartsson D, Helgason A, Rafnar T, Bergthorsson JT, Agnarsson BA, Baker A, Sigurdsson A, Benediktsdottir KR, Jakobsdottir M, Xu J, Blondal T, Kostic J, Sun J, Ghosh S, Stacey SN, Mouy M, Saemundsdottir J, Backman VM, Kristjansson K, Tres A, Partin AW, Albers-Akkers MT, Godino-Ivan Marcos J, Walsh PC, Swinkels DW, Navarrete S, Isaacs SD, Aben KK, Graif T, Cashy J, Ruiz-Echarri M, Wiley KE, Suarez BK, Witjes JA, Frigge M, Ober C, Jonsson E, Einarsson GV, Mayordomo JI, Kiemeney LA, Isaacs WB, Catalona WJ, Barkardottir RB, Gulcher JR, Thorsteinsdottir U, Kong A, Stefansson K (2007a) Genome-wide association study identifies a second prostate cancer susceptibility variant at 8q24. Nat Genet 39(5):631–647

Gudmundsson J, Sulem P, Steinthorsdottir V, Bergthorsson JT, Thorleifsson G, Manolescu A, Rafnar T, Gudbjartsson D, Agnarsson BA, Baker A, Sigurdsson A, Benediktsdottir KR, Jakobsdottir M, Blondal T, Stacey SN, Helgason A, Gunnarsdottir S, Olafsdottir A, Kristinsson KT, Birgisdottir B, Ghosh S, Thorlacius S, Magnusdottir D, Stefansdottir G, Kristjansson K, Bagger Y, Wilensky RL, Reilly MP, Morris AD, Kimber CH, Adeyemo A, Chen Y, Zhou J, So WY, Tong PC, Ng MC, Hansen T, Andersen G, Borch-Johnsen K, Jorgensen T, Tres A, Fuertes F, Ruiz-Echarri M, Asin L, Saez B, van Boven E, Klaver S, Swinkels DW, Aben KK, Graif T, Cashy J, Suarez BK, van Vierssen Trip O, Frigge ML, Ober C, Hofker MH, Wijmenga C, Christiansen C, Rader DJ, Palmer CN, Rotimi C, Chan JC, Pedersen O, Sigurdsson G, Benediktsson R, Jonsson E, Einarsson GV, Mayordomo JI, Catalona WJ, Kiemeney LA, Barkardottir RB, Gulcher JR, Thorsteinsdottir U, Kong A, Stefansson K (2007b) Two variants on chromosome 17 confer prostate cancer risk, and the one in TCF2 protects against type 2 diabetes. Nat Genet. doi:10.1038/ng2062

Haiman CA, Patterson N, Freedman ML, Myers SR, Pike MC, Waliszewska A, Neubauer J, Tandon A, Schirmer C, McDonald GJ, Greenway SC, Stram DO, Le Marchand L, Kolonel LN, Frasco M, Wong D, Pooler LC, Ardlie K, Oakley-Girvan I, Whittemore AS, Cooney KA, John EM, Ingles SA, Altshuler D, Henderson BE, Reich D (2007) Multiple regions within 8q24 independently affect risk for prostate cancer. Nat Genet 39(5):638–644

Johannesdottir G, Gudmundsson J, Bergthorsson JT, Arason A, Agnarsson BA, Eiriksdottir G, Johannsson OT, Borg A, Ingvarsson S, Easton DF, Egilsson V, Barkardottir RB. (1996) High prevalence of the 999del5 mutation in icelandic breast and ovarian cancer patients. Cancer Res 56(16):3663–3665

Kasper JS, Giovannucci E. (2006) A meta-analysis of diabetes mellitus and the risk of prostate cancer. Cancer Epidemiol Biomarkers Prev 15(11):2056–2062

Lange EM, Gillanders EM, Davis CC, Brown WM, Campbell JK, Jones M, Gildea D, Riedesel E, Albertus J, Freas-Lutz D, Markey C, Giri V, Dimmer JB, Montie JE, Trent JM, Cooney KA. (2003) Genome-wide scan for prostate cancer susceptibility genes using families from the University of Michigan prostate cancer genetics project finds evidence for linkage on chromosome 17 near BRCA1. Prostate 57(4):326–334

Lange EM, Robbins CM, Gillanders EM, Zheng SL, Xu J, Wang Y, White KA, Chang BL, Ho LA, Trent JM, Carpten JD, Isaacs WB, Cooney KA. (2007) Fine-mapping the putative chromosome 17q21–22 prostate cancer susceptibility gene to a 10 cM region based on linkage analysis. Hum Genet 121(1):49–55

Schaid DJ. (2004) The complex genetic epidemiology of prostate cancer. Hum Mol Genet 13(1):R103– R121

Schumacher FR, Feigelson HS, Cox DG, Haiman CA, Albanes D, Buring J, Calle EE, Chanock SJ, Colditz GA, Diver WR, Dunning AM, Freedman ML, Gaziano JM, Giovannucci E, Hankinson SE, Hayes RB, Henderson BE, Hoover RN, Kaaks R, Key T, Kolonel LN, Kraft P,

Le Marchand L, Ma J, Pike MC, Riboli E, Stampfer MJ, Stram DO, Thomas G, Thun MJ, Travis R, Virtamo J, Andriole G, Gelmann E, Willett WC, Hunter DJ. (2007) A common 8q24 variant in prostate and breast cancer from a large nested case-control study. Cancer Res 67(7):2951–2956

Severi G, Hayes VM, Padilla EJ, English DR, Southey MC, Sutherland RL, Hopper JL, Giles GG. (2007) The common variant rs1447295 on chromosome 8q24 and prostate cancer risk: results from an Australian population-based case-control study. Cancer Epidemiol Biomarkers Prev 16(3):610–612

Sigurdsson S, Thorlacius S, Tomasson J, Tryggvadottir L, Benediktsdottir K, Eyfjord JE, Jonsson E (1997) BRCA2 mutation in Icelandic prostate cancer patients. J Mol Med 75(10):758–761

Simard J, Dumont M, Labuda D, Sinnett D, Meloche C, El-Alfy M, Berger L, Lees E, Labrie F, Tavtigian SV (2003) Prostate cancer susceptibility genes: lessons learned and challenges posed. Endocr Relat Cancer 10(2):225–259

Suuriniemi M, Agalliu I, Schaid DJ, Johanneson B, McDonnell SK, Iwasaki L, Stanford JL, Ostrander EA (2007) Confirmation of a positive association between prostate cancer risk and a locus at chromosome 8q24. Cancer Epidemiol Biomarkers Prev 16(4):809–814

Thorlacius S, Olafsdottir G, Tryggvadottir L, Neuhausen S, Jonasson JG, Tavtigian SV, Tulinius H, Ogmundsdottir HM, Eyfjord JE (1996) A single BRCA2 mutation in male and female breast cancer families from Iceland with varied cancer phenotypes. Nat Genet 13(1):117–119

Tryggvadottir L, Vidarsdottir L, Thorgeirsson T, Jonasson JG, Olafsdottir EJ, Olafsdottir GH, Rafnar T, Thorlacius S, Jonsson E, Eyfjord JE, Tulinius H. 2007. Prostate cancer progression and survival in BRCA2 mutation carriers. J Natl Cancer Inst 99(12):929–935

Tulinius H, Egilsson V, Olafsdottir GH, Sigvaldason H (1992) Risk of prostate, ovarian, and endometrial cancer among relatives of women with breast cancer. BMJ 305(6858):855–857

Tulinius H, Olafsdottir GH, Sigvaldason H, Arason A, Barkardottir RB, Egilsson V, Ogmundsdottir HM, Tryggvadottir L, Gudlaugsdottir S, Eyfjord JE. (2002) The effect of a single BRCA2 mutation on cancer in Iceland. J Med Genet 39(7):457–462

Wang L, McDonnell SK, Slusser JP, Hebbring SJ, Cunningham JM, Jacobsen SJ, Cerhan JR, Blute ML, Schaid DJ, Thibodeau SN (2007) Two common chromosome 8q24 variants are associated with increased risk for prostate cancer. Cancer Res 67(7):2944–2950

Xu J, Dimitrov L, Chang BL, Adams TS, Turner AR, Meyers DA, Eeles RA, Easton DF, Foulkes WD, Simard J, Giles GG, Hopper JL, Mahle L, Moller P, Bishop T, Evans C, Edwards S, Meitz J, Bullock S, Hope Q, Hsieh CL, Halpern J, Balise RN, Oakley-Girvan I, Whittemore AS, Ewing CM, Gielzak M, Isaacs SD, Walsh PC, Wiley KE, Isaacs WB, Thibodeau SN, McDonnell SK, Cunningham JM, Zarfas KE, Hebbring S, Schaid DJ, Friedrichsen DM, Deutsch K, Kolb S, Badzioch M, Jarvik GP, Janer M, Hood L, Ostrander EA, Stanford JL, Lange EM, Beebe-Dimmer JL, Mohai CE, Cooney KA, Ikonen T, Baffoe-Bonnie A, Fredriksson H, Matikainen MP, Tammela TL, Bailey-Wilson J, Schleutker J, Maier C, Herkommer K, Hoegel JJ, Vogel W, Paiss T, Wiklund F, Emanuelsson M, Stenman E, Jonsson BA, Gronberg H, Camp NJ, Farnham J, Cannon-Albright LA, Seminara D (2005) A combined genomewide linkage scan of 1,233 families for prostate cancer-susceptibility genes conducted by the international consortium for prostate cancer genetics. Am J Hum Genet 77(2):219–229

Yeager M, Orr N, Hayes RB, Jacobs KB, Kraft P, Wacholder S, Minichiello MJ, Fearnhead P, Yu K, Chatterjee N, Wang Z, Welch R, Staats BJ, Calle EE, Feigelson HS, Thun MJ, Rodriguez C, Albanes D, Virtamo J, Weinstein S, Schumacher FR, Giovannucci E, Willett WC, Cancel-Tassin G, Cussenot O, Valeri A, Andriole GL, Gelmann EP, Tucker M, Gerhard DS, Fraumeni JF, Jr, Hoover R, Hunter DJ, Chanock SJ, Thomas G. 2007. Genome-wide association study of prostate cancer identifies a second risk locus at 8q24. Nat Genet 39(5):645–649

9.2 Genetics in Poland

Cezary Cybulski and Jan Lubiński

9.2.1 Introduction

Prostate cancer constitutes approximately 11% of all male cancer cases diagnosed in Poland, being the second leading cancer in Polish men. In 2005, there were 7,095 new cases of prostate cancer diagnosed in Poland and the prostate cancer incidence rate (per 100,000) was 27.3. The lifetime risk of being diagnosed with prostate cancer is approximately 3.5% for men in Poland. This is significantly lower than in other European countries. The mean age of diagnosis of prostate cancer is approximately 68 years, and 6.5% of these cases are diagnosed before age 55.

Epidemiologic data suggest that an inherited susceptibility plays a role in the etiology of prostate cancer in the Polish population – familial clustering of prostate cancer is seen in 13% of all prostate cancer cases, and the frequency of hereditary prostate cancer among unselected cases of prostate cancer is approximately 2%. The research conducted over the last decade has led to identification of DNA variants conferring an increased risk of prostate cancer in Polish men. Germline mutations in genes in the DNA damage signaling pathway, such as *NBS1*, *BRCA1*, and *CHEK2*, confer an increased prostate cancer risk in the Polish men. However, inherited variation in *RNASEL*, and *MSR1* genes do not seem to contribute to prostate cancer development in this country.

9.2.2 *NBS1* Gene

Nijmegen breakage syndrome (NBS) is characterized by spontaneous chromosomal instability, immunodeficiency, and a predisposition to cancer. This is an autosomal recessive condition and the product of the causative gene, *NBS1*, now known as *NBN*,

C. Cybulski and J. Lubiński (✉)
Department of Genetics and Pathomorphology, Pomeranian Medical University,
PL−70-111 Szczecin, al. Powstanco Wlkp. 72, Pomerania, Poland
lubinski@sci.pam.szczecin.pl

is part of the DNA damage repair signaling pathway (Varon et al. 1998). A 5-bp deletion in exon 6 of *NBS1* (657del5) is present in the majority of NBS patients from Eastern Europe. This variant is present in approximately 0.6% individuals (heterozygous carriers) from the general population of Poland.

It has been suggested that heterozygous carriers of the founder mutation in the gene *NBS1 (NBN)* (657del5 allele) may be at increased risk of cancer at various sites. We documented the role of the 657del5 allele in the etiology of prostate cancer (Cybulski et al. 2004a). We showed an excess of the *NBS1* founder mutation in a series of 340 unselected prostate cancer cases compared with the general public (2.6% vs. 0.6%; OR = 4.5; *P* = 0.002). The prevalence of the mutant founder allele was high particularly among men with familial prostate cancer (9%) (OR = 16; *P* < 0.0001), and within these families, the *NBS1* mutation segregated with the disease (Fig. 9.2.1). In addition, the wild-type *NBS1* allele was lost in the majority of the prostate cancers from 657del5 mutation carriers. Therefore, it appears that *NBS1*

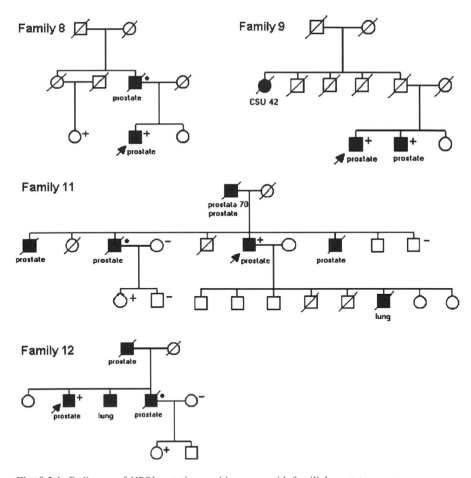

Fig. 9.2.1 Pedigrees of *NBS1* mutation-positive cases with familial prostate cancer

functions as a classical tumor suppressor gene for prostate cancer that increases the risk of prostate cancer by 4.5-fold. This risk may be higher (16-fold increased) in *NBS1* mutation carriers with a positive family history of prostate cancer. The *NBS1* founder allele may be responsible for ~2% of prostate cancers and ~9% of families with two or more cases of prostate cancer in Poland. Given the geographic distribution of reported clinical cases of NBS, the 657del5 mutation also may be an important contributor to prostate cancer in patients of Slavic origin from other countries.

9.2.3 *BRCA1* Gene

The studies of DNA damage signaling pathway exhibit an important role of BRCA1 multisubunit protein complex, referred to as the BRCA1– associated genome surveillance complex genome surveillance complex. It is well established that germline mutations in the *BRCA1* gene confer high risk of breast and ovarian cancer. However, some epidemiological and association studies have suggested an increased risk of prostate cancer in Ashkenazi Jewish men with a *BRCA1* mutation (185delAG or 5382insC) (see subchapter by Foulkes and Notte, this volume). Other studies, in non-Jewish populations, have found little or no evidence of an increased risk for prostate cancer in *BRCA1* mutation carriers (Thompson and Easton 2002; Gayther et al. 2000; Sinclair et al. 2000; Ikonen et al. 2003).

In Poland, there are three common founder alleles in *BRCA1* (C61G, 4153delA, and 5382insC - named with original nomenclature), which, in total, account for 90% of all *BRCA1* mutations. We observed increased risks for prostate cancer associated with the BRCA1 4153delA and the C61G mutations (Table 9.2.1) (Cybulski et al. 2008). One of these two mutations was seen in significant excess in men with unselected prostate cancer (OR = 3.6; P = 0.05). The two mutations were seen in excess in men with familial prostate cancer (OR = 12; P = 0.0004). The C61G mutation alone was associated with familial prostate cancer (OR = 13.4; P = 0.008). Furthermore, two of the three C61G carriers from a series of unselected cases had strong family histories of prostate cancer (which contained four and five men, respectively with prostate cancer). Segregation analysis suggested that five of the

Table 9.2.1 Comparison of the frequency of *BRCA1* mutations in 1,793 patients with prostate cancer and 4,570 controls

Mutation	Number of carriers (frequency)		OR	95% CI	P
	Cases (n = 1,793)	Controls (n = 4,570)			
BRCA1	8 (0.45%)	22 (0.48%)	0.9	0.4–2.1	1.0
C61G	3 (0.17%)	3 (0.07%)	2.6	0.5–12.7	0.5
4153delA	4 (0.22%)	2 (0.04%)	5.1	0.9–27.9	0.1
5382insC	1 (0.06%)	17 (0.37%)	0.15	0.02–1.1	0.06
C61G or 4153delA[a]	7 (0.39%)	5 (0.11%)	3.6	1.1–11.3	0.045

OR is not corrected for ascertainment

[a] When 5382insC is excluded, as unlikely pathogenic for prostate cancer in the Polish population

nine men with prostate cancer in these families carried the C61G variant (Fig. 9.2.2). These data support the idea that the C61G mutation confers an increased risk of prostate cancer in Poland. A positive association between prostate cancer and the 4153delA variant alone was also seen, but the evidence is less compelling. Although this alteration was more common in unselected and in familial cases than in controls (OR 5.1 and 10, respectively), these differences were not statistically significant (Table 9.2.1).

In contrast, the 5382insC mutation does not seem to confer an increased risk of prostate cancer in Poland. This mutation was under-represented in cases compared

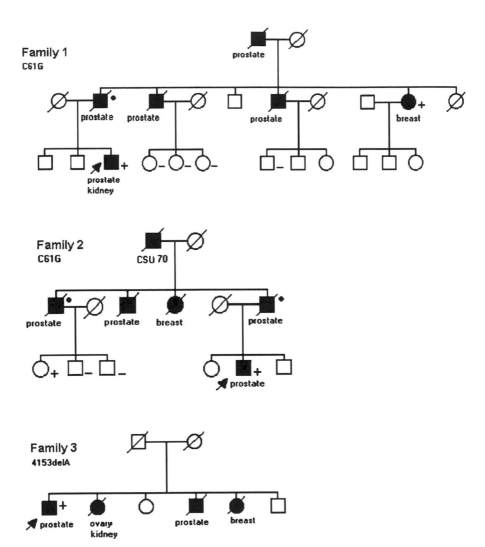

Fig. 9.2.2 Pedigrees of *BRCA1* mutation-positive cases with familial prostate cancer

Table 9.2.2 Comparison of the frequency of *CHEK2* mutations in prostate cancer patients and in control group

Mutation	Group	Number of carriers/ number of tested (frequency)	OR	95% CI	P
del5395	Controls	24/5,496 (0.4%)	1.0		
	Unselected cases	15/1,864 (0.8%)	1.9	0.97–3.5	0.009
	Familial cases	4/249 (1.6 %)	3.7	1.3–10.8	0.03
1100delC	Controls	12/5,496 (0.2%)	1.0		
	Unselected cases	14/1,864 (0.8%)	3.5	1.6–7.5	0.002
	Familial cases	3/249 (1.2%)	5.6	1.6–19.9	0.02
IVS2 + 1G > A	Controls	22/5,496 (0.4%)	1.0		
	Unselected cases	15/1,864 (0.8%)	2.0	1.05–3.9	0.052
	Familial cases	5/249 (2.0%)	5.1	1.9–13.6	0.002
Protein truncating mutation[a]	Controls	58/5,496 (1.1%)	1.0		
	Unselected cases	44/1,864 (2.4%)	2.3	1.5–3.4	<0.0001
	Familial cases	12/249 (4.8%)	4.7	2.5–9.0	<0.0001
I157T	Controls	264/5,496 (4.8%)	1.0		
	Unselected cases	142/1,864 (7.6%)	1.6	1.3–2.0	<0.0001
	Familial cases	30/249 (12.0%)	2.7	1.8–4.1	<0.0001
CHEK2[b]	Controls	321/5,496 (5.8%)	1.0		
	Unselected cases	184/1,864 (9.9%)	1.8	1.5–2.1	<0.0001
	Familial cases	42/249 (16.9%)	3.3	2.3–4.6	<0.0001

ORs are not corrected for ascertainment

[a] One of the three truncating mutations (del5395, IVS2 + 1G > A, 1100delC)

[b] Any CHEK2 mutation (del5395, IVS2 + 1G > A, 1100delC, I157T)

to controls (0.06 vs. 0.37%). Only one (12.5%) of the eight prostate cancer cases with a *BRCA1* mutation carried the 5382insC mutation, whereas this mutation constituted 77% of all *BRCA1* mutations seen in the control group ($P = 0.003$). It is therefore possible that the risk of prostate cancer is dependent on the type and/or location of the *BRCA1* mutation. Mutations in the 3′ end of *BRCA1* (such as the 5382insC) may confer lower risk of prostate cancer than mutations located elsewhere (such as the C61G and 4153delA). The C61G and 4153delA founder alleles might be responsible for ~0.3% of prostate cancers and ~1% of families with two or more cases of prostate cancer in Poland.

9.2.4 CHEK2 Gene

CHEK2 is a multiorgan cancer susceptibility gene whose product functions as a barrier to tumorigenesis by maintaining genomic stability (Meijers-Heijboer et al. 2002). Rare germ-line mutations are associated with a slightly increased risk of a cancer at a number of sites, including breast, prostate, colon, kidney, and thyroid, bladder, ovarian (low-grade), and the hematopoietic system (chronic lymphocytic leukemia.) (Meijers-Heijboer et al. 2002; Cybulski et al. 2004b; Złowocka et al. 2008; Szymanska-Pasternak et al. 2006; Rudd et al. 2006; Antoni et al. 2007). In addition, somatic mutations have been reported in some tumors, particularly prostate cancer (Wu et al. 2006).

In Poland there are four founder alleles of the *CHEK2* gene, which in aggregate are present in 6% of the population. Three of these result in a truncated CHEK2 protein (del5395, 1100delC, IVS2 + 1G>A), and the other is a missense substitution of an isoleucine for a threonine (I157T). We observed increased risks for prostate cancer associated with all *CHEK2* mutations (Table 9.2.2) (Cybulski et al. 2006; Cybulski et al. 2000c). The truncating mutations were associated with a 2.3-fold increase in the risk of prostate cancer and the missense I157T mutation increased the risk by 1.6-fold. The risk is higher for carriers of a *CHEK2* mutation with a positive family history of prostate cancer - 4.7 for carriers of the truncating mutations and 2.7 for carriers of the missense I157T mutation. *CHEK2* mutations account for ~7% of prostate cancers and ~12% of families with two or more cases of prostate cancer in Poland.

9.2.5   RNASEL and MSR1 Genes

RNASEL and *MSR1* genes were identified as prostate cancer susceptibility genes through linkage studies of prostate cancer families. We sequenced the entire coding region of *RNASEL* and *MSR1* gene in Polish men with familial prostate cancer. Four DNA variants were detected including the R462Q and D541E in *RNASEL* gene, the P275A and R293X in *MSR1* gene. None of these variants was found to be associated with increased prostate cancer risk in Polish men (Table 9.2.3) (Cybulski et al. 2007).

Table 9.2.3 Comparison of the frequency of variants in *RNASEL* and *MSR1* genes in 737 patients with prostate cancer and 511 individuals from control group

Gene	Variant	Genotype	Number of carriers (frequency)		OR	95% CI	P
			Cases ($n = 737$)	Controls ($n = 511$)			
RNASEL	1385G>A(R462Q)	GG	245 (33.3%)	177 (34.6%)	0.9	0.7–1.2	0.6
		GA	376 (51.0%)	252 (49.3%)	1.1	0.9–1.3	0.6
		AA	116 (15.7%)	82 (16.1%)	1.0	0.7–1.3	0.9
	1623T>G (D541E)	TT	111 (15.1%)	84 (16.4%)	0.9	0.7–1.2	0.5
		TG	372 (50.5%)	259 (50.7%)	1.0	0.8–1.2	1.0
		GG	254 (34.4%)	168 (32.9%)	1.1	0.8–1.4	0.6
MSR1	945C>G (P275A)	CC	663 (90.0%)	474 (92.8%)	0.7	0.5–1.1	0.1
		CG	74 (10.0%)	37 (7.2%)	1.4	0.9–2.2	0.1
	999C>T (R293X)	CC	725 (98.4%)	503 (98.4%)	1.0	0.4–2.4	1.0
		CT	12 (1.6%)	8 (1.6%)	1.0	0.4–2.6	1.0

ORs are not corrected for ascertainment

9.2.6   Region 8q24

Several recent association studies implicate three neighboring regions of chromosome 8q24 as the site of prostate cancer susceptibility loci. One region contains both a microsatellite marker DG8S737 and a single nucleotide polymorphism rs1447295. Both have been consistently associated with prostate cancer risk in several populations. Interestingly, neither polymorphism appears to be connected with any particular gene nor is the mechanistic basis of prostate cancer susceptibility yet clear. These variants confer an increased risk of prostate cancer in the Polish population, as well (Table 9.2.4). The A allele of rs1447295, present 19.1% of healthy men in the population, is associated with 1.4 increase in the risk of prostate cancer and accounts for ~7% of prostate cancers in Poland. The −8 allele of DG8S737, present 9.1% of healthy men in the population, is associated with 1.6-fold increase in the risk of prostate cancer and accounts for ~5% of prostate cancers in Poland.

9.2.7   Conclusion

Groups of individuals with an increased risk of prostate cancer in the Polish population can be identified by testing of specific variants in *NBS1*, *BRCA1*, and *CHEK2* genes and 8q24 region. It seems that analysis of *RNASEL* and *MSR1* genes is not justified in this purpose. The list of known genetic markers of high risk of prostate cancer (in addition to strong family history of prostate cancer and germline mutations in *BRCA2* gene) may be extended by specific mutations in *NBS1*, *BRCA1*, and *CHEK2* genes in men with a positive family history of prostate cancer in at least

Table 9.2.4 Association of variants on chromosome 8q24 with prostate cancer risk in a series of 690 unselected prostate cancer cases and 602 cancer-free men

Marker	Risk allele	Subjects	Total N	Genotype N (%)		OR	95% CI	p-value
				AA	AC	AA or AC vs. CC		
RS1447295	A	Controls	602	3 (0.5)	115 (19.1)	1.0		
		Unselected cases	690	19 (2.7)	156 (22.6)	1.4	1.1–1.8	0.01
		Familial cases	103	6 (5.8)	28 (27.2)	2.0	1.3–3.2	0.004
				−8–8	−8X[a]	−8–8 or −8X vs. XX		
DG8S737	−8	Controls	602	1 (0.2)	55 (9.1)	1.0		
		Unselected cases	690	3 (0.4)	96 (14.0)	1.6	1.1–2.3	0.006
		Familial cases	103	1 (1.0)	26 (25.2)	3.5	2.1–5.8	<0.0001

ORs are not corrected for ascertainment
[a] The X defines the group of alleles in DG8S737 other than the −8 allele

one first or second degree relative (the risk increased ~5–15-fold). The establishment of management protocols, including effective methods of prevention, surveillance, and treatment for carriers of these mutations require further studies. We estimate that all known susceptibility alleles are responsible for approximately 20% of cases of prostate cancer in Poland.

References

Antoni L, Sodha N, Collins I, Garrett MD (2007) CHK2 kinase: cancer susceptibility and cancer therapy – two sides of the same coin? Nat Rev Cancer 7(12):925–936

Cybulski C, Górski B, Debniak T, Gliniewicz B, Mierzejewski M, Masojć B, Jakubowska A, Matyjasik J, Złowocka E, Sikorski A, Narod SA, Lubiński J (2004a) NBS1 is a prostate cancer susceptibility gene. Cancer Res 64(4):1215–1219

Cybulski C, Górski B, Huzarski T, Masojć B, Mierzejewski M, Debniak T, Teodorczyk U, Byrski T, Gronwald J, Matyjasik J, Zlowocka E, Lenner M, Grabowska E, Nej K, Castaneda J, Medrek K, Szymańska A, Szymańska J, Kurzawski G, Suchy J, Oszurek O, Witek A, Narod SA, Lubiński J (2004b) CHEK2 is a multiorgan cancer susceptibility gene. Am J Hum Genet 75(6):1131–1135

Cybulski C, Huzarski T, Górski B, Masojć B, Mierzejewski M, Debniak T, Gliniewicz B, Matyjasik J, Złowocka E, Kurzawski G, Sikorski A, Posmyk M, Szwiec M, Czajka R, Narod SA, Lubiński J (2004c) A novel founder CHEK2 mutation is associated with increased prostate cancer risk. Cancer Res 64(8):2677–2679

Cybulski C, Wokołorczyk D, Huzarski T, Byrski T, Gronwald J, Górski B, Debniak T, Masojć B, Jakubowska A, Gliniewicz B, Sikorski A, Stawicka M, Godlewski D, Kwias Z, Antczak A, Krajka K, Lauer W, Sosnowski M, Sikorska-Radek P, Bar K, Klijer R, Zdrojowy R, Małkiewicz B, Borkowski A, Borkowski T, Szwiec M, Narod SA, Lubiński J (2006) A large germline deletion in the Chek2 kinase gene is associated with an increased risk of prostate cancer. J Med Genet 43(11):863–866

Cybulski C, Wokołorczyk D, Jakubowska A, Gliniewicz B, Sikorski A, Huzarski T, Debniak T, Narod SA, Lubiński J (2007) DNA variation in MSR1, RNASEL and E-cadherin genes and prostate cancer in Poland. Urol Int 79(1):44–49

Cybulski C, Górski B, Gronwald J, Huzarski T, Byrski T, Dębniak T, Jakubowska A, Wokołorczyk D, Gliniewicz B, Sikorski A, Stawicka S, Godlewski D, Kwias Z, Antczak A, Krajka K, Lauer W, Sosnowski M, Sikorska-Radek P, Bar K, Klijer R, Romuald Z, Małkiewicz B, Borkowski A, Borkowski T, Szwiec M, Posmyk M, Narod SA, Lubiński J 2008 BRCA1 mutations and prostate cancer in Poland. Eur J Cancer Prev 17(1):62–66

Gayther SA, de Foy KA, Harrington P et al (2000) The Cancer Research Campaign/British Prostate Group United Kingdom Familial Prostate Cancer Study Collaborators. The frequency of germ-line mutations in the breast cancer predisposition genes BRCA1 and BRCA2 in familial prostate cancer. Cancer Res 60:4513–4518

Ikonen, T, Matikainen, MP, Syrjakoski, K, Mononen, N, Koivisto, PA, Rokman, A, Seppala, EH, Kallioniemi, OP, Tammela, TL, Schleutker, J (2003) BRCA1 and BRCA2 mutations have no major role in predisposition to prostate cancer in Finland. J Med Genet 40:e98

Meijers-Heijboer H, van den Ouweland A, Klijn J, Wasielewski M, de Snoo A, Oldenburg R, Hollestelle A, Houben M, Crepin E, van Veghel-Plandsoen M, Elstrodt F, van Duijn C, Bartels C, Meijers C, Schutte M, McGuffog L, Thompson D, Easton D, Sodha N, Seal S, Barfoot R, Mangion J, Chang-Claude J, Eccles D, Eeles R, Evans DG, Houlston R, Murday V, Narod S, Peretz T, Peto J, Phelan C, Zhang HX, Szabo C, Devilee P, Goldgar D, Futreal PA, Nathanson KL, Weber B, Rahman N, Stratton MR; CHEK2-Breast Cancer Consortium. (2002) Low-penetrance susceptibility to breast cancer due to CHEK2(*)1100delC in noncarriers of BRCA1 or BRCA2 mutations. Nat Genet 31(1):55–59

Rudd MF, Sellick GS, Webb EL, Catovsky D, Houlston RS (2006) Variants in the ATM-BRCA2-CHEK2 axis predispose to chronic lymphocytic leukemia. Blood 108(2):638–644

Sinclair, CS, Berry, R, Schaid, D, Thibodeau, SN, Couch, FJ (2000) BRCA1 and BRCA2 have a limited role in familial prostate cancer. Cancer Res 60:1371–1375

Szymanska-Pasternak J, Szymanska A, Medrek K, Imyanitov EN, Cybulski C, Gorski B, Magnowski P, Dziuba I, Gugala K, Debniak B, Gozdz S, Sokolenko AP, Krylova NY, Lobeiko OS, Narod SA, Lubinski J (2006) CHEK2 variants predispose to benign, borderline and low-grade invasive ovarian tumors. Gynecol Oncol 102(3):429–431

Thompson D, Easton DF and The Breast Cancer Linkage Consortium (2002) Cancer Incidence in BRCA1 mutation carriers. J Natl Cancer Inst 94:1358–1365

Varon R, Vissinga C, Platzer M, Cerosaletti KM, Chrzanowska KH, Saar K, Beckmann G, Seemanova E, Cooper PR, Nowak NJ et al (1998) Nibrin, a novel DNA double-strand break repair protein, is mutated in Nijmegen breakage syndrome. Cell 93:467–476

Wu X, Dong X, Liu W, Chen J (2006) Characterization of CHEK2 mutations in prostate cancer. Hum Mutat. 27(8):742–747

Złowocka E, Cybulski C, Górski B, Debniak T, Słojewski M, Wokołorczyk D, Serrano-Fernández P, Matyjasik J, van de Wetering T, Sikorski A, Scott RJ, Lubiński J (2008) Germline mutations in the CHEK2 kinase gene are associated with an increased risk of bladder cancer. Int J Cancer 122(3):583–586

9.3 Prostate Cancer in Ashkenazi Jewish Men

William D. Foulkes and Sabrina Notte

9.3.1 Introduction

In this section, we discuss the genetic contribution to prostate cancer in the Ashkenazi Jewish population. Note that most, if not all, of the studies referred to herein have been carried out in Ashkenazi Jewish populations living in North America or Israel.

Ethnic groups who have been genetically isolated from other local populations may have a differential risk of developing certain diseases that is due to inherited factors. Some of the observed excess risk may be due to genetic factors that arise only once in each population but have been allowed to become frequent, usually as a result of chance fluctuations in allele frequencies. In this situation, no selection has taken place, and this process is known as genetic drift.

Founder alleles are alleles that have reached an appreciable (but not defined) frequency in a given genetically isolated population by either genetic drift or selection and this leads to the formation of "founder populations." Ethnic groups that exhibit these effects include French Canadians and Ashkenazi Jews. In some countries, such as Poland and Iceland, founder effects predominate in several genes, including the breast cancer susceptibility genes *BRCA1* and/or *BRCA2*.

The word Ashkenazi is Hebrew for "German" and refers to Jews from Germany, Poland, Lithuania, Ukraine, Russia and other regions of eastern europe. As a result of forced and unforced migrations, and more recently, the effects of the Second World War and the Holocaust, Ashkenazi Jews today live throughout the world. Most, however, live in North America or Israel. It has been known for some time that populations whose ancestors are of Eastern European (Ashkenazi) Jewish background are at higher risk for certain inherited conditions such as Tay-Sachs, Gaucher, and many other recessive diseases (Ostrer 2001). This is mainly because the founder alleles have drifted to a high frequency, in the absence of selection. Alternatively, heterozy-

W.D. Foulkes (✉) and S. Notte
Cancer Genetics Program, Departments of Oncology and Human Genetics, McGill University,
546 Pine Avenue West, Montreal, QC, Canada H2W 1S6
e-mail: william.foulkes@mcgill.ca

gous carriers may have some advantage (as is the case for sickle cell trait in those at risk for malaria) but in the case of the diseases that are common in the Ashkenazim, it is less clear what might be the nature of these advantages (Risch et al. 1995). Some dominantly inherited disorders are also mainly attributable to a small number of founder mutations. The best example of this is hereditary breast and ovarian cancer, where approximately 95% of all *BRCA1* and *BRCA2* mutations can be accounted for by just three mutations – two in *BRCA1* and one in *BRCA2* (Roa et al. 1996; Phelan et al. 2002; Kauff et al. 2002).

The question of the contribution of genetic factors to the etiology of prostate cancer in the Ashkenazim remains largely unanswered, but some data do exist, and this will be summarized below. In particular, several genes, and specific mutations within these genes, have been examined specifically in the Ashkenazi Jewish population to question their implications in the development of both hereditary and sporadic prostate cancer. Also, genome-wide association studies have been conducted, although thus far with a very small number of Ashkenazi Jewish cases (Kote-Jarai et al. 2008), see Chap. 8.

9.3.2   BRCA1

BRCA1 mutations have been previously associated with a large proportion of hereditary breast and ovarian cancers in the Ashkenazi Jewish population. Two founder mutations in *BRCA1* (usually known as 187delAG and 5385insC) are found in ~1.2% of the Ashkenazi Jewish population (Struewing et al. 1995; Roa et al. 1996; Struewing et al. 1997). These two mutations account for 95% or more of all *BRCA1* mutations found in this population (Phelan et al. 2002; Kauff et al. 2002). Five to ten percent of Ashkenazi Jewish women with breast cancer (Warner et al. 1999) and ~20% of those with ovarian cancer (Moslehi et al. 2000) carry one or other of these two mutations. By age 70, a female carrier of a *BRCA1* mutation has an ~65% risk of developing breast cancer and an ~39% lifetime risk of developing ovarian cancer (Antoniou et al. 2003). Because of these very high frequencies, researchers have studied the role of *BRCA1* mutations in the risk of developing prostate cancer among Ashkenazi Jews. These studies have painted a mixed picture. First, in the general (not specifically Jewish) population, several linkage studies have suggested that male carriers of a *BRCA1* mutation with a threefold increased risk of prostate cancer (Ford et al. 1994). Later studies from the same group, based on mutation analysis of at least the breast and/or ovarian cancer cases linked to *BRCA1*, found that the risk was much less (Thompson and Easton 2002). In the latter study, there was no evidence of increased risk for men over age 65, and the risk for those under 65 was increased by less than twofold, and with borderline statistical significance. Notably, while linkage studies in hereditary prostate cancer families have indicated the presence of a broad linkage peak near the position of *BRCA1* on chromosome 17q (Lange et al. 2003), subsequent mutation analysis of *BRCA1* did not reveal truncating mutations that could account for the signal (Zuhlke et al. 2004). Therefore in the non-Jewish population, the evidence for the involvement of *BRCA1* in prostate cancer susceptibility is limited, but does indicate the possibility of increased risk, especially for those diagnosed under age 65.

In studies focused on Ashkenazi Jewish men, results similarly suggested a minor role, if any, for *BRCA1* in prostate carcinogenesis. The Johns Hopkins group studied 18 Ashkenazi Jewish hereditary prostate cancer families, each having at least three first-degree relatives affected with prostate cancer and did not identify any *BRCA1* mutation carriers (Wilkens et al. 1999). Around the same time, another group from the United States, this time studying 83 sporadic cases of early-onset prostate cancer, identified only one 187delAG mutation carrier (Nastiuk et al. 1999). In the same year, a study from Israel found that among 95 prostate cancer cases of Ashkenazi origin, the rate of the predominant Jewish *BRCA1* mutations differed significantly from that of the general population, but only for the mutation 5385insC (2/60 cases, 3.3%). 187delG was seen in 2/87 cases (2.3%) (Vazina et al. 2000). A similar Israeli study found only 2 *BRCA1* carriers in 87 Ashkenazi Jewish men with prostate cancer (Hubert et al. 1999). Our group in Canada did not find any *BRCA1* carriers among 146 men with prostate cancer (Hamel et al. 2003). Finally, a population-based study from Israel found some evidence for an increased risk of prostate cancer in association with the 187delAG mutation (14/940 in cases vs. 6/872 in controls – Ashkenazi Jews from the Washington study who were over 50 and had no personal history of prostate cancer (OR 2.18, not significant) (Giusti et al. 2003), but no pathological features that would allow one to predict who might be a carrier of a mutation. Finally, a study from Memorial Hospital found that 5/251 (2.0%) Ashkenazi Jewish men with prostate cancer had a mutation in *BRCA1*. This prevalence is not different from the 12/1,472 seen in controls (age-adjusted OR 2.2, *P* = 0.16) (Kirchhoff et al. 2004) (Table 9.3.1). Thus the picture for *BRCA1* and prostate cancer is uncertain – there maybe some increased risk associated with a *BRCA1* mutation, but it is unlikely that this risk is more than twofold increased compared with controls.

9.3.3   BRCA2

In contrast to the rather unclear picture with respect to *BRCA1* and prostate cancer risk, in non-Jewish men with prostate cancer, it is quite clear that *BRCA2* is an important prostate cancer risk gene. This is discussed in more detail in Chap. 8. Suffice it to say that BRCA2 is the sole established high-risk prostate cancer gene at the current time, with risks in excess of fivefold overall, and much higher risks at younger ages (Edwards et al. 2003).

In Ashkenazi Jewish men, there does appear to be an increased risk for prostate cancer in association with the founder mutation 6174delT, although this view remains controversial and is based on very little data, some of which is conflicting (Table 9.3.1). The most convincing (and most positive study) found that, after adjusting for age, *BRCA2*:6174delT was associated with an odds ratio for prostate cancer of 4.8 [95% CI 1.9–12.3 (Kirchhoff et al. 2004)]. Nearly all of the studies

Table 9.3.1 Comparison of frequencies of mutations in *BRCA1* and *BRCA2* in Ashkenazi Jewish men with prostate cancer and ethnically matched controls (unadjusted)

Study	Type of study	Prevalence of BRCA1 mutations in cases	Prevalence of BRCA2 mutations in cases	OR in association with BRCA2 mutation versus BRCA1	Prevalence in controls	OR for BRCA1/2 combined versus controls
Hubert et al. (1999)	Hospital-based case-control study from Israel	2/87	1/87	NS, underpowered	2/87	1.5 (95% CI: 0.16–18.6)
Vazina et al. (2000)	Hospital-based case-control study from Israel	2/87	2/60	NS, underpowered	–	–
Hamel et al. (2003)	Hospital-based cases from Montreal	0/146	2/146	NS, underpowered	–	–
Kirchhoff et al. (2004)	Hospital-based cases, male controls were unaffected AJ males from Washington D.C. (Struewing et al. 1997)	2/251	8/251	4.1 (95% CI: 0.8–40)	28/1,472	2.1 (95% CI:0.9–4.6)
Giusti et al. (2003)	Population-based cases from Israel, controls from two previous studies of mutation frequencies in Jewish populations (Struewing et al. 1997; Gruber et al. 2002), limited to males >50 years	16/940	14/940	0.87 (95% CI: 0.4–1.9)	21/1,344	2.07 (95% CI: 1.1–3.8)

Only those studies that analyzed all three founder *BRCA1/2* mutations in Ashkenazi Jewish men with prostate cancer are included here discussed in the section above on BRCA1 have also looked at the founder mutation *BRCA2*:6174delT as well, and hence a direct comparison can be made between studies of *BRCA1* and *BRCA2*. These are summarized in Table 9.3.1. Overall, *BRCA2* mutations are only slightly more common in Ashkenazi Jewish men with prostate cancer compared to *BRCA1* mutations. Perhaps the reason for this somewhat surprising result is that most of the mutations found to increase the risk of prostate cancer in the study of Edwards et al. (2003) lie outside the ovarian cancer cluster region, within which 6174delT lies. Notably, studies of Ashkenazi Jewish hereditary prostate cancer families have failed to identify *BRCA2*: 6174delT mutations in those affected by prostate cancer (Wilkens et al. 1999). Therefore, Ashkenazi Jewish males may not be as at much of an increased risk for prostate cancer as are males carrying other mutations in *BRCA2*. Importantly, at this time there is no evidence that Ashkenazi Jewish men with prostate cancer who carry the *BRCA2*:6174delT allele are at lower risk of aggressive disease than are men with prostate cancer who carry other *BRCA2* mutations.

Some studies have combined data regarding both *BRCA1* and *BRCA2* mutations to provide an overall assessment of the contribution of these founder mutations to prostate cancer in Ashkenazi Jewish men. In a study based on volunteers from the Washington D.C. area, the estimated risk of prostate cancer among Ashkenazi Jewish carriers of *BRCA1* or *BRCA2* mutations was 16% by the age of 70 (95% confidence interval 4–30) and 39% by the age of 80 (Struewing et al. 1997). In noncarriers, the risk was 3.8%. Notably, the risk of prostate cancer to age 70 among *BRCA1* carriers was much higher than among *BRCA2* carriers (25% vs. 5%), but age 80, there was no difference in risk. Five of twenty (25%) individuals carrying the BRCA1:5385insC mutation reported a family history of prostate cancer in first-degree relatives. This was significantly greater than the number of noncarriers reporting such a history (364/4,759, 8%). The figure was 12% for those carrying 187delAG (not significantly different from controls). A similarly indirect study of the role of *BRCA1/2* in prostate cancer focused on the incidence of prostate cancer in the first-degree relatives of Ashkenazi Jewish women with breast cancer who carry *BRCA1* mutations. In this study, Narod and colleagues found that there was a significant threefold excess of prostate cancer in the male relatives of 48 such women diagnosed in Toronto or Montreal, compared with unaffected control Ashkenazi Jewish women from Toronto who were not tested for *BRCA1/2* (Warner et al. 1999). The diagnoses of prostate cancer were not confirmed in either study.

9.3.4 Ribonuclease L

There have been conflicting data surrounding the role of the ribonuclease L (*RNASEL*) gene in predisposing to prostate cancer among Ashkenazi Jewish men. *RNASEL* is an interesting candidate because of its association with infection. It was first proposed as a prostate cancer susceptibility gene by Carpten et al. (2002), where germ-line mutations in this gene were found to segregate with two *HPC1*-linked families. It was a particularly interesting candidate because it lies on chromosome 1q, within a region previously linked to hereditary prostate cancer (*HPC1*) (Smith et al. 1996). Subsequent work from many other laboratories have not really clarified the situation, as, for example, some have found increased risk in association with certain missense mutations in *RNASEL*, whereas others have found the very same variants are associated with a decreased risk of prostate cancer (Wang et al. 2002; Casey et al. 2002; Rokman et al. 2002; Chen et al. 2003). Taken together, the data suggest that *RNASEL* has a limited role in prostate cancer susceptibility. It seems possible that *RNASEL* is a low-to-moderate penetrance prostate cancer susceptibility gene but it is clearly not *HPC1*, and following very large-scale linkage studies (Xu et al. 2005) there is considerable doubt that "*HPC1*," as such, exists.

As for previous studies in breast cancer, it was hoped that the discovery of a founder mutation in *RNASEL* in the Ashkenazi Jewish population that was linked to increased risk of prostate cancer would bolster the argument in favor of an important role for this gene in prostate cancer. Thus the finding of an Israeli group who identified *RNASEL*: 471delAAAG in Ashkenazi Jewish men with prostate cancer was an interesting observation (Rennert et al. 2002). Notably, the mutation frequency was 4% in 150 healthy young women, 6.9% in men prostate cancer, and 2.4% in elderly male controls. Unfortunately, subsequent studies did not support this initial finding. For example, our group reported no significant role for *RNASEL* genetic alterations in prostate cancer in Ashkenazi Jews (Kotar et al. 2003). In addition, among 190 Ashkenazi Jewish men with prostate cancer, only one individual tested positive for this mutation (Dagan et al. 2006). In a further study from the original group that initially described the variant, no difference in frequency of this allele between Ashkenazi Jewish prostate cancer cases and ethnically matched controls was found (Orr-Urtreger et al. 2006). Thus it appears that this founder mutation has little or no role in the incidence of prostate cancer in Ashkenazi Jewish men.

9.3.5   CHEK2

The *CHEK2* gene plays a key role in DNA damage repair. Alterations in this gene have been previously investigated and found to be associated with cancer. For example, the 1100delC alteration confers an increased risk of breast cancer International CHEK2 Collaborative Group, (2004), and other alleles predispose to prostate cancer in non-Jewish populations (see Chap. 9.2). Notably, King and colleagues identified a *CHEK2* variant, S428F, that is, over-represented in Ashkenazi Jewish women with breast cancer, and is rare outside of this population (Shaag et al. 2005). It is associated with a less than twofold increased risk for breast cancer.

As a result of the identification of the *CHEK2* founder mutation S248F, it was logical to look for the contribution of this and possibly other founder mutations to prostate cancer in Ashkenazi Jewish males. A large collaborative study resequenced CHEK2 in prostate cancer cases and identified seven single nucleotide polymorphisms (R3W, E394F, Y424H, S428F, D438Y, P509S, and P509L). Note that the above-mentioned *CHEK2* S428F mutation was found not to be at an increased significant frequency in Ashkenazi Jewish men with prostate cancer. The frequency of each variant was then determined in 76 Ashkenazi Jewish families collected by members of the International Consortium for Prostate Cancer Genetics (ICPCG) where ≥2 men were affected by prostate cancer. Only one variant, Y424H in exon 11, was identified in more than two families. Exon 11 was then screened in nine additional Ashkenazi Jewish ICPCG families (a total of 85 families). The Y424H variant occurred in nine affected cases from four different families; however, it did not completely segregate with the disease. Following bioinformatics analysis, functional assays, and frequency comparisons between cases and controls, it was concluded that specifically *CHEK2*: Y242H has a minor role in prostate cancer susceptibility in Ashkenazi Jewish men. Furthermore, this study indicated that overall, *CHEK2* does not appear to have an important part to play in the etiology of prostate cancer in Ashkenazi Jewish men (Tischkowitz et al. 2008).

9.3.6   MSR1

Similar to *RNASEL*, Macrophage Scavenger Receptor 1 (*MSR1*) is an attractive candidate prostate cancer susceptibility locus because of its links to infections, and hence to prostatitis and prostate cancer risk. Early studies (Xu et al. 2002) suggested a strong association between common variants in *MSR1* and prostate cancer risk, but subsequent studies (Wang et al. 2003; Seppala et al. 2003), some of which included a small number of Ashkenazi Jewish men with prostate cancer (Hope et al. 2005) or were restricted to Jews (Bar-Shira et al. 2006), did not support these initial findings. The exception, perhaps, is in African-American men (Miller et al. 2003) where associations between certain *MSR1* variants and prostate cancer risk has been demonstrated. A meta-analysis of all studies concluded that *MSR1* had a limited role in prostate cancer susceptibility, especially if African-Americans were excluded (Sun et al. 2006).

9.3.7   Chromosome 7 Locus

Using a genome-wide approach, Ostrander and colleagues identified a region of chromosome 7q that was linked to risk of prostate cancer in Ashkenazi Jewish hereditary prostate cancer families (Friedrichsen et al. 2004). Using 36 multiplex prostate cancer families, the highest nonparametric linkage score was 3.01 at marker D7S634 (corresponding to a genome-wide *P* value of.006). Our group was unable to identify a common haplotype on chromosome 7q that was over-represented in Jewish men with prostate cancer compared with controls (Hamel, Foulkes, and others, unpublished data), and no further studies have been published that support these initial findings.

9.3.8 Additional Genome-Wide Studies

Eeles et al. recently conducted a genome-wide study (GWAS) and identified genetic variants on chromosomes 3, 6, 7, 10, 11, 19, and X that were associated with increased risk for prostate cancer. These findings, including the replication study that included a small group of Ashkenazi Jewish men, are discussed in detail in Chap. 8 and therefore will not be discussed here.

9.3.9 Other Loci

Several other loci such as *CAPB* on chromosome 1p36, linkage to chromosome 8p22–23, *HPC2/ELAC2* on chromosome 17p, HPC20 on chromosome 20q13, and *HPCX* on chromosome Xq27–28 are believed to exist (Schaid 2004). None of these loci have been specifically studied in Ashkenazi Jewish populations and therefore are not discussed in this subchapter. Two specific genes have been studied in Ashkenazi Jews, namely, Hypoxia-Inducible Factor-1 α (*HIF-1α*), and Aurora Kinase A (*AURKA*). For *HIF-1α*, one group from Israel found that the 1772T variant (missense mutation 1772C > T, resulting in P582S) was present on 90 of 502 alleles in Ashkenazi Jewish cases and in 55 of 400 Ashkenazi Jewish controls. This difference is not significant (OR 1.37, 95% CI: 0.9–2.0, $P = 0.10$) and there was a borderline effect in a smaller series of non-Ashkenazi prostate cancer cases and controls (Orr-Urtreger et al. 2007). The group chose this variant because it prevents HIF-1α protein degradation and enhances transcriptional activity of HIF. While other variants may be important, these findings do not suggest that this variant is a significant determinant of prostate cancer risk.

The same investigative team also studied a specific variant of *AURKA*, Ile31 resulting from T91A, that had been previously associated with cancer risk. While they found that increased expression of AURKA was associated with the presence of the variant, they did not report the frequency of this polymorphism in Ashkenazi Jewish prostate cancer cases and controls (Matarasso et al. 2007). The variant has been studied in non-Jewish series, and no effect on risk was seen (Feik et al. 2008).

9.3.10 Conclusions

Although a significant amount of research has been conducted using a candidate gene approach for identifying prostate cancer susceptibility loci in Ashkenazi Jewish men, further genome-wide approaches may reveal surprises. It is quite possible that newly identified risk alleles may point in different directions in genetically isolated populations. If this is found to be true, this will significantly complicate public health efforts in risk prediction based on genetic profiles. Nevertheless, it is likely that moderately common, low penetrance alleles for prostate cancer that are relevant to the Ashkenazi Jewish population will be identified in the coming years.

References

Antoniou A, Pharoah PD, Narod S, Risch HA, Eyfjord JE, Hopper JL, Loman N, Olsson H, Johannsson O, Borg A, Pasini B, Radice P, Manoukian S, Eccles DM, Tang N, Olah E, Anton-Culver H, Warner E, Lubinski J, Gronwald J, Gorski B, Tulinius H, Thorlacius S, Eerola H, Nevanlinna H, Syrjakoski K, Kallioniemi OP, Thompson D, Evans C, Peto J, Lalloo F, Evans DG, Easton DF (2003) Average risks of breast and ovarian cancer associated with BRCA1 or BRCA2 Mutations detected in case series unselected for family history: A combined analysis of 22 studies. Am J Hum Genet 72, 1117–1130
Bar-Shira A, Matarasso N, Rosner S, Bercovich D, Matzkin H, Orr-Urtreger A (2006) Mutation screening and association study of the candidate prostate cancer susceptibility genes MSR1, PTEN, and KLF6. Prostate 66, 1052–1060
Carpten J, Nupponen N, Isaacs S, Sood R, Robbins C, Xu J, Faruque M, Moses T, Ewing C, Gillanders E, Hu P, Bujnovszky P, Makalowska I, Baffoe-Bonnie A, Faith D, Smith J, Stephan D, Wiley K, Brownstein M, Gildea D, Kelly B, Jenkins R, Hostetter G, Matikainen M, Schleutker J, Klinger K, Connors T, Xiang Y, Wang Z, De Marzo A, Papadopoulos N, Kallioniemi OP, Burk R, Meyers D, Gronberg H, Meltzer P, Silverman R, Bailey-Wilson J, Walsh P, Isaacs W, Trent J (2002) Germline mutations in the ribonuclease L gene in families showing linkage with HPC1. Nat Genet 30, 181–184
Casey G, Neville PJ, Plummer SJ, Xiang Y, Krumroy LM, Klein EA, Catalona WJ, Nupponen N, Carpten JD, Trent JM, Silverman RH, Witte JS (2002) RNASEL Arg462Gln variant is implicated in up to 13% of prostate cancer cases. Nat Genet 32, 581–583
Chen H, Griffin AR, Wu YQ, Tomsho LP, Zuhlke KA, Lange EM, Gruber SB, Cooney KA (2003) RNASEL mutations in hereditary prostate cancer. J Med Genet 40, e21
Dagan E, Laitman Y, Levanon N, Feuer A, Sidi AA, Baniel J, Korach Y, Ben BG, Friedman E, Gershoni-Baruch R (2006) The 471delAAAG mutation and C353T polymorphism in the RNASEL gene in sporadic and inherited cancer in Israel. Fam Cancer 5, 389–395
Edwards SM, Kote-Jarai Z, Meitz J, Hamoudi R, Hope Q, Osin P, Jackson R, Southgate C, Singh R, Falconer A, Dearnaley DP, Ardern-Jones A, Murkin A, Dowe A, Kelly J, Williams S, Oram R, Stevens M, Teare DM, Ponder BA, Gayther SA, Easton DF, Eeles RA (2003) Two percent of men with early-onset prostate cancer harbor germline mutations in the BRCA2 gene. Am J Hum Genet 72, 1–12
Feik E, Baierl A, Madersbacher S, Schatzl G, Maj-Hes A, Berges R, Micksche M, Gsur A (2008) Common genetic polymorphisms of AURKA and prostate cancer risk. Cancer Causes Control 20, 147–152
Ford D, Easton DF, Bishop DT, Narod SA, Goldgar DE (1994) Risks of cancer in BRCA1-mutation carriers. Breast Cancer Linkage Consortium. Lancet 343, 692–695
Friedrichsen DM, Stanford JL, Isaacs SD, Janer M, Chang BL, Deutsch K, Gillanders E, Kolb S, Wiley KE, Badzioch MD, Zheng SL, Walsh PC, Jarvik GP, Hood L, Trent JM, Isaacs WB, Ostrander EA, Xu J (2004) Identification of a prostate cancer susceptibility locus on chromosome 7q11–21 in Jewish families. Proc Natl Acad Sci USA 101, 1939–1944
Giusti RM, Rutter JL, Duray PH, Freedman LS, Konichezky M, Fisher-Fischbein J, Greene MH, Maslansky B, Fischbein A, Gruber SB, Rennert G, Ronchetti RD, Hewitt SM, Struewing JP, Iscovich J (2003) A twofold increase in BRCA mutation related prostate cancer among Ashkenazi Israelis is not associated with distinctive histopathology. J Med Genet 40, 787–792
Gruber SB, Ellis NA, Rennert G, Offit K, Scott KK, Almog R, Kolachana P, Bonner JD, Kirchhoff T, Tomsho LP, Nafa K, Pierce H, Low M, Satagopan J, Rennert H, Huang H, Greenson JK,

Groden J, Rapaport B, Shia J, Johnson S, Gregersen PK, Harris CC, Boyd J (2002) BLM heterozygosity and the risk of colorectal cancer. Science 297, 2013

Hamel N, Kotar K, Foulkes WD (2003) Founder mutations in BRCA1/2 are not frequent in Canadian Ashkenazi Jewish men with prostate cancer. BMC Med Genet 4, 7

Hope Q, Bullock S, Evans C, Meitz J, Hamel N, Edwards SM, Severi G, Dearnaley D, Jhavar S, Southgate C, Falconer A, Dowe A, Muir K, Houlston RS, Engert JC, Roquis D, Sinnett D, Simard J, Heimdal K, Moller P, Maehle L, Badzioch M, Eeles RA, Easton DF, English DR, Southey MC, Hopper JL, Foulkes WD, Giles GG (2005) Macrophage scavenger receptor 1 999C > T (R293X) mutation and risk of prostate cancer. Cancer Epidemiol Biomarkers Prev 14, 397–402

Hubert A, Peretz T, Manor O, Kaduri L, Wienberg N, Lerer I, Sagi M, Abeliovich D (1999) The Jewish Ashkenazi founder mutations in the BRCA1/BRCA2 genes are not found at an increased frequency in Ashkenazi patients with prostate cancer. Am J Hum Genet 65, 921–924

International CHEK2 collaborative group (2004) CHEK2*1100delC and susceptibility to breast cancer: a collaborative analysis involving 10,860 breast cancer cases and 9,065 controls from 10 studies. Am J Hum Genet 74, 1175–1182

Kauff ND, Perez-Segura P, Robson ME, Scheuer L, Siegel B, Schluger A, Rapaport B, Frank TS, Nafa K, Ellis NA, Parmigiani G, Offit K (2002) Incidence of non-founder BRCA1 and BRCA2 mutations in high risk Ashkenazi breast and ovarian cancer families. J Med Genet 39, 611–614

Kirchhoff T, Kauff ND, Mitra N, Nafa K, Huang H, Palmer C, Gulati T, Wadsworth E, Donat S, Robson ME, Ellis NA, Offit K (2004) BRCA mutations and risk of prostate cancer in Ashkenazi Jews. Clin Cancer Res 10, 2918–2921

Kotar K, Hamel N, Thiffault I, Foulkes WD (2003) The RNASEL 471delAAAG allele and prostate cancer in Ashkenazi Jewish men. J Med Genet 40, e22

Kote-Jarai Z, Easton DF, Stanford JL, Ostrander EA, Schleutker J, Ingles SA, Schaid D, Thibodeau S, Dork T, Neal D, Cox A, Maier C, Vogel W, Guy M, Muir K, Lophatananon A, Kedda MA, Spurdle A, Steginga S, John EM, Giles G, Hopper J, Chappuis PO, Hutter P, Foulkes WD, Hamel N, Salinas CA, Koopmeiners JS, Karyadi DM, Johanneson B, Wahlfors T, Tammela TL, Stern MC, Corral R, McDonnell SK, Schurmann P, Meyer A, Kuefer R, Leongamornlert DA, Tymrakiewicz M, Liu JF, O'Mara T, Gardiner RA, Aitken J, Joshi AD, Severi G, English DR, Southey M, Edwards SM, Al Olama AA, Eeles RA (2008) Multiple novel prostate cancer predisposition loci confirmed by an international study: the PRACTICAL Consortium. Cancer Epidemiol Biomarkers Prev 17, 2052–2061

Lange EM, Gillanders EM, Davis CC, Brown WM, Campbell JK, Jones M, Gildea D, Riedesel E, Albertus J, Freas-Lutz D, Markey C, Giri V, Dimmer JB, Montie JE, Trent JM, Cooney KA (2003) Genome-wide scan for prostate cancer susceptibility genes using families from the University of Michigan prostate cancer genetics project finds evidence for linkage on chromosome 17 near BRCA1. Prostate 57, 326–334

Matarasso N, Bar-Shira A, Rozovski U, Rosner S, Orr-Urtreger A (2007) Functional analysis of the Aurora Kinase A Ile31 allelic variant in human prostate. Neoplasia 9, 707–715

Miller DC, Zheng SL, Dunn RL, Sarma AV, Montie JE, Lange EM, Meyers DA, Xu J, Cooney KA (2003) Germ-line mutations of the macrophage scavenger receptor 1 gene: association with prostate cancer risk in African-American men. Cancer Res 63, 3486–3489

Moslehi R, Chu W, Karlan B, Fishman D, Risch H, Fields A, Smotkin D, Ben-David Y, Rosenblatt J, Russo D, Schwartz P, Tung N, Warner E, Rosen B, Friedman J, Brunet JS, Narod SA (2000) BRCA1 and BRCA2 mutation analysis of 208 Ashkenazi Jewish women with ovarian cancer. Am J Hum Genet 66, 1259–1272

Nastiuk KL, Mansukhani M, Terry MB, Kularatne P, Rubin MA, Melamed J, Gammon MD, Ittmann M, Krolewski JJ (1999) Common mutations in BRCA1 and BRCA2 do not contribute to early prostate cancer in Jewish men. Prostate 40, 172–177

Orr-Urtreger A, Bar-Shira A, Bercovich D, Matarasso N, Rozovsky U, Rosner S, Soloviov S, Rennert G, Kadouri L, Hubert A, Rennert H, Matzkin H (2006) RNASEL mutation screening and association study in Ashkenazi and non-Ashkenazi prostate cancer patients. Cancer Epidemiol Biomarkers Prev 15, 474–479

Orr-Urtreger A, Bar-Shira A, Matzkin H, Mabjeesh NJ (2007) The homozygous P582S mutation in the oxygen-dependent degradation domain of HIF-1 alpha is associated with increased risk for prostate cancer. Prostate 67, 8–13

Ostrer H (2001) A genetic profile of contemporary Jewish populations. Nat Rev Genet 2, 891–898

Phelan CM, Kwan E, Jack E, Li S, Morgan C, Aube J, Hanna D, Narod SA (2002) A low frequency of non-founder BRCA1 mutations in Ashkenazi Jewish breast-ovarian cancer families. Hum Mutat 20, 352–357

Rennert H, Bercovich D, Hubert A, Abeliovich D, Rozovsky U, Bar-Shira A, Soloviov S, Schreiber L, Matzkin H, Rennert G, Kadouri L, Peretz T, Yaron Y, Orr-Urtreger A (2002) A novel founder mutation in the RNASEL gene, 471delAAAG, is associated with prostate cancer in Ashkenazi Jews. Am J Hum Genet 71, 981–984

Risch N, de Leon D, Ozelius L, Kramer P, Almasy L, Singer B, Fahn S, Breakefield X, Bressman S (1995) Genetic analysis of idiopathic torsion dystonia in Ashkenazi Jews and their recent descent from a small founder population. Nat Genet 9, 152–159

Roa BB, Boyd AA, Volcik K, Richards CS (1996) Ashkenazi Jewish population frequencies for common mutations in *BRCA1* and *BRCA2*. Nat Genet 14, 185–187

Rokman A, Ikonen T, Seppala EH, Nupponen N, Autio V, Mononen N, Bailey-Wilson J, Trent J, Carpten J, Matikainen MP, Koivisto PA, Tammela TL, Kallioniemi OP, Schleutker J (2002) Germline alterations of the RNASEL gene, a candidate HPC1 gene at 1q25, in patients and families with prostate cancer. Am J Hum Genet 70, 1299–1304

Schaid DJ (2004) The complex genetic epidemiology of prostate cancer. Hum Mol Genet 13 Spec No 1, R103–R121

Seppala EH, Ikonen T, Autio V, Rokman A, Mononen N, Matikainen MP, Tammela TL, Schleutker J (2003) Germ-line alterations in MSR1 gene and prostate cancer risk. Clin Cancer Res 9, 5252–5256

Shaag A, Walsh T, Renbaum P, Kirchhoff T, Nafa K, Shiovitz S, Mandell JB, Welcsh P, Lee MK, Ellis N, Offit K, Levy-Lahad E, King MC (2005) Functional and genomic approaches reveal an ancient CHEK2 allele associated with breast cancer in the Ashkenazi Jewish population. Hum Mol Genet 14, 555–563

Smith JR, Freije D, Carpten JD, Gronberg H, Xu J, Isaacs SD, Brownstein MJ, Bova GS, Guo H, Bujnovszky P, Nusskern DR, Damber JE, Bergh A, Emanuelsson M, Kallioniemi OP, Walker-Daniels J, Bailey-Wilson JE, Beaty TH, Meyers DA, Walsh PC, Collins FS, Trent JM, Isaacs WB (1996) Major susceptibility locus for prostate cancer on chromosome 1 suggested by a genome-wide search. Science 274, 1371–1374

Struewing JP, Abeliovich D, Peretz T, Avishai N, Kaback MM, Collins FS, Brody LC (1995) The carrier frequency of the BRCA1 185delAG mutation is approximately 1 percent in Ashkenazi Jewish individuals. Nat Genet 11, 198–200

Struewing JP, Hartge P, Wacholder S, Baker SM, Berlin M, McAdams M, Timmerman MM, Brody LC, Tucker MA (1997) The risk of cancer associated with specific mutations of BRCA1 and BRCA2 among Ashkenazi Jews. N Engl J Med 336, 1401–1408

Sun J, Hsu FC, Turner AR, Zheng SL, Chang BL, Liu W, Isaacs WB, Xu J (2006) Meta-analysis of association of rare mutations and common sequence variants in the MSR1 gene and prostate cancer risk. Prostate 66, 728–737

Thompson D, Easton DF (2002) Cancer Incidence in BRCA1 mutation carriers. J Natl Cancer Inst 94, 1358–1365

Tischkowitz MD, Yilmaz A, Chen LQ, Karyadi DM, Novak D, Kirchhoff T, Hamel N, Tavtigian SV, Kolb S, Bismar TA, Aloyz R, Nelson PS, Hood L, Narod SA, White KA, Ostrander EA, Isaacs WB, Offit K, Cooney KA, Stanford JL, Foulkes WD (2008) Identification and characterization of novel SNPs in CHEK2 in Ashkenazi Jewish men with prostate cancer. Cancer Lett 270,173–180.

Vazina A, Baniel J, Yaacobi Y, Shtriker A, Engelstein D, Leibovitz I, Zehavi M, Sidi AA, Ramon Y, Tischler T, Livne PM, Friedman E (2000) The rate of the founder Jewish mutations in BRCA1 and BRCA2 in prostate cancer patients in Israel. Br J Cancer 83, 463–466

Wang L, McDonnell SK, Elkins DA, Slager SL, Christensen E, Marks AF, Cunningham JM, Peterson BJ, Jacobsen SJ, Cerhan JR, Blute ML, Schaid DJ, Thibodeau SN (2002) Analysis of the RNASEL gene in familial and sporadic prostate cancer. Am J Hum Genet 71, 116–123

Wang L, McDonnell SK, Cunningham JM, Hebbring S, Jacobsen SJ, Cerhan JR, Slager SL, Blute ML, Schaid DJ, Thibodeau SN (2003) No association of germline alteration of MSR1 with prostate cancer risk. Nat Genet 35, 128–129

Warner E, Foulkes W, Goodwin P, Meschino W, Blondal J, Paterson C, Ozcelik H, Goss P, Allingham-Hawkins D, Hamel N, Di Prospero L, Contiga V, Serruya C, Klein M, Moslehi R, Honeyford J, Liede A, Glendon C, Brunet JS, Narod S (1999) Prevalence and penetrance of BRCA1 and BRCA2 gene mutations in unselected Ashkenazi Jewish women with breast cancer. J Natl Cancer Inst 91, 1241–1247

Wilkens EP, Freije D, Xu J, Nusskern DR, Suzuki H, Isaacs SD, Wiley K, Bujnovsky P, Meyers DA, Walsh PC, Isaacs WB (1999) No evidence for a role of BRCA1 or BRCA2 mutations in Ashkenazi Jewish families with hereditary prostate cancer. Prostate 39, 280–284

Xu J, Zheng SL, Komiya A, Mychaleckyj JC, Isaacs SD, Hu JJ, Sterling D, Lange EM, Hawkins GA, Turner A, Ewing CM, Faith DA, Johnson JR, Suzuki H, Bujnovszky P, Wiley KE, DeMarzo AM, Bova GS, Chang B, Hall MC, McCullough DL, Partin AW, Kassabian VS, Carpten JD, Bailey-Wilson JE, Trent JM, Ohar J, Bleecker ER, Walsh PC, Isaacs WB, Meyers DA (2002) Germline mutations and sequence variants of the macrophage scavenger receptor 1 gene are associated with prostate cancer risk. Nat Genet 32, 321–325

Xu J, Dimitrov L, Chang BL, Adams TS, Turner AR, Meyers DA, Eeles RA, Easton DF, Foulkes WD, Simard J, Giles GG, Hopper JL, Mahle L, Moller P, Bishop T, Evans C, Edwards S, Meitz J, Bullock S, Hope Q, Hsieh CL, Halpern J, Balise RN, Oakley-Girvan I, Whittemore AS, Ewing CM, Gielzak M, Isaacs SD, Walsh PC, Wiley KE, Isaacs WB, Thibodeau SN, McDonnell SK, Cunningham JM, Zarfas KE, Hebbring S, Schaid DJ, Friedrichsen DM, Deutsch K, Kolb S, Badzioch M, Jarvik GP, Janer M, Hood L, Ostrander EA, Stanford JL, Lange EM, Beebe-Dimmer JL, Mohai CE, Cooney KA, Ikonen T, Baffoe-Bonnie A, Fredriksson H, Matikainen MP, Tammela TL, Bailey-Wilson J, Schleutker J, Maier C, Herkommer K, Hoegel JJ, Vogel W, Paiss T, Wiklund F, Emanuelsson M, Stenman E, Jonsson BA, Gronberg H, Camp NJ, Farnham J, Cannon-Albright LA, Seminara D (2005) A combined genomewide linkage scan of 1,233 families for prostate cancer-susceptibility genes conducted by the international consortium for prostate cancer genetics. Am J Hum Genet 77, 219–229

Zuhlke KA, Madeoy JJ, Beebe-Dimmer J, White KA, Griffin A, Lange EM, Gruber SB, Ostrander EA, Cooney KA (2004) Truncating BRCA1 mutations are uncommon in a cohort of hereditary prostate cancer families with evidence of linkage to 17q markers. Clin Cancer Res 10, 5975–5980

9.4 African-American Populations: Inherited Susceptibility for Prostate Cancer

Agnes B. Baffoe-Bonnie and Isaac J. Powell

9.4.1 Introduction

Decades of epidemiological observation suggest that along with increasing age and a positive family history, sub-Saharan African ancestry is an important risk factor for prostate cancer (PCa) (Powell 2007). In the United States, the incidence of prostate cancer is approximately 60% higher in African-American men (AAM) than in European-American men (EAM) and the mortality rate from the disease is more than twice as high (Powell and Meyskens 2001; Zeigler-Johnson 2001; Clegg et al. 2002; Narain, Cher et al. 2002; Cunningham et al. 2003). While environmental factors may account for some of this observed difference, the possibility of a genetic contribution deserved serious consideration. In the early 1990s, studies of families with multiple affected males, mostly from the Caucasian population, indicated that a subset may harbor a dominant susceptibility gene for hereditary prostate cancer (HPC) (Carter et al., 1992,1993). In 1996, the two African-American families included in the linkage mapping of the susceptibility locus *HPC1* (1q24–25) showed linkage to this region with a combined LOD score of 1.4 (Smith et al. 1996). This report led to a nationwide concerted effort to assemble African-American families informative for linkage.

9.4.2 Evidence that Genetic Factors Play a Critical Role in Prostate Cancer Outcomes Among African-Americans

The fact that cancer is a genetic disease is well accepted. It may be epigenetic or genetic susceptibility accounting for the phenotypic presentation but evidence certainly suggests that cancer, and specifically PCa, is genetically based.

A.B. Baffoe-Bonnie (✉) and I.J. Powell
Fox Chase Cancer Center, 333 Cottman Avenue, Philadelphia, PA 19111. Inherited Disease Research Branch National Human Genome Research Institute, National Institutes of Health, 333 Cassell Drive, Suite 1200 Baltimore, MD 21224. Now at Merck Research Laboratories, Department of Epidemiology, North Wales, PA 19454
agnes_baffoe-bonnie@merck.com

We propose that higher incidence and earlier age presentation of PCa among African-American men (AAM) is based on genetic factors. Higher disease recurrence rates and earlier failure following radical prostatectomy also point to a more aggressive variant of PCa in AAM (Moul et al. 1996; Iselin et al. 1998). Even when patients are stratified into risk categories based on their clinical tumor stage, Prostate Specific Antigen (PSA) value at diagnosis, and Gleason grade, AA ancestry remains an independent predictor of disease recurrence following radical prostatectomy, suggesting that outcome differences following this intervention are not just a matter of more advanced disease at presentation (Grossfeld et al. 2002; Powell et al. 2002).

Over the last 20 years, evidence that prostate cancer may be caused by multiple genes, possibly interacting with endocrine and environmental factors, has continued to grow (Rebbeck et al. 1998; Crawford 2003; Gronberg 2003; Powell et al. 2004; Schaid 2004). Linkage studies have identified susceptibility loci for prostate cancer at several chromosomal locations: including *HPC1* at chromosome 1q23–25, *HPC2* at chromosome 17p, *HPC20* at chromosome 20q13, *HPCX* at chromosome Xq27–28, linkage to chromosome 8p22–23, *PCAP* at chromosome 1q42–43, and *CAPB* at chromosome 1p36, and several strong candidate genes including *RNASEL*, *ELAC2*, and *MSR1* have been mapped (Schaid 2004). Kittles et al. recently reported that a variant in the *EphB2* gene on Chromosome 1p is found to be associated with PCa among AAM with a family history of PCa but not found among European-American men (EAM) (Kittles et al. 2006).

While few clinically meaningful associations of genetic polymorphisms with prostate cancer risk have thus far been demonstrated, the results of a recent meta-analysis suggest that *CYP17* polymorphisms may play a role in the susceptibility to prostate cancer of men of sub-Saharan African, but not European, descent (Ntais et al. 2003). In a study that examined the relationship between genetic variants in *CYP3A4* and disease-free survival in a diverse population of men undergoing radical prostatectomy, EAM presented with 8% variant G allele while AAM were observed to have an 81% variant G allele frequency. The variant G allele was associated with greater disease progression in men with pathologically locally advanced prostate cancer than men diagnosed with the normal or wild-type A allele (Powell et al. 2004). In a case-control study, the variant G allele was strongly associated with aggressive PCa among AAM (Bangsi et al. 2006). Other studies have shown that altered expression of the *BCL-2* gene may be an important genetic factor underlying the greater aggressiveness of prostate cancer in AAM (deVere White et al. 1998). This gene plays a central role in preventing cancer cells from dying (i.e., via its anti-apoptotic effect), and its up-regulation in AAM may be responsible for causing prostate cancer cells to flourish when they would normally perish, and for conferring resistance to anticancer therapies. The linkage between increased cancer proliferation and *BCL-2* positively seen in prostate tumors of AAM, but not EAM, may contribute to the aggressive behavior of prostate cancer in AAM (deVere White et al. 1998).

9.4.3   The African-American Hereditary Prostate Cancer Study (1997–2000)

The African-American Hereditary Prostate Cancer Study (AAHPC) was a national collaboration funded by the National Institutes of Health to recruit African-American families to a hereditary prostate cancer study under the NIH CONTRACT No1-HG-75418. In 1997, the investigators at the NHGRI in collaboration with Howard University and a predominantly African-American group of urologists involved in prostate cancer research established the AAHPC Study Network primarily to increase the number of HPC families for genetic studies (Royal et al. 2000; Powell et al. 2001). This network of Collaborative Recruitment Centers (CRCs) was geographically located in major metropolitan areas highly populated with African-American families, including Atlanta, Georgia; Chicago, Illinois; Detroit, Michigan; Houston, Texas; New York, New York; Columbia, South Carolina and Washington, D.C. Provisions for the recruitment of African-American families from other geographical locations were made through a national referral strategy. The AAHPC study was designed to confirm the suggested linkage to *HPC1* in African-American families, as well as to conduct a genome-wide search for other loci associated with hereditary prostate cancer. The proposed AAHPC inclusion criteria were as follows (a) African-American families with four or more members diagnosed with PCa, (b) the average age at diagnosis of the affected members in the family preferably ≤65 years (but no greater than 70 years); (c) at least three affected and three unaffected members must donate a sample of blood for genotyping.

9.4.4   Clinical Characteristics of African-American Men in the AAHPC Study

Seventy percent of the 92 families analyzed had 4 to 6 affected men with prostate cancer ($n = 108$), while the remaining 30% (28/92) had more than six affected men per family with a range of 7–11 ($n = 46$) (Ahaghotu et al. 2004). For all families, the mean number of affected men per family was 5.5, with a mean age at diagnosis of 61.0 (±8.4) years. For the ">6" group, the mean number of affected per family was 8.5, with a mean age at diagnosis of 59.9 (±9.4) years. The median age was 62 years across groups. The mean PSA level for affected males at diagnosis for all families was 19.3 (± 30.7) ng/ml, 21.2 (±34.6) ng/ml for the "4–6" group, and 13.9 (± 13.3) ng/ml for the >6 group. Without the two extreme high PSA values of 210 and 253 ng/ml in the "4–6" group, the mean PSA level was 17.3 (± 19.0) for that group, 13.9 (± 13.3) and 16.4 (±17.7) for the ">6" group and for all families, respectively. PSA at diagnosis did not show significant difference between the two groups ($P = 0.578$). PSA levels were also stratified into three categories similarly to those used in previous studies (Goode et al. 2001) and compared between the

"4–6" and ">6" groups. There was no significant difference in PSA values in the two groups ($P = 0.158$). Based on the Gleason score, 77.2% (119/154) had a range of "2–6" compared with 11.0% with higher grades "7–10" of histology. There was no difference between "4–6" and ">6" group in terms of Gleason score ($P = 0.7519$). In all families, 68.2% (105/154) of affected men presented with organ-confined disease (T1-T2/No/Mo) at diagnosis compared with 10.4% (16/154) with more advanced disease (T3-T4/No/Mo). The families with >6 affected men had a significantly higher proportion of node-positive prostate cancer (21.7%) compared with 8.4% among families with 4–6 affected men ($P = 0.01$). The presence of distant metastases at diagnosis also differed between these two groups, with 23.9% (11/46) in the ">6" group vs. 2.1% (3/108) in the "4–6" group ($P < 0.0001$). Radical prostatectomy was the preferred primary therapy for 66.2% of all affected men (102/154) followed by 20.8% (32/154) who chose radiation therapy. The proportion of affected men receiving definitive therapy, 87.0% (134/154) was much higher compared to those choosing watchful waiting (2.0%) or hormonal therapy (11.0%).

9.4.5   Genome-Wide Linkage of 77 Families from the AAHPC

The genetic basis for prostate cancer susceptibility has been difficult to elucidate despite a decade of research by the International Consortium on Prostate Cancer Genetics (ICPCG) (Ostrander and Stanford 2000). In an effort to focus on high-risk AA families, Baffoe-Bonnie et al. (2007) reported that of the 77 AAHPC families analyzed 65 (84.4%) had an early age at diagnosis of ≤65 years (Baffoe-Bonnie et al. 2007). All families fulfilled the criteria of ≥4 affected. A subsequent ~10 cM genome-wide linkage analysis included 254 affected and 274 unaffected genotyped.

Linkage analysis revealed three chromosomal regions with GENEHUNTER multipoint HLOD scores ≥1.3 for all 77 families at 11q22, 17p11, and Xq21. One family yielded genome-wide significant evidence of linkage (LOD = 3.5) to the 17p11 region with seven other families having LOD scores of ≥2.3 in this region. Twenty-nine families with no-male-to-male (NMM) transmission gave a peak HLOD of 1.62 ($\alpha = 0.33$) at the Xq21 locus. For the 16 families with ">6 affected," two novel LOD score peaks ≥0.91 occurred at 2p21 and 2q12. These chromosomal regions in the genome warrant further follow up based on the hypothesis of multiple susceptibility genes with modest effects, or several major genes segregating in small subsets of families (Baffoe-Bonnie et al. 2007).

9.4.6   Compelling Evidence for a Prostate Cancer Gene at 22q12.3 – ICPCG

Previously, an analysis of 14 extended, high-risk Utah pedigrees localized in the chromosome 22q linkage region to 3.2 Mb at 22q12.3–13.1 (flanked on each side by three recombinants) contained 31 annotated genes (Camp et al. 2006). In this large, multi-centered, ICPCG collaborative study, Camp et al. (2007) performed statistical recombinant mapping in 54 pedigrees selected to be informative for recombinant mapping from nine member groups of the International Consortium for Prostate Cancer Genetics (ICPCG). These 54 pedigrees included five pedigrees from the African-American Hereditary Prostate Cancer (AAHPC) consortium and pedigrees from seven other ICPCG member groups. The additional 40 pedigrees were selected from a total pool of 1,213 such that each pedigree was required to contain both at least four prostate cancer (PCa) cases and exhibit evidence for linkage to the chromosome 22q region. The recombinant events in these 40 independent pedigrees confirmed the previously proposed region. Further, when all 54 pedigrees were considered, the three-recombinant consensus region was narrowed down by more than a megabase to 2.2 Mb at chromosome 22q12.3 flanked by D22S281 and D22S683. This narrower region eliminated 20 annotated genes from that previously proposed, leaving only 11 genes. This region at 22q12.3 is the most consistently identified and smallest linkage region for PCa (Camp et al. 2006, 2007).

9.4.7   Genetic Variants at the 8q24 Locus in African-American Men

Recently, the chromosome 8q genomic region has been reported to be highly associated with prostate cancer susceptibility risk, using family-based linkage studies, association studies, and studies of tumors among different Caucasian populations (Amundadottir et al. 2006; Haiman et al. 2007; Schumacher et al. 2007; Suuriniemi et al. 2007; Wang et al. 2007) (See Chap. 9.1). A whole-genome admixture mapping scan in African-Americans, a 3.8 Mb interval at this 8q24 locus was found to be significantly associated with susceptibility to PCa (Freedman et al. 2006), showing that other SNPs apart from the rs1447295 might be important in PCa in African-Americans. Since the mixture between Europeans and West African populations is estimated to have occurred within the past 15 generations, stretches of DNA (extending millions of base pairs) with contiguous European and African ancestry have not had much time to break up because of recombination (Smith et al. 2004). Thus whole-genome admixture mapping, the process by which the genome of populations of mixed ancestry, such as African-Americans, is performed to search for regions where the proportion of DNA inherited from either the ancestral African or European population is unusual compared with the genome-wide average (Smith et al. 2004). Admixture mapping, therefore, employs a relatively smaller number of markers for a whole-genome scan (a couple of thousand) compared to the hundreds of thousands often necessary in non-admixed populations (Smith et al. 2004; McKeigue 1997).

More prostate cancer studies are being conducted and a recent study including African-Americans suggested that newer SNPs within this region might be associated (specifically rs16901979) (Gudmundsson et al. 2007). The increased risk associated with African ancestry is greater in men diagnosed before 72 years of age

(P < 0.0003) and may contribute to the epidemiological observation that the higher risk for prostate cancer in African-Americans is greatest in younger men (and attenuates with older age). The same region was recently identified through linkage analysis of prostate cancer, followed by fine-mapping. Freedman and colleagues (Haiman et al. 2007) replicated this association (P < 4.2 × 10^{-9}) but found that the previously described alleles did not explain more than a fraction of the admixture signal.

9.4.8   Conclusion

Due to the noted disparities of the burden of disease between African-American men and other ethnic groups, we suggest that the genetics of initiation and progression of PCa may be different among AAM, accounting for the clinical differences reported. With the advent of appropriate panels of markers and analytical methods, prostate cancer genomic research has included whole-genome admixture scans because of its marked difference in incidence rates across populations. With few clinically meaningful genetic polymorphisms detected among AAM with prostate cancer, the recent confirmation of the highly significant association at 8q24 appears most interesting.

Prostate cancer genetic research in African-American men must continue as long as we lack explanations for the earlier age of diagnosis, aggressiveness of disease, familial aggregation in multiplex families, higher incidence and mortality rates, increased disease recurrence rates, and earlier failure after radical prostatectomy. Many gaps remain as the reported linkage peaks in AA families are still awaiting fine-mapping and the alleles identified to date through genome-wide scans are insufficient to explain more than a small fraction of the admixture signal. The causative alleles remain to be identified in regions including the "still-unidentified risk gene for prostate cancer at 8q24," and as Freedman et al. (2006) suggest, "intense work is needed to find it."

Furthermore, the collaborative studies by the AAHPC and the ICPCG illustrate the value of consortium efforts and the continued utility of genetic linkage analysis using informative pedigrees to localize genes for a disease as complex and heterogeneous as prostate cancer.

Note Added in Proof

Several papers have been published since this article was written. In summary, the associations previously observed in African-American populations on chromosome 8q24 have been confirmed in many studies to date (for example Bock et al. Human Genet July 1, 2009 (epublication) and Xu et al. (2009) Cancer Epidemiol Biomarkers Prevent 18, 2145-49, and references therein.

References

Ahaghotu C, Baffoe-Bonnie A et al (2004) Clinical characteristics of African-American men with hereditary prostate cancer: the AAHPC Study. Prostate Cancer Prostatic Dis 7(2):165–169

Amundadottir LT, Sulem P et al (2006) A common variant associated with prostate cancer in European and African populations. Nat Genet 38(6):652–658

Baffoe-Bonnie AB, Kittles RA et al (2007) Genome-wide linkage of 77 families from the African American Hereditary Prostate Cancer Study (AAHPC). Prostate 67(1):22–31.

Bangsi D, Zhou J et al (2006) Impact of a genetic variant in CYP3A4 on risk and clinical presentation of prostate cancer among white and African-American men. Urol Oncol 24(1):21–27.

Bock CH, Schwartz AG, Ruterbusch JJ, Levin AM, Neslund-Dudas C, Land SJ,Wenzlaff AS, Reich D, McKeigue P, Chen W, Heath EI, Powell IJ, Kittles RA, Rybicki BA. Hum Genet. 2009 Jul 1. [Epub ahead of print]

Xu J, Kibel AS, Hu JJ, Turner AR, Pruett K, Zheng SL, Sun J, Isaacs SD, Wiley KE, Kim ST, Hsu FC, Wu W, Torti FM, Walsh PC, Chang BL, Isaacs WB. Cancer Epidemiol Biomarkers Prev. 2009 Jul;18(7):2145-9.

Camp NJ, Farnham JM et al (2006). Localization of a prostate cancer predisposition gene to an 880-kb region on chromosome 22q12.3 in Utah high-risk pedigrees. Cancer Res 66(20): 10205–10212

Camp NJ, Cannon-Albright LA et al; International Consortium for Prostate Cancer Genetics (2007) Compelling evidence for a prostate cancer gene at 22q12.3 by the International Consortium for Prostate Cancer Genetics. Hum Mol Genet 1;16 (11):1271–1278

Carter BS, Beaty TH et al (1992) Mendelian inheritance of familial prostate cancer. Proc Natl Acad Sci U S A 89(8):3367–3371

Carter BS, Bova GS et al (1993) Hereditary prostate cancer: epidemiologic and clinical features. J Urol 150(3):797–802

Clegg L, Li FP, Hankey BF, Chu K, Edwards BK (2002). Cancer survival among US whites and minorities: a SEER (Surveillance, Epidemiology, and End Results) Program population-based study. Arch Intern Med 162(17):1985–1993

Crawford ED (2003) Epidemiology of prostate cancer. Urology 62(6 Suppl 1):3–12

Cunningham GR, Ashton CM et al (2003) Familial aggregation of prostate cancer in African-Americans and white Americans. Prostate 56(4):256–262

deVere White R, Deitch A et al (1998) Racial differences in clinically localized prostate cancers of black and white men. J Urol 159(6):1979–1982

Freedman ML, Haiman CA et al (2006) Admixture mapping identifies 8q24 as a prostate cancer risk locus in African-American men. Proc Natl Acad Sci U S A 103(38):14068–14073

Goode EL, Stanford JL et al (2001) Clinical characteristics of prostate cancer in an analysis of linkage to four putative susceptibility loci. Clin Cancer Res 7(9):2739–2749

Gronberg H (2003) Prostate cancer epidemiology. Lancet 361(9360):859–864

Grossfeld GD, Latini DM et al (2002). Is ethnicity an independent predictor of prostate cancer recurrence after radical prostatectomy? J Urol 168(6):2510–2515

Gudmundsson J, Sulem P et al (2007) Genome-wide association study identifies a second prostate cancer susceptibility variant at 8q24. Nat Genet 39:631–637

Haiman CA, Patterson N et al (2007) Multiple regions within 8q24 independently affect risk for prostate cancer. Nat Genet 39(5):638–644

Iselin CE, Box JW et al (1998) Surgical control of clinically localized prostate carcinoma is equivalent in African-American and white males. Cancer 83(11):2353–2360

Kittles RA, Baffoe-Bonnie AB et al. (2006) A common nonsense mutation in EphB2 is associated with prostate cancer risk in African American men with a positive family history. J Med Genet 43(6): 507–511

McKeigue PM (1997) Mapping genes underlying ethnic differences in disease risk by linkage disequilibrium in recently admixed populations. Am J Hum Genet 60:188–196

Moul, JW, Douglas TH et al (1996) Black race is an adverse prognostic factor for prostate cancer recurrence following radical prostatectomy in an equal access health care setting. J Urol 155(5):1667–1673

Narain V, Cher ML et al (2002) Prostate cancer diagnosis, staging and survival. Cancer Metastasis Rev 21(1):17–27

Ntais C, Polycarpou A et al (2003) Association of the CYP17 gene polymorphism with the risk of prostate cancer: a meta-analysis. Cancer Epidemiol Biomarkers Prev 12(2):120–126

Ostrander EA and Stanford JL (2000) Genetics of prostate cancer: too many loci, too few genes. Am J Hum Genet 67(6):1367–1375

Powell IJ (2007) Epidemiology and pathophysiology of prostate cancer in African-American men. J Urol 177(2):444–449

Powell IJ Meyskens FL Jr. (2001) African American men and hereditary/familial prostate cancer: Intermediate-risk populations for chemoprevention trials. Urology 57(4 Suppl 1):178–181

Powell IJ, Carpten J et al (2001) African-American heredity prostate cancer study: a model for genetic research. J Natl Med Assoc 93(12 Suppl): 25S–28S

Powell IJ, Dey J et al (2002) Disease-free survival difference between African Americans and whites after radical prostatectomy for local prostate cancer: a multivariable analysis. Urology 59(6):907–912

Powell IJ, Zhou J. et al (2004) CYP3A4 genetic variant and disease-free survival among white and black men after radical prostatectomy. J Urol 172(5 Pt 1):1848–1852

Rebbeck TR, Jaffe JM et al (1998) Modification of clinical presentation of prostate tumors by a novel genetic variant in CYP3A4. J Natl Cancer Inst 90(16):1225–1229

Royal C, Baffoe-Bonnie A et al. (2000) Recruitment experience in the first phase of the African American Hereditary Prostate Cancer (AAHPC) study. Ann Epidemiol 10(8 Suppl):S68–S77

Schaid, D. (2004) The complex genetic epidemiology of prostate cancer. Hum Mol Genet 13:R103–R121 [Epub ahead of print].

Schumacher FR, Feigelson HS et al (2007) A common 8q24 variant in prostate and breast cancer from a large nested case-control study. Cancer Res 67(7):2951–2956

Smith, JR, Freije D et al (1996) Major susceptibility locus for prostate cancer on chromosome 1 suggested by a genome-wide search. Science 274(5291):1371–1374

Smith MW, Patterson N et al (2004) A high-density admixture map for disease gene discovery in African Americans. Am J Hum Genet 74(5):1001–1013

Suuriniemi M, Agalliu I et al (2007) Confirmation of a positive association between prostate cancer risk and a locus at chromosome 8q24. Cancer Epidemiol Biomarkers Prev 16(4):809–814

Wang L, McDonnell SK et al (2007) Two common chromosome 8q24 variants are associated with increased risk for prostate cancer. Cancer Res 67(7):2944–2950

Zeigler-Johnson, C. (2001) CYP3A4: a potential prostate cancer risk factor for high-risk groups. Clin J Oncol Nurs 5(4):153–154

Chapter 10
Inherited Susceptibility of Aggressive Prostate Cancer

Audrey H. Schnell and John S. Witte

10.1 Introduction

The severity of prostate cancer varies widely, ranging from latent disease and having essentially no impact on morbidity, to an aggressive course of disease with high morbidity and potential mortality. Deciphering the risk factors for prostate cancer and aggressive forms of the disease is crucial for improving screening, prevention, and treatment of this common but complex disease. Established risk factors for overall prostate cancer include older age, African-American ethnicity, a positive family history of prostate cancer, and a few genetic loci. The potential relationship between these risk factors and more aggressive disease remains to be clearly understood. Moreover, a number of genetic linkage and association studies support an inherited susceptibility to aggressive prostate cancer.

Prostate cancer is the second most common cancer in American men after skin cancer (Carter et al. 2006; SEER Cancer Statistics Review 1975–2004 2007). The only established risk factors for prostate cancer are increasing age, African-American (AA) ethnicity, and a positive family history of prostate cancer. The risk of prostate cancer increases with older ages with most cases diagnosed after age 65. African-Americans have the highest incidence of prostate cancer, Asians the lowest, whereas Caucasians have in-between rates (SEER Cancer Statistics Review 1975–2004 2007). Some studies have also found a higher mortality rate in AA men (Albano et al. 2007; Powell 2007) (see Chap. 9.4). The risk of prostate cancer also increases with the occurrence of the disease in first-degree relatives and increases with increasing numbers of affected family members (Gann 2002; Giovannucci et al. 2007; Noe et al. 2007). There is a twofold risk to men who have one affected first-degree relative and increases to 11-fold with three affected family members (Steinberg et al. 1990). A number of studies have investigated the risk of prostate cancer in families with other cancers (e.g., breast), but the occurrence of other

J.S. Witte (✉)
Epidemiology & Biostatistics, and Urology, University of California, San Francisco, Box 0794, San Francisco, CA, 94143-0794, USA
e-mail: wittej@humgen.ucsf.edu

W.D. Foulkes and K.A. Cooney (eds.), *Male Reproductive Cancers:*
Epidemiology, Pathology and Genetics, Cancer Genetics,
DOI 10.1007/978-1-4419-0449-2_10, © Springer Science+Business Media, LLC 2010

cancers has not been established as risk factors (Peters et al. 2001; Verhage et al. 2004). Studies have also looked at environmental factors such as diet and occupational exposures, but these have not been consistently associated with disease (Carter et al. 2006; SEER Cancer Statistics Review 1975–2004 2007).

One can classify prostate cancer cases as "sporadic," "familial," or "hereditary" based on the disease patterns occurring in a family. Prostate cancers classified as sporadic are those where there are no other known family members with prostate cancer. Using this label, however, can be problematic in light of the potential latent disease and late onset of prostate cancer (i.e., in apparently disease-free family members). Moreover, sporadic prostate cancer (SPCa) cases may be due to an inherited susceptibility. Hereditary prostate cancer (HPCa) classifies families with at least three generations affected with prostate cancer, or three first-degree relatives affected or two relatives affected before age 55 years (Bova et al. 1998). Familial prostate cancer (FPCa) is a more general category and is used when at least one additional family member is affected with the disease.

The occurrence of prostate cancer in other family members can impact the association of family history and aggressiveness in that men with a positive family history may be more likely to seek out screening than "sporadic" cases leading to an earlier diagnosis. Moreover, diagnostic patterns have changed since the widespread adoption of Prostate Specific Antigen (PSA) testing as a screening tool for prostate cancer. PSA testing is likely responsible for the increase in the early detection of prostate cancer (Epstein 2006), giving rise to diagnoses at earlier ages and stage. The effect of these factors must be taken into account when examining family history and aggressiveness.

While great efforts have attempted to identify the causal genetic variants for prostate cancer, until recently there have been few consistently replicated results. This may be due to different ascertainment methods, diagnostic criteria, populations, and small sample sizes (i.e., low power) across studies. It may also reflect the heterogeneous nature of prostate cancer. Therefore, when searching for disease-causing genes it is important to define homogeneous subgroups of cases such as disease aggressiveness. This is complicated by the numerous potential definitions of disease aggressiveness. Should aggressiveness be defined by stage or grade at diagnosis, speed of progression, recurrence after treatment, mortality, or some combination of these factors? In particular, measures of aggressiveness (e.g., stage and grade at diagnosis) have likely been affected by earlier diagnosis of prostate cancer due to improvements in screening.

10.2 Assessment of Prostate Cancer Aggressiveness

Deciphering the genetic basis of prostate cancer aggressiveness requires careful consideration of the different clinical and pathological measures used to define "aggressiveness." We review each of the different measures of prostate cancer aggressiveness here.

10.2.1   Staging

Staging refers to the localization or spread of the cancer. Clinical staging of prostate cancer is most often based on the TNM system (Tumor, Nodes, Metastasis) using biopsy specimens and digital rectal exams (DRE). Stage T1 is based on the differentiation of the cells in the primary tumor (T). Stage T2 is based on the findings from the DRE and T3 is assigned when cells extend into areas surrounding the prostate gland. Stage T4, N, and M are based on the extent of cell spread (Bostwick et al. 1994). When using stage to reflect aggressiveness, it is typically defined as regional spread or beyond, but this varies across studies.

10.2.2   Grading

Histologic examination of the tissue specimen allows grading of the differentiation level of the tumor. The Gleason Score (GS) is based on the level of differentiation of the glandular cells and is made by the pathologist based on either biopsy or radical prostatectomy (RP) samples. The primary and secondary Gleason patterns describe the two most common patterns seen by the pathologist. The GS is a composite score equal to the sum of two Gleason grades – the primary pattern, consisting of the majority of the tumor, and the secondary pattern, relating to the minority of the tumor. The grade can range from 1 to 5 with 5 being the most severe. Grades 1 and 2 closely resemble the normal prostate with grade 2 being slightly less differentiated than grade 1. Grade 3 is the most common and in this grade, the cells remain recognizable as glandular tissue. Grades 4 and 5 represent increasingly poor differentiation of tumor cells and increased severity. While grade 3 is not significantly worse than grade 2, grade 4 is significantly worse than 3 such that the qualitative difference of the raise in grades is not uniform (i.e., the transition from grade 3 to 4 is worse than from 1 to 2). Grade 5 is the most severe and the presentation is not as variable as grade 4, having no recognizable glandular tissue. The primary score is doubled if the secondary pattern comprises less than 3% of the total tumor (Bostwick 1994). Recent studies have indicated that a GS of 7 comprised of a primary grade 3 is less aggressive than a score of 7 with a primary grade of 4 (Tollefson et al. 2006). Issues surrounding GS are discussed in extensive detail in Chap. 3.

10.2.2.1   Reliability of Gleason Score

There have been a number of studies on the inter-rater reliability and reproducibility of GS. The general conclusion is that reliability is higher for a specialist in prostate cancer pathology and that training among non-specialists improves the agreement (Allsbrook et al. 2001a, 2001b; Freeman et al. 2004; Griffiths et al. 2006; Oyama et al. 2005). When general pathologists were compared to specialists, the most common disagreement was an under-grading by the non-specialist. The areas which produced the most variability were in grades 4 and 5. The difficult cases typically stem from a biopsy with limited volume, and for certain patterns such as cribriform. Most disagreements come from under-grading and disagreement is naturally higher in difficult cases (Allsbrook et al. 2001a, 2001b).

Studies that compare GS obtained from biopsy to the GS obtained from RP found correlations between 31% and 58% and depended on factors such as tumor size and number of specimens obtained on biopsy (Altay et al. 2001; Djavan et al. 1998; Fukagai et al. 2001; Hsieh et al. 2005; Montironi et al. 2005). In spite of these issues, the GS has remained a standard measurement of aggressiveness (Epstein et al. 2005; Humphrey 2004; Menon 1997) and is the predominant predictor of several measures related to patient outcome including prostate cancer-specific survival (Boyle et al. 2003; Humphrey 2004).

10.2.3 Other Measures of Aggressiveness

Other criteria for "aggressive" prostate cancer include biochemical recurrence following treatment and fatality due to prostate cancer. Measures of recurrence include postoperative PSA doubling time (PSADT) and biochemical recurrence time (RT). Postoperative PSADT appears to be predictive of recurrence of disease and correlates with lymph node involvement (Molitierno et al. 2006; Pound et al. 1999).

10.3 Non-genetic Risk Factors for Aggressive Prostate Cancer

Before considering genetic risk factors for aggressiveness, we discuss non-genetic factors. For a detailed discussion of epidemiological studies of risk factors relating to aggressiveness, please see Chap. 1.

10.3.1 Age and Ethnicity

Increasing age is a well-documented risk factor for prostate cancer and age of onset is often the most correlated trait among family members with prostate cancer (Goode et al. 2001). While one might hypothesize that younger age is a risk factor for more aggressive disease, this does not appear to be the case (Antunes et al. 2005; Billis et al. 2005; D'amico et al. 2003). African-American ethnicity is associated with higher incidence, but the relationship between AA ethnicity and aggressiveness is less clear (Albano et al. 2007; Giovannucci et al. 2007; Powell 2007). However, a recent summary of the literature by Powell (2007) noted evidence for more aggressive prostate cancer in AA men as opposed to European American men, especially at younger ages based on incidence, fatality and also a higher stage for prostate cancer not detected until autopsy (see Chap. 9.4).

10.3.2   Smoking, Alcohol, Physical Exercise, Obesity, and Diet

Smoking has been investigated as a risk factor for mortality from prostate cancer. Recent studies are contradictory, but indicate that smoking may be associated with more aggressive disease including increased prostate cancer mortality for both current and ever smokers (Coughlin et al. 1996; Giovannucci et al. 1999; Hiatt et al. 1994; Plaskon et al. 2003; Rodriguez et al. 1997a; Rohrmann et al. 2007). Some studies also observed a dose response relationship between smoking amounts and prostate cancer mortality (Cerhan et al. 1997; Coughlin et al. 1996; Plaskon et al. 2003; Rohrmann et al. 2007; Villeneuve et al. 1999). A proposed mechanism for this relationship is smoking's affect on hormone levels (Plaskon et al. 2003).

Higher physical activity levels may decrease the risk of prostate cancer aggressiveness. Two large prospective studies have shown physical activity to be associated with aggressive prostate cancer. Nilsen et al. (2006) recently conducted a large prospective study in Norway of physical activity and risk of prostate cancer especially in relation to aggressive disease as defined by metastases at diagnosis and death from prostate cancer. While no association was seen for physical activity and occurrence of prostate cancer, a statistically significant association between physical activity and decreased risk of prostate cancer mortality was observed. Taking into account frequency, length, and intensity of physical exercise, there was a trend toward decreasing risk with increasing levels of these measures of physical activity. Possible mechanisms for this decreased risk include an exercise effect on hormone levels including insulin. In a similar large prospective study in the USA, Patel et al. (2005) found comparable results.

Recent studies have sought to clarify the conflicting results from studies of prostate cancer and obesity. The complex interaction of BMI, weight, height, and obesity, as well as the ages and duration of obesity, is intertwined and findings have been inconsistent and contradictory (Dal Maso et al. 2004; Nilsen and Vatten 1999; Schuurman et al. 2000). In recent reviews of the literature, Buschemeyer and Freedland (2007) and Freedland and Platz (2007) conclude that obesity is inversely related to non-aggressive prostate cancer but positively associated with aggressive prostate cancer, as categorized by stage and grade and mortality. This may be due to prostate cancer being more difficult to detect in obese men from physical examination, as well as other possible biological causes (Freedland and Platz 2007). Obese men have a greater risk of mortality from prostate cancer (Rodriguez et al. 2001; Snowdon et al. 1984).

There is some evidence for an association of diets high in saturated fat and aggressive disease (Slattery et al. 1990; Snowdon et al. 1984). Slattery et al. (1990) saw a positive association, although weak, between a diet high in saturated fat as an adult and aggressive disease that was not seen in non-aggressive cases.

This association was the same for all age groups. Snowdon et al. (1984) saw an association between risk of fatal disease and a high consumption of milk, cheese, egg, and meat. West et al. (1991) saw an association that was strongest for diets high in fat that was significant for older men with aggressive tumors. Neuhouser et al. (2007) found an association between high dairy intake and a reduced risk of aggressive prostate cancer defined by a GS ≥ 7 and/or grade III/IV. Chavarro et al. (2007) looked at fatty acid levels and aggressive prostate cancer using the same cutoff for GS and including metastases or death from prostate cancer in their definition of aggressive prostate cancer. The authors found long-chain n-3 fatty acids and linoleic acid to be associated with a reduced risk of aggressive prostate cancer.

Of interest, a recent study (The Health Professional Follow Up Study) found that non-genetic risk factors did not show the same pattern of risk for fatal, advanced stage, higher grade, high-grade/low stage and low-grade/advanced stage categories (Giovannucci et al. 2007). This has implications for the findings from many studies that combine categories to define aggressive disease. Family history was a statistically significant risk factor for all measures of aggressiveness while other risk factors showed different and sometimes complicated patterns. Of note, the findings related to GS were not altered using a cutoff of ≥ 8 or ≥ 7.

10.4 Family History and Prostate Cancer Aggressiveness

Studies examining the relationship between family history and aggressive prostate cancer have been inconsistent (Azzouzi et al. 2003; Bauer et al. 1998; Bova et al. 1998; Gronberg et al. 1998; Hanlon and Hanks 1998; Kupelian et al. 1997a, 1997b, 1999; Rodriguez et al. 1997b; Sacco et al. 2005). A recent study (Kupelian et al. 2006) suggests that this inconsistency may be, at least in part, related to differences resulting from the introduction of PSA screening.

Kupelian et al. (1999, 1997a, 1997b) showed a positive association between a positive family history of prostate cancer in cases diagnosed from 1987 to 1996 and biochemical failure, local failure, and distant metastases after RP or radiation therapy (RT). Others looking at family history and biochemical failure found no association after RP or RT (Azzouzi et al. 2003; Bauer et al. 1998; Bova et al. 1998; Hanlon and Hanks 1998; Sacco et al. 2005). In two studies that looked at fatality as the outcome and compared familial to sporadic prostate cancer, one found an association (Rodriguez et al. 1997b) and one did not (Gronberg et al. 1998). Rodriguez et al. (1997b) used a large population-based cohort ascertained between 1987 and 1997 and linked the cases to death certificates. The authors saw an association between positive family history and prostate cancer mortality compared to sporadic cases (RR = 1.60; CI = 1.31–1.97). The risk of death from prostate cancer was even higher for men with more than one affected relative. Gronberg et al. (1998) used a smaller Swedish cohort sample diagnosed between 1959 and 1963 and found no difference in overall mortality or prostate cancer-specific mortality between familial and sporadic prostate cancer cases.

Spangler et al. (2005) looked at family history (divided into any, moderate, and high) in relation to clinical characteristics including stage and grade in incident cases diagnosed from 1995 to 2002. They observed no association between family history and clinical characteristics. However, when they stratified by early (<60) versus late (≥60) age at onset, tumor stage and extra capsular extension were positively associated with early onset and positive family history. A recent study by Giovannucci et al. (2007) examined several risk factors including family history for different classifications of prostate cancer severity including fatality, grade, stage, and advanced in men diagnosed from 1986 to 2002 accounting for PSA screening era. A family history of prostate cancer was positively associated with both high and low categories of all the author's different classifications of aggressive disease.

Rouprêt et al. (2006) studied men 50 year old or younger diagnosed with prostate cancer between 1994 and 2004 who underwent RP. Comparing sporadic cases to cases with a family history of prostate cancer, the authors found no difference in clinical characteristics or in time to biochemical failure between these two groups. Siddiqui et al. (2006) compared SPCa, FPCa, and HPCa RP cases from 1987 to 1997 for disease-free survival and found no differences among the classifications. Another report by Roemeling et al. (2006) studied 19,970 men aged 55 to 74 year old screened for prostate cancer from December 1993 through December 1999 in the Netherlands. The study confirmed an increase risk of prostate cancer in men who had a brother or father with prostate cancer, but found no differences in clinical characteristics or disease-free survival time between men with and without a positive family history.

Kupelian et al. (2006) found that a family history was positively associated with biochemical disease-free survival only in those subjects treated in or prior to 1993 and with a younger age at diagnosis. Note that in Rodriguez et al. (1997b), which found convincing evidence of an association between family history and fatality, the subjects came from the pre-treatment era of 1982–1991. As family history is a known risk factor for prostate cancer, the authors conclude that the current focus on early detection for men with a family history may lead to diagnosis of cancer at an earlier and therefore more favorable time.

10.5 Segregation Analysis

Segregation analysis is a method of establishing the genetic inheritance of disease using family data. Different models with various restrictions (e.g., dominant or recessive inheritance) are compared to a model where all parameters in the model are estimated in order to see what model(s) best fit the data. There have been several segregation analyses of prostate cancer. The studies used various ascertainment schemes with some being population based and others using selection criteria based on age at diagnosis and others requiring multiplex families. Subjects came from various countries including the USA, Canada, Australia, the Netherlands, and

Finland. Some studies have found a dominant mode of inheritance prostate cancer with varying allele frequencies (Carter et al. 1992; Cui et al. 2001; Gong et al. 2002; Gronberg et al. 1997; Schaid et al. 1998; Valeri et al. 2003; Verhage et al. 2001). Others found a dominant mode for young age at diagnosis and an X-linked model for older age at diagnosis (Cui et al. 2001). Early findings of X-linked inheritance were largely discounted after accounting for trends in diagnosis over time that explained the excess risk to brothers over fathers previously thought to be indicative of X-linkage (Gong et al. 2002). However, a recent study (Pakkanen et al. 2007) found a recessive mode of inheritance and an increased risk associated with having an affected father even after accounting for trends in diagnosis. A number of studies have indicated a multifactorial or polygenic nature of prostate cancer genetics (Conlon et al. 2003; Gong et al. 2002; Valeri et al. 2003).

These segregation analyses had varying designs, including different ascertainment and populations. Nevertheless, their results suggest that prostate cancer is a heterogeneous disease that may be due to several genes, as well as environmental factors. These studies have all looked at prostate cancer using either age at diagnosis or affection status as the trait of interest. To date, there have been no segregation analyses of aggressive prostate cancer.

10.6   Linkage Analysis

When loci are relatively close together on the same chromosome, recombination during meiosis is uncommon and the loci are said to be "linked." Linkage analysis examines the co-segregation of genetic markers and a disease trait within families to see if the markers and the trait co-segregate in families. If co-segregation is detected, this is taken to mean that the disease-causing variant(s) is nearby the marker(s). This subject is discussed in great detail in Chap. 7.

Linkage analyses of prostate cancer have been inconclusive, with many initially positive findings across the genome. Given the high prevalence of prostate cancer, one of the problems that linkage studies face is that some members of families with prostate cancer are likely to be phenocopies (i.e., the same phenotype but with a non-genetic cause). Although the linkage results from some studies have been replicated, overall the results have been inconsistent. The earliest studies focused on HPCa families and age of onset as sub-groupings of prostate cancer. Many of the these studies showed linkage to 1q22-23, 1q42-43, and the X chromosome; however, these findings were not consistently replicated (Cooney et al. 1997; Eeles et al. 1998; Gibbs et al. 1999; Goode et al. 2000; Gronberg et al. 1999; Hsieh et al. 1997; Singh 2000; Smith et al. 1996; Suarez et al. 2000; Whittemore et al. 1999; Xu 2000; Xu et al. 2001a, 2003, 2005). These findings are discussed elsewhere in this volume, especially in Chaps.7 and 8.

Several recent studies have shown evidence for linkage to 22q particularly in families with multiple cases (Camp et al. 2006, 2007; Xu et al. 2005). In addition, at least three studies have shown linkage to Chromosome 17. Xu et al. (2005) found suggestive linkage using families with multiple affected family members (≥5). Similarly, Lange et al. (2007) saw the highest LOD score on Chromosome 17 in families with multiple affected members (≥4) and a younger average (≤65) age at diagnosis. Gudmundsson et al. (2007b) in a genome-wide association (GWA) study followed up on the linkage results for chromosome 17 and found two variants (rs7501939 and rs4430796) that were independently associated with prostate cancer risk (see Chap. 9.1).

In addition to looking at prostate cancer itself as the trait of interest in linkage analyses, one can also study linkage to disease aggressiveness – either as a quantitative trait or as a covariate. Such studies have been less common, but similarly equivocal (Chang et al. 2005; Christensen et al. 2007; Goddard et al. 2001; Goode et al. 2001; Neville et al. 2003; Schaid 2006; Schaid et al. 2007; Slager et al. 2003, 2006; Stanford et al. 2006; Whittemore and Halpern 2006; Witte et al. 2000, 2003). To date, there have been at least 14 studies that have used aggressiveness either as the main trait or as a covariate.

There are differences among the studies in terms of definition of aggressiveness and methods. Most linkage analyses of disease aggressiveness have used GS as a quantitative trait, but some have used a broader definition of aggressiveness, including advanced stage, higher PSA value, metastasis, or fatality from prostate cancer. Several studies looked at additional sub-groupings based on number of affected family members, age at diagnosis/onset, male-to-male transmission or included these as covariates (Christensen et al. 2007; Goddard et al. 2001; Goode et al. 2001; Schaid et al. 2006; Stanford et al. 2006). Many studies analyzed the data using affected sib or relative pair methods, but at least one study used a parametric approach with a dominant mode of inheritance (Chang et al. 2005) and one specified both a dominant and recessive mode of inheritance (Stanford et al. 2006).

The strongest evidence of linkage for aggressive disease has been found on chromosomes 1, 7, and 19, with evidence of linkage also reported for chromosomes 2, 3, 4, 5, 6, 10, 11, 16, 18, 21, and 22 (Chang et al. 2005; Christensen et al. 2007; Goddard et al. 2001; Goode et al. 2001; Lange et al. 2006; Neville et al. 2002, 2003; Paiss et al. 2003; Schaid et al. 2006, 2007; Slager et al. 2003, 2006; Stanford et al. 2006; Witte et al. 2000, 2003).

Witte et al. (2000) was the first linkage analysis that used GS as a measure for prostate cancer aggressiveness. Using 326 sib-pairs the authors performed a genome-wide model-free linkage analysis. Linkage peaks were detected on chromosomes 5q31.3–33.3, 7q32.3, and 19q12. Other studies since then have also reported linkage to 7q using GS as a measure of aggressiveness (Neville et al. 2002; Paiss et al. 2003; Schaid et al. 2006, 2007; Witte et al. 2003) and using a broader measure of aggressiveness that also included advanced stage (Schaid et al. 2006). Neville et al. (2002), building on the initial work of Witte et al. (2000), added finely spaced markers to the linkage analysis and identified a region on chromosome 7 between markers D7S2452 and D7S640 that was strongly associated with aggressive disease ($p < 0.001$). In addition, allelic imbalance (AI) was detected in prostate tumors within the same chromosomal region. Associations between AI and age at diagnosis, tumor grade (Gleason score), stage, and family history were also observed. AI correlated with higher GS ($p = 0.012$) and lymph node metastasis ($p = 0.017$), adding further evidence for a gene for aggressive prostate cancer in this region. In a replication and pooled analysis of their initial work, Witte et al. (2003) detected even stronger evidence of linkage to 7q32 ($p = 0.0002$).

In the same region, Paiss et al. (2003) also observed a linkage peak (chromosome 7q31–33), using GS as a covariate among a study of German families. The peak LOD score was 1.98 ($p = 0.002$), and this was observed when the highest weights were given to families with two or more affected individuals and late age of onset. When aggressiveness was not included in the model, the linkage to 7q31–32 was no longer statistically significant. Association studies of candidate genes within this region have also detected intriguing results (discussed further below). More recently, Schaid et al. (2006) detected linkage to the chromosome 7q21.11 region, with a maximum LOD score of 4.1 in families selected on the basis of having three or more affected males with aggressive disease and without male-to-male transmission. However, a number of other studies of GS did not detect linkage to this region (Slager et al. 2003; Christensen et al. 2007; Lange et al. 2003; Stanford et al. 2006).

Some studies have shown linkage to aggressiveness on chromosome 19q (Neville et al. 2003; Schaid et al. 2007; Slager et al. 2003; Whittemore and Halpern 2006; Witte et al. 2003, 2000). The strongest evidence was reported by Slager et al. (2003) at 19q13 ($p = 0.0001$). Similar to the aforementioned results for 7q31–32, Neville et al. (2003) saw a high level of AI in this region. Interestingly, Whittemore and Halpern (2006) saw the highest LOD score (2.81; $p = 0.01$) when both aggressiveness and an age at diagnosis earlier than 66.5 years were included in the model. In this study, men were classified as having aggressive prostate cancer if they had a GS > 6, high initial PSA or death where prostate cancer was the main or secondary cause. Nevertheless, other genome-wide scans failed to observe linkage in this region (Christensen et al. 2007; Lange et al. 2006; Schaid et al. 2006; Slager et al. 2006; Stanford et al. 2006).

HPC1, *PCAP*, and Xq12 have also shown promising, but inconsistent results. For example, *HPC1* (1q24–25) and *PCAP* (1q42.243), which have both been identified as linkage regions in previous analyses of prostate cancer, have also exhibited linkage in some of the studies incorporating aggressiveness. Goddard et al. (2001) using GS as a covariate observed linkage to both regions where only a weak signal was seen for overall prostate cancer. For *PCAP*, the best model also included a covariate for male-to-male transmission. Goode et al. (2001) observed a peak for *HPC1* especially in aggressive (defined by high stage or grade) families not linked to other regions and for families with a later age at diagnosis (≥65). *HPC1* and PCAP have not shown linkage to aggressive prostate cancer in other genome-wide linkage studies (Christensen et al. 2007; Lange et al. 2006; Schaid et al. 2006, 2007). Finally, linkage has been detected between aggressive prostate cancer and regions on the X chromosome previously linked to prostate cancer development. For example, Goddard et al. (2001) reported a LOD score of 3.06 at Xq12–13 ($p = 0.00053$) and Chang et al. (2005) saw evidence of linkage at Xq27–28

($p = 0.0006$). Even in light of these studies, there is limited overlap between the linkage areas observed for prostate cancer and aggressive prostate cancer.

10.7 Association Studies

While linkage analysis methods can be successful at detecting high risk, relatively rare disease-causing loci, association studies may have more power to detect common causal variants (Risch and Merikangas 1996). In addition, association studies may allow for getting closer to a disease-causing variant as smaller chromosomal areas are examined with higher resolution. With the reduction in cost of large-scale single nucleotide polymorphism (SNP) genotyping, association studies are increasingly common and are quickly expanding from focused candidate gene studies to genome-wide association studies.

Association studies are based on a case-control design, with cases typically coming from a hospital or disease registry. Controls are either unrelated (population or hospital/registry based) or cases' family members (e.g., parents or siblings). The occurrence of a given allele in cases versus controls is compared to see if an "association" exists between genes and disease.

The selection of cases is worth noting as some studies recruit them from a well-defined population while others may simply collect a convenience sample. It is important to keep this in mind when considering study results, especially where they differ. The same scrutiny should be applied to other selection issues as well, such as how aggressiveness is defined.

10.7.1 Candidate Gene Association Studies and Aggressiveness

Numerous variants have been associated with aggressive prostate cancer. These have primarily been in candidate genes with high-priority biologic rationale, such as involvement with the androgen pathway. We review a handful of these results here. Germ-line disease-associated *BRCA2* mutations form a special group, and are discussed in Chap. 8.

10.7.1.1 Androgen Receptors

Initial studies showed a positive association between androgen receptors (*AR* – CAG and/or GCC repeats) and aggressiveness defined by higher stage, grade, or disease-free progression, but later studies did not show an association with either repeat (Cicek et al. 2004; Edwards et al. 1999; Ingles et al. 1998; Li et al. 2001; Mir et al. 2002). One study saw an association with the instability, but not the size, of the CAG repeat and progression of BPH to prostate cancer (Tayeb et al. 2004).

A large comprehensive study by Freedman et al. (2005) did not find any association between the CAG repeat and advanced disease.

Cicek et al. (2004) found an association with the *SRD5A2* V89L variant that was most pronounced in men with an early age of onset or more aggressive disease. No association was seen for the A49T variant. However, Jaffe et al. (2000) found the opposite: the A49T variant was associated with more advanced disease and there was no association for the V89L variant. Two other studies found no association with aggressiveness and *SRD5A2* (Mononen et al. 2001; Onen et al. 2007). Studies have found no association between *CYP17* and aggressive prostate cancer (Cicek et al. 2004; Cussenot et al. 2007; Loukola et al. 2004; Onen et al. 2007).

Studies have implicated a *CYP3A4* variant as being associated with more aggressive disease, especially in AA men (Paris et al. 1999; Plummer et al. 2003; Rebbeck et al. 1998). Rebbeck et al. (1998) found *CYP3A4-V* (A to G mutation) in Caucasian men to be positively associated with worse tumor grade and stage with the strongest association seen in men with no family history and a later age of onset. African-American men have been found to be more often homozygous for *CYP3A4* G allele (*CYP3A4*1B*) than their peers and homozygosity was associated with more advanced disease especially in men with a later age of onset. The G allele was also found to be associated with men with BPH that progressed to prostate cancer (Tayeb et al. 2002). Powell et al. (2004) found no association between grade and the G allele, but the G allele was associated with worse disease-free survival following RP in Caucasians. Loukola et al. (2004) found four *CYP3A4* SNPs (*CYP3A4*1B* was one) and one haplotype to be inversely associated with lower grade and stage in Caucasians, the association in AA men was not significant, but the numbers were small.

Zeigler-Johnson et al. (2004) and Plummer et al. (2003) also saw inverse relationship with *CYP3A4*1B* and less aggressive prostate cancer in Caucasians, that was positively associated with risk in more aggressive prostate cancer. Plummer et al. (2003) also found the *CYP3A5*1* variant to be associated in Caucasians with less aggressive disease but Zeigler-Johnson et al. (2004) did not replicate this finding. Bangsi et al. (2006) saw no association with *CYP3A4* and aggressiveness in Caucasians, possibly due to small numbers. In AA men the G allele was however associated with more aggressive but not with less aggressive prostate cancer. One of the most recent although a small study, looked at *CYP3A4* (*CYP3A4*1B*) and found no association with biochemical failure or survival following RT in Caucasian or AA men (Roach et al. 2007). It has been hypothesized that the association with *CYP3A4* in AA men may be due to population stratification (Kittles et al. 2002).

Cicek et al. (2005) found that *CYP1B1* had no overall association with prostate cancer, but was associated in men with more aggressive disease. In the same study, the authors found no association with *CYP11a*, but *PSA/KLK3* was associated with less aggressive disease. Nock et al. (2006) found a combination of *CYP1B1*, *hOGG1*, *XRCC1*, and *COMT* to be inversely associated in men with more aggressive prostate cancer, but not less aggressive. Cussenot et al. (2007) investigated *CYP17*, *CYP19*, *CYP1B1*, and *COMT*, all genes involved in estrogen metabolism, and found *CYP1B1 V* allele to be associated with more aggressive disease.

10.7.1.2 Vitamin D Receptors

There have been many studies of vitamin D receptors (*VDR*) (e.g., alleles revealed by digestion with FokI, PolyA, BsmI, ApaI, and TaqI restriction enzymes) on chromosome 12, including looking at interactions with other factors. There is little evidence of an association between *VDR* TaqI and aggressive prostate cancer. Hamasaki et al. (2001) found the TT genotype associated with locally advanced or metastatic disease in cases when compared to controls in a Japanese population (OR = 2.52; p = 0.009), but not for local disease compared to controls. The same pattern was seen for higher grade (OR = 5.38; p = 0.002), but not lower grade in cases versus controls. Other studies, including those in a Japanese population, saw no significant association between TaqI and aggressive prostate cancer (Cicek et al. 2006; Habuchi et al. 2000; Huang et al. 2004; Tayeb et al. 2003; Williams et al. 2004).

Kibel et al. (1998) and Cicek et al. (2006) reported no association between *VDR*-poly A and aggressive prostate cancer. Ingles et al. (1998) reported an association between carrying a long repeat of Poly A and more aggressive cases (local vs. advanced). Poly A was not associated (by itself) with local or advanced disease in AA men (Ingles et al. 1998). There was no association in two studies in an Asian population with ApaI or TaqI and advanced stage or grade, but an association with BsmI was found (Habuchi et al. 2000; Huang et al. 2004). Williams et al. (2004) saw no overall association of BsmI and clinical features, but found the B allele did show evidence of reduced risk of recurrence in Caucasian men who had locally advanced disease. Ingles et al. (1998) found that the B allele was associated with reduced risk of advanced prostate cancer in AA men but only men also carrying a long poly(A) allele.

Not surprisingly, the results from studies of FokI have also been mixed. Most studies have found no association between FokI and aggressive prostate cancer (Cicek et al. 2006; Mikhak et al. 2007; Mishra et al. 2005). Only one study has seen an association with advanced disease and ApaI, other studies have been negative (Cicek et al. 2006; Huang et al. 2004; Maistro et al. 2004). No studies have shown an association with the Cdxz polymorphism (Cicek et al. 2006; Mikhak et al. 2007) and aggressive prostate cancer.

A recent meta-analysis reported no association between the *VDR* polymorphisms and risk of prostate cancer. The authors could not, however, rule out an association with sub-types or with ethnic differences (Berndt et al. 2006). It seems possible that vitamin D's affects are through interactions with other environmental variables (Rukin et al. 2007). Li et al. (2007) found plasma vitamin D status interacted with the ff genotype of the FokI polymorphism such that men with this combination had an increased risk of aggressive prostate cancer (OR = 2.5, 95% CI = 1.1–5.8). Mikhak et al. (2007) saw no individual association with the Cdx2, FokI, and BsmI polymorphisms, but did see a reduced risk of aggressive prostate cancer for two haplotypes. In addition, the Cdx2 A allele interacted with low plasma 1,25-dihydroxyvitamin D levels showing a greater risk of aggressiveness (higher GS) in cases compared to non-carriers with high levels. Li et al. also saw an interaction with FokI and plasma vitamin D levels such that the ff genotype was associated with lower or higher risk of prostate cancer and aggressive prostate cancer depending on the 25(OH) vitamin D levels.

10.7.1.3   Other Candidate Genes

Familial clustering of breast and prostate cancer has been observed and male relatives of breast cancer probands, in particular, probands carrying a *BRCA* mutation, appear to have an increased risk of prostate cancer (Loman et al. 2003; Rodriguez et al. 1998; Sigurdsson et al. 1997; Tulinius et al. 1992, 2002). The majority of studies have found that men who carry a *BRCA2* mutation themselves are at increased risk for prostate cancer compared to non-carriers.(Horsburgh et al. 2005; Kirchhoff et al. 2004; Struewing et al. 1997; Tryggvadottir et al. 2007). Most but not all of the studies that looked for an excess frequency of *BRCA2* mutations in prostate cancer cases have been negative (Edwards et al. 2003; Hamel et al. 2003; Hubert et al. 1999; Ikonen et al. 2003; Loman et al. 2003; Nastiuk et al. 1999; Vazina et al. 2000; Wilkens et al. 1999).

BRCA2 may play a role in aggressive disease. Recently, Tryggvadottir et al. (2007) reported on Icelandic male relatives of breast cancer probands. *BRCA2* status (999del5 mutation) was ascertained for men with prostate cancer. *BRCA2* carriers had more advanced disease compared to non-carriers. Agalliu et al. (2007) found an association between the *BRCA2* mutations (4625_4629delACATT, 4074_4075delGT) and early onset prostate cancer.

Other examples of potential candidate genes include *CKDN1A*, *CDKN1B* (Kibel et al. 2003), and vascular endothelial growth factor (*VEGF*) (Sfar et al. 2006, 2007) in the angiogenesis pathway and have been most strongly associated in men with more aggressive disease (metastasis or death).

Recent studies have also explored inflammation mechanisms and advanced prostate cancer risk. One study found a positive association with a Toll-like receptor (*TLR 4*) SNP (rs10759932) and an inverse association for *COX2* (rs2745557) in cases with advanced disease compared to controls (Cheng et al. 2007a, 2007b).

Finally, association studies of candidate genes within the chromosome 7q linkage region have also been undertaken. Podocalyxin-like (*PODXL*) was associated with more advanced disease (Casey et al. 2006). The candidate genes testis-derived transcript (*TES* – 7q31.2) and Caveolin-1 (*CAV1* – 7q31.1) have also been followed up with association studies. Haeusler et al. (2005) reported an association with one SNP (rs1543293; $p = 0.02$) in cases with higher stage, but not in all cases and not for other measures of aggressiveness (age of onset, grade, or survival). CAV1 has also been associated with aggressiveness based on expression data and possible differences between Caucasians and AA men (Karam et al. 2007; Yang et al. 2000). Liu et al. (2007) in a case control study looked at seven tagging SNPs (tSNPs) for the testis-derived transcript gene (*TES*). *TES* has been shown to be a promising candidate based on linkage and AI studies and from mRNA expression data. No associations were found when looking at the entire study population composed of

Caucasians and AA men. However, when only the AA men were analyzed, there was a significant protective effect of 3 SNPs (rs2402056, rs1004109, and rs4730721).

10.7.2   Chromosome 8q24

While there have been few consistently replicated associations between genetic variants and prostate cancer, several studies have now demonstrated and replicated a positive finding for 8q24 (Cheng et al. 2008). While only one previous linkage study had highlighted this specific area (albeit weakly), this region is known to be one of the most commonly duplicated regions of the human genome in prostate cancer tumors (Cher et al. 1994; Emmert-Buck et al. 1995; Haggman et al. 1997; Kalapurakal et al. 1999; Lutchman et al. 1999; Macgrogan et al. 1994; Matsuyama et al. 2001; Perinchery et al. 1999; Sato et al. 1999; Wiklund et al. 2003; Xu et al. 2001b).

Focusing on the 8q24 region from an initial linkage study of families from Iceland, Amundadottir et al. (2006) detected and replicated a statistically significant association between the A allele of the SNP rs1447295 and overall prostate cancer (OR = 1.51, $p = 1.0 \times 10^{-11}$). They also detected an association with the -8 allele of the marker DG8S737 in this region (OR = 1.62, $p = 2.7 \times 10^{-11}$). The highest risk was seen in men who had both the A allele of rs1447295 and the -8 allele of DG8S737. Among African-American men, rs1447295 was not statistically significantly associated with prostate cancer, although DG8S737 was (OR = 1.60, $p = 0.0022$). There was also a weak but intriguing association ($p = 0.07$) between the -8 allele and more aggressive disease (GS = 7–10) in comparison with less-aggressive prostate cancer (GS < 7).

The 8q24 region was also localized by an admixture mapping study in AA men: 1,597 prostate cancer cases and 873 controls (Freedman et al. 2006). In particular, the authors found a significant LOD score (7.1) within 8q24, but DG8S737 or rs1447295 could not account for their admixture signal, suggesting that there are other prostate cancer susceptibility loci at 8q24. Of note, among this study the highest LOD score (8.39) was for cases diagnosed at 72 years of age or younger. Although rs1447295 was significantly associated with prostate cancer among Japanese Americans, Native Hawaiians, Latino Americans, and European Americans in this study, there was no association between rs1447295 and family history of prostate cancer or GS dichotomized at ≥8 (a different cutoff than used in others studies) (Freedman et al. 2006).

Following the results of Amundadottir et al. (2006), Gudmundsson et al. (2007a) found an association with the A allele of rs1447295 (OR = 1.71; $p = 1.6 \times 10^{-14}$). They also found a statistically significant association with allele A of another SNP in the 8q24 region, rs16901979, after adjusting for rs1447295 (1.63, $p = 2.4 \times 10^{-6}$) suggesting that this is a second locus. They were able to replicate this finding in three additional groups (from the Netherlands, Spain, and USA) and in a separate sample of AA men (OR = 1.34, p = 0.0049). Using the Icelandic sample, which was population based, each copy of the A allele was associated with decreasing age at diagnosis. The authors also found a significant association for DG8S737-8 in AA cases (OR = 1.34, CI = 1.09–1.64).

Yeager et al. (2007) found an association with rs6983267 that they were able to replicate adding in four additional sets of cases and controls – all of European ancestry. Both rs6983267 and rs1447295 were independently associated with disease. The OR for individuals who carry both risk alleles was 3.17 (p = 9.18 × 10^{-22}). There was no significant association with aggressiveness or age at diagnosis.

Haiman et al. (2007) performed fine mapping of this region and identified five new SNPs in addition to replicating previous results, including rs6983267. The authors found rs16901979 to be strongly associated with prostate cancer (p = 1.5 × 10^{-18}). When all SNPs were examined together using stepwise logistic regression, seven SNPs were found to be positively and independently associated with prostate cancer risk. These SNPs were evaluated concerning stage and grade, as well as family history (first-degree relative) and younger age at diagnosis (<68). DG8S737-8 was positively associated with tumor grade (GS > 7). In AA men, rs6983561 and rs13254738 were significantly associated with younger age at diagnosis. There was suggestive evidence of an association between rs6983561 with both negative family history (no first-degree relative with prostate cancer) and stage.

Severi et al. (2007) detected an association between the 8q24 SNP rs1447295 and prostate cancer (OR = 1.52, p = 0.0005). They found no association with stage, age at diagnosis, or aggressiveness. The authors concluded that there was no association with grade as the findings were similar for high and low aggressiveness groups defined by GS of 7–10 and 5 or 6. However, their sample was composed only of men diagnosed at <70 years of age and with GS ≥ 5. Suuriniemi et al. (2007) found an association for the rs1447295 A allele, but not DG8S737-8. Their results for DG8S737 indicated a significant association with the -10 allele and not the -8, differing from Amundadottir et al. (2006); however, both markers were associated with prostate cancer in men with higher GS (4 + 3 and 8–10) compared to men with lower scores (2–6 and 3 + 4). These authors also looked specifically at HPCa and found no association. Wang et al. (2007) found the A allele of rs1447295 to be significantly more prevalent in familial cases (OR = 1.93; p = 0.0004) and in aggressive cases (OR = 1.87; p = 0.00005) but not sporadic cases when compared to controls. However, there was no difference when cases were divided into high and low aggressiveness as defined by <7 or ≥7. The -10/A combination showed the largest risk for FPCa and the -8/A the largest for aggressive prostate cancer. Looking specifically at familial cases, there was no association with aggressiveness. Their sample was collected with emphasis on aggressive cases defined by GS ≥ 8. Schumacher et al. (2007) carried out one of the largest case control studies and again replicated the rs1447295 association with prostate cancer in Caucasians (p = 8.64 × 10^{-13}). The association was seen in AA men who were diagnosed at early ages (≤ 65). There was no association with GS, stage, or mortality.

In a study specifically designed to evaluate 8q24 and advanced disease (GS ≥ 7, PSA ≥ 10, or stage > T2c) Cheng et al. (2008) found three previously reported variants (rs10090154, rs16901979, and rs6983267) significantly and independently associated with advanced prostate cancer. Of interest, these three variants each resided in one of the three 8q24 regions previously associated with prostate cancer. These variants were not associated with age at diagnosis and no evidence of heterogeneity across age groups was observed. In addition, the authors conduced a meta-analysis and found four variants (rs1447295, dg8s737, rs16901979, and rs6983267) demonstrating highly significant association with prostate cancer risk across a wide array of study designs and populations of European and African Ancestry.

Overall, the results for association studies of 8q24 are extremely encouraging, though the causal variant and biological mechanism underlying these findings, and their implications for aggressive disease, remain unclear at the time of this writing.

10.8   Conclusion and Future Work

In summary, there is limited evidence that aggressive prostate cancer is more common in HPCa or FPCa families. While age of onset is often the most correlated trait in families, this is not the case for measures of aggressiveness. Yet, measures of aggressiveness continue to prove to be a meaningful classification for this heterogeneous disease. There is reason to believe that the relationship of casual factors to prostate cancer may depend on how aggressiveness is defined, and this could be one of the reasons for the inconsistent findings and lack of replication in genetic epidemiologic studies.

There remains much work in deciphering the genetic basis of disease aggressiveness. The recent consistent findings for 8q24 are encouraging, although it remains unclear whether they are relevant to prostate cancer in general or also to aggressiveness. Future studies will entail larger collaborative efforts with sufficient power to assess the genetic basis of more aggressive disease. Detecting such markers could help improve our understanding of prostate cancer biology, and allow for more focused screening and treatment of this common but complex disease.

References

Agalliu I, Karlins E, Kwon EM, Iwasaki LM, Diamond A, Ostrander EA, Stanford JL (2007) Rare germline mutations in the BRCA2 gene are associated with early-onset prostate cancer. Br J Cancer 97:826–831

Albano JD, Ward E, Jemal A, Anderson R, Cokkinides VE, Murray T, Henley J et al (2007) Cancer mortality in the United States by education level and race. J Natl Cancer Inst 99:1384–1394

Allsbrook WC Jr, Mangold KA, Johnson MH, Lane RB, Lane CG, Epstein JI (2001a) Interobserver reproducibility of Gleason grading of prostatic carcinoma: general pathologist. Hum Pathol 32:81–88

Allsbrook WC Jr, Mangold KA, Johnson MH, Lane RB, Lane CG, Amin MB, Bostwick DG et al (2001b) Interobserver reproducibility of Gleason grading of prostatic carcinoma: urologic pathologists. Hum Pathol 32:74–80

Altay B, Kefi A, Nazli O, Killi R, Semerci B, Akar I (2001) Comparison of Gleason scores from sextant prostate biopsies and radical prostatectomy specimens. Urol Int 67:14–18

Amundadottir LT, Sulem P, Gudmundsson J, Helgason A, Baker A, Agnarsson BA, Sigurdsson A et al (2006) A common variant associated with prostate cancer in European and African populations. Nat Genet 38:652–658

Antunes AA, Leite KR, Dall'Oglio MF, Crippa A, Nesrallah LJ, Srougi M (2005) Prostate biopsy: is age important for determining the pathological features in prostate cancer? Int Braz J Urol 31:331–337

Azzouzi AR, Valeri A, Cormier L, Fournier G, Mangin P, Cussenot O (2003) Familial prostate cancer cases before and after radical prostatectomy do not show any aggressiveness compared with sporadic cases. Urology 61:1193–1197

Bangsi D, Zhou J, Sun Y, Patel NP, Darga LL, Heilbrun LK, Powell IJ et al (2006) Impact of a genetic variant in CYP3A4 on risk and clinical presentation of prostate cancer among white and African-American men. Urol Oncol 24:21–27

Bauer JJ, Srivastava S, Connelly RR, Sesterhenn IA, Preston DM, McLeod DG, Moul JW (1998) Significance of familial history of prostate cancer to traditional prognostic variables, genetic biomarkers, and recurrence after radical prostatectomy. Urology 51:970–976

Berndt SI, Dodson JL, Huang WY, Nicodemus KK (2006) A systematic review of vitamin D receptor gene polymorphisms and prostate cancer risk. J Urol 175:1613–1623

Billis A, Magna LA, Lira MM, Moreira LR, Okamura H, Paz AR, Perina RC, et al (2005) Relationship of age to outcome and clinicopathologic findings in men submitted to radical prostatectomy. Int Braz J Urol 31:534–539; discussion 9-40

Bostwick DG (1994) Grading prostate cancer. Am J Clin Pathol 102:S38–S56

Bostwick DG, Myers RP, Oesterling JE (1994) Staging of prostate cancer. Semin Surg Oncol 10:60–72

Bova GS, Partin AW, Isaacs SD, Carter BS, Beaty TL, Isaacs WB, Walsh PC (1998) Biological aggressiveness of hereditary prostate cancer: long-term evaluation following radical prostatectomy. J Urol 160:660–663

Boyle P, Severi G, Giles GG (2003) The epidemiology of prostate cancer. Urol Clin North Am 30:209–217

Buschemeyer WC 3rd, Freedland SJ (2007) Obesity and prostate cancer: epidemiology and clinical implications. Eur Urol 52(2):331–343

Camp NJ, Farnham JM, Cannon-Albright LA (2006) Localization of a prostate cancer predisposition gene to an 880-kb region on chromosome 22q12.3 in Utah high-risk pedigrees. Cancer Res 66:10205–10212

Camp NJ, Cannon-Albright LA, Farnham JM, Baffoe-Bonnie AB, George A, Powell I, Bailey-Wilson JE et al (2007) Compelling evidence for a prostate cancer gene at 22q12.3 by the International Consortium for Prostate Cancer Genetics. Hum Mol Genet 16:1271–1278

Carter BS, Beaty TH, Steinberg GD, Childs B, Walsh PC (1992) Mendelian inheritance of familial prostate cancer. Proc Natl Acad Sci USA 89:3367–3371

Carter HB, Ferrucci L, Kettermann A, Landis P, Wright EJ, Epstein JI, Trock BJ et al (2006) Detection of life-threatening prostate cancer with prostate-specific antigen velocity during a window of curability. J Natl Cancer Inst 98:1521–1527

Casey G, Neville PJ, Liu X, Plummer SJ, Cicek MS, Krumroy LM, Curran AP et al (2006) Podocalyxin variants and risk of prostate cancer and tumor aggressiveness. Hum Mol Genet 15:735–741

Cerhan JR, Torner JC, Lynch CF, Rubenstein LM, Lemke JH, Cohen MB, Lubaroff DM et al (1997) Association of smoking, body mass, and physical activity with risk of prostate cancer in the Iowa 65+ Rural Health Study (United States). Cancer Causes Control 8:229–238

Chang BL, Isaacs SD, Wiley KE, Gillanders EM, Zheng SL, Meyers DA, Walsh PC et al (2005) Genome-wide screen for prostate cancer susceptibility genes in men with clinically significant disease. Prostate 64:356–361

Chavarro JE, Stampfer MJ, Li H, Campos H, Kurth T, Ma J (2007) A prospective study of poly-unsaturated fatty acid levels in blood and prostate cancer risk. Cancer Epidemiol Biomarkers Prev 16(7):1364–1370

Cheng I, Plummer SJ, Casey G, Witte JS (2007a) Toll-like receptor 4 genetic variation and advanced prostate cancer risk. Cancer Epidemiol Biomarkers Prev 16:352–355

Cheng I, Liu X, Plummer SJ, Krumroy LM, Casey G, Witte JS (2007b) COX2 genetic variation, NSAIDs, and advanced prostate cancer risk. Br J Cancer 97:557–561

Cheng I, Plummer SJ, Jorgenson E, Liu X, Rybicki BA, Casey G, Witte JS (2008) 8q24 and prostate cancer: associated with advanced disease and meta-analysis. Eur J Hum Genet 16(4):496–505

Cher ML, MacGrogan D, Bookstein R, Brown JA, Jenkins RB, Jensen RH (1994) Comparative genomic hybridization, allelic imbalance, and fluorescence in situ hybridization on chromosome 8 in prostate cancer. Genes Chromosomes Cancer 11:153–162

Christensen GB, Camp NJ, Farnham JM, Cannon-Albright LA (2007) Genome-wide linkage analysis for aggressive prostate cancer in Utah high-risk pedigrees. Prostate 67: 605–613

Cicek MS, Liu X, Casey G, Witte JS (2005) Role of androgen metabolism genes CYP1B1, PSA/KLK3, and CYP11alpha in prostate cancer risk and aggressiveness. Cancer Epidemiol Biomarkers Prev 14:2173–2177

Cicek MS, Liu X, Schumacher FR, Casey G, Witte JS (2006) Vitamin D receptor genotypes/haplotypes and prostate cancer risk. Cancer Epidemiol Biomarkers Prev 15:2549–2552

Cicek MS, Conti DV, Curran A, Neville PJ, Paris PL, Casey G, Witte JS (2004) Association of prostate cancer risk and aggressiveness to androgen pathway genes: SRD5A2, CYP17, and the AR. Prostate 59:69–76

Conlon EM, Goode EL, Gibbs M, Stanford JL, Badzioch M, Janer M, Kolb S et al (2003) Oligogenic segregation analysis of hereditary prostate cancer pedigrees: evidence for multiple loci affecting age at onset. Int J Cancer 105:630–635

Cooney KA, McCarthy JD, Lange E, Huang L, Miesfeldt S, Montie JE, Oesterling JE et al (1997) Prostate cancer susceptibility locus on chromosome 1q: a confirmatory study. J Natl Cancer Inst 89:955–959

Coughlin SS, Neaton JD, Sengupta A (1996) Cigarette smoking as a predictor of death from prostate cancer in 348, 874 men screened for the Multiple Risk Factor Intervention Trial. Am J Epidemiol 143:1002–1006

Cui J, Staples MP, Hopper JL, English DR, McCredie MR, Giles GG (2001) Segregation analyses of 1, 476 population-based Australian families affected by prostate cancer. Am J Hum Genet 68:1207–1218

Cussenot O, Azzouzi AR, Nicolaiew N, Fromont G, Mangin P, Cormier L, Fournier G et al (2007) Combination of polymorphisms from genes related to estrogen metabolism and risk of prostate cancers: the hidden face of estrogens. J Clin Oncol 25:3596–3602

D'Amico AV, Moul J, Carroll PR, Sun L, Lubeck D, Chen MH (2003) Cancer-specific mortality after surgery or radiation for patients with clinically localized prostate cancer managed during the prostate-specific antigen era. J Clin Oncol 21:2163–2172

Dal Maso L, Zucchetto A, La Vecchia C, Montella M, Conti E, Canzonieri V, Talamini R et al (2004) Prostate cancer and body size at different ages: an Italian multicentre case-control study. Br J Cancer 90:2176–2180

Djavan B, Kadesky K, Klopukh B, Marberger M, Roehrborn CG (1998) Gleason scores from prostate biopsies obtained with 18-gauge biopsy needles poorly predict Gleason scores of radical prostatectomy specimens. Eur Urol 33:261–270

Edwards SM, Badzioch MD, Minter R, Hamoudi R, Collins N, Ardern-Jones A, Dowe A et al (1999) Androgen receptor polymorphisms: association with prostate cancer risk, relapse and overall survival. Int J Cancer 84:458–465

Edwards SM, Kote-Jarai Z, Meitz J, Hamoudi R, Hope Q, Osin P, Jackson R et al (2003) Two percent of men with early-onset prostate cancer harbor germline mutations in the BRCA2 gene. Am J Hum Genet 72:1–12

Eeles RA, Durocher F, Edwards S, Teare D, Badzioch M, Hamoudi R, Gill S et al (1998) Linkage analysis of chromosome 1q markers in 136 prostate cancer families. The Cancer Research Campaign/British Prostate Group U.K. Familial Prostate Cancer Study Collaborators. Am J Hum Genet 62:653–658

Emmert-Buck MR, Vocke CD, Pozzatti RO, Duray PH, Jennings SB, Florence CD, Zhuang Z et al (1995) Allelic loss on chromosome 8p12–21 in microdissected prostatic intraepithelial neoplasia. Cancer Res 55:2959–2962

Epstein JI (2006) What's new in prostate cancer disease assessment in 2006? Curr Opin Urol 16:146–151

Epstein JI, Allsbrook WC Jr, Amin MB, Egevad LL (2005) The 2005 International Society of Urological Pathology (ISUP) Consensus Conference on Gleason Grading of Prostatic Carcinoma. Am J Surg Pathol 29:1228–1242

Freedland SJ, Platz EA (2007) Obesity and prostate cancer: making sense out of apparently conflicting data. Epidemiol Rev 29:88–97

Freedman ML, Pearce CL, Penney KL, Hirschhorn JN, Kolonel LN, Henderson BE, Altshuler D (2005) Systematic evaluation of genetic variation at the androgen receptor locus and risk of prostate cancer in a multiethnic cohort study. Am J Hum Genet 76:82–90

Freedman ML, Haiman CA, Patterson N, McDonald GJ, Tandon A, Waliszewska A, Penney K et al (2006) Admixture mapping identifies 8q24 as a prostate cancer risk locus in African-American men. Proc Natl Acad Sci USA 103:14068–14073

Freeman VL, Coard KC, Wojcik E, Durazo-Arvizu R (2004) Use of the Gleason system in international comparisons of prostatic adenocarcinomas in blacks. Prostate 58:169–173

Fukagai T, Namiki T, Namiki H, Carlile RG, Shimada M, Yoshida H (2001) Discrepancies between Gleason scores of needle biopsy and radical prostatectomy specimens. Pathol Int 51:364–370

Gann PH (2002) Risk factors for prostate cancer. Rev Urol 4(Suppl 5):S3–S10

Gibbs M, Chakrabarti L, Stanford JL, Goode EL, Kolb S, Schuster EF, Buckley VA et al (1999) Analysis of chromosome 1q42.2–43 in 152 families with high risk of prostate cancer. Am J Hum Genet 64:1087–1095

Giovannucci E, Liu Y, Platz EA, Stampfer MJ, Willett WC (2007) Risk factors for prostate cancer incidence and progression in the health professionals follow-up study. Int J Cancer 121:1571–1578

Giovannucci E, Rimm EB, Ascherio A, Colditz GA, Spiegelman D, Stampfer MJ, Willett WC (1999) Smoking and risk of total and fatal prostate cancer in United States health professionals. Cancer Epidemiol Biomarkers Prev 8:277–282

Goddard KA, Witte JS, Suarez BK, Catalona WJ, Olson JM (2001) Model-free linkage analysis with covariates confirms linkage of prostate cancer to chromosomes 1 and 4. Am J Hum Genet 68:1197–1206

Gong G, Oakley-Girvan I, Wu AH, Kolonel LN, John EM, West DW, Felberg A et al (2002) Segregation analysis of prostate cancer in 1, 719 white, African-American and Asian-American families in the United States and Canada. Cancer Causes Control 13:471–482

Goode EL, Stanford JL, Peters MA, Janer M, Gibbs M, Kolb S, Badzioch MD et al (2001) Clinical characteristics of prostate cancer in an analysis of linkage to four putative susceptibility loci. Clin Cancer Res 7:2739–2749

Goode EL, Stanford JL, Chakrabarti L, Gibbs M, Kolb S, McIndoe RA, Buckley VA et al (2000) Linkage analysis of 150 high-risk prostate cancer families at 1q24–25. Genet Epidemiol 18:251–275

Griffiths DF, Melia J, McWilliam LJ, Ball RY, Grigor K, Harnden P, Jarmulowicz M et al (2006) A study of Gleason score interpretation in different groups of UK pathologists; techniques for improving reproducibility. Histopathology 48:655–662

Gronberg H, Damber L, Damber JE, Iselius L (1997) Segregation analysis of prostate cancer in Sweden: support for dominant inheritance. Am J Epidemiol 146:552–557

Gronberg H, Damber L, Tavelin B, Damber JE (1998) No difference in survival between sporadic, familial and hereditary prostate cancer. Br J Urol 82:564–567

Gronberg H, Smith J, Emanuelsson M, Jonsson BA, Bergh A, Carpten J, Isaacs W et al (1999) In Swedish families with hereditary prostate cancer, linkage to the HPC1 locus on chromosome 1q24–25 is restricted to families with early-onset prostate cancer. Am J Hum Genet 65:134–140

Gudmundsson J, Sulem P, Manolescu A, Amundadottir LT, Gudbjartsson D, Helgason A, Rafnar T et al (2007a) Genome-wide association study identifies a second prostate cancer susceptibility variant at 8q24. Nat Genet 39:631–637

Gudmundsson J, Sulem P, Steinthorsdottir V, Bergthorsson JT, Thorleifsson G, Manolescu A, Rafnar T et al (2007b) Two variants on chromosome 17 confer prostate cancer risk, and the one in TCF2 protects against type 2 diabetes. Nat Genet 39:977–983

Habuchi T, Suzuki T, Sasaki R, Wang L, Sato K, Satoh S, Akao T et al (2000) Association of vitamin D receptor gene polymorphism with prostate cancer and benign prostatic hyperplasia in a Japanese population. Cancer Res 60:305–308

Haeusler J, Hoegel J, Bachmann N, Herkommer K, Paiss T, Vogel W, Maier C (2005) Association of a CAV-1 haplotype to familial aggressive prostate cancer. Prostate 65:171–177

Haggman MJ, Wojno KJ, Pearsall CP, Macoska JA (1997) Allelic loss of 8p sequences in prostatic intraepithelial neoplasia and carcinoma. Urology 50:643–647

Haiman CA, Patterson N, Freedman ML, Myers SR, Pike MC, Waliszewska A, Neubauer J et al (2007) Multiple regions within 8q24 independently affect risk for prostate cancer. Nat Genet 39:638–44

Hamasaki T, Inatomi H, Katoh T, Ikuyama T, Matsumoto T (2001) Clinical and pathological significance of vitamin D receptor gene polymorphism for prostate cancer which is associated with a higher mortality in Japanese. Endocr J 48:543–549

Hamel N, Kotar K, Foulkes WD (2003) Founder mutations in BRCA1/2 are not frequent in Canadian Ashkenazi Jewish men with prostate cancer. BMC Med Genet 4:7

Hanlon AL, Hanks GE (1998) Patterns of inheritance and outcome in patients treated with external beam radiation for prostate cancer. Urology 52:735–738

Hiatt RA, Armstrong MA, Klatsky AL, Sidney S (1994) Alcohol consumption, smoking, and other risk factors and prostate cancer in a large health plan cohort in California (United States). Cancer Causes Control 5:66–72

Horsburgh S, Matthew A, Bristow R, Trachtenberg J (2005) Male BRCA1 and BRCA2 mutation carriers: a pilot study investigating medical characteristics of patients participating in a prostate cancer prevention clinic. Prostate 65:124–129

Hsieh CL, Oakley-Girvan I, Gallagher RP, Wu AH, Kolonel LN, Teh CZ, Halpern J et al (1997) Re: prostate cancer susceptibility locus on chromosome 1q: a confirmatory study. J Natl Cancer Inst 89:1893–1894

Hsieh TF, Chang CH, Chen WC, Chou CL, Chen CC, Wu HC (2005) Correlation of Gleason scores between needle-core biopsy and radical prostatectomy specimens in patients with prostate cancer. J Chin Med Assoc 68:167–171

Huang SP, Chou YH, Wayne Chang WS, Wu MT, Chen YY, Yu CC, Wu TT et al (2004) Association between vitamin D receptor polymorphisms and prostate cancer risk in a Taiwanese population. Cancer Lett 207:69–77

Hubert A, Peretz T, Manor O, Kaduri L, Wienberg N, Lerer I, Sagi M et al (1999) The Jewish Ashkenazi founder mutations in the BRCA1/BRCA2 genes are not found at an increased frequency in Ashkenazi patients with prostate cancer. Am J Hum Genet 65:921–924

Humphrey PA (2004) Gleason grading and prognostic factors in carcinoma of the prostate. Mod Pathol 17:292–306

Ikonen T, Matikainen MP, Syrjakoski K, Mononen N, Koivisto PA, Rokman A, Seppala EH et al (2003) BRCA1 and BRCA2 mutations have no major role in predisposition to prostate cancer in Finland. J Med Genet 40:e98

Ingles SA, Coetzee GA, Ross RK, Henderson BE, Kolonel LN, Crocitto L, Wang W et al (1998) Association of prostate cancer with vitamin D receptor haplotypes in African-Americans. Cancer Res 58:1620–1623

Jaffe JM, Malkowicz SB, Walker AH, MacBride S, Peschel R, Tomaszewski J, Van Arsdalen K et al (2000) Association of SRD5A2 genotype and pathological characteristics of prostate tumors. Cancer Res 60:1626–1630

Kalapurakal JA, Jacob AN, Kim PY, Najjar DD, Hsieh YC, Ginsberg P, Daskal I et al (1999) Racial differences in prostate cancer related to loss of heterozygosity on chromosome 8p12–23. Int J Radiat Oncol Biol Phys 45:835–840

Karam JA, Lotan Y, Roehrborn CG, Ashfaq R, Karakiewicz PI, Shariat SF (2007) Caveolin-1 overexpression is associated with aggressive prostate cancer recurrence. Prostate 67:614–622

Kibel AS, Isaacs SD, Isaacs WB, Bova GS (1998) Vitamin D receptor polymorphisms and lethal prostate cancer. J Urol 160:1405–1409

Kibel AS, Suarez BK, Belani J, Oh J, Webster R, Brophy-Ebbers M, Guo C et al (2003) CDKN1A and CDKN1B polymorphisms and risk of advanced prostate carcinoma. Cancer Res 63:2033–2036

Kirchhoff T, Kauff ND, Mitra N, Nafa K, Huang H, Palmer C, Gulati T et al (2004) BRCA mutations and risk of prostate cancer in Ashkenazi Jews. Clin Cancer Res 10:2918–2921

Kittles RA, Chen W, Panguluri RK, Ahaghotu C, Jackson A, Adebamowo CA, Griffin R et al (2002) CYP3A4-V and prostate cancer in African Americans: causal or confounding association because of population stratification? Hum Genet 110:553–560

Kupelian PA, Klein EA, Witte JS (1999) Re: Biological aggressiveness of hereditary prostate cancer: long-term evaluation following radical prostatectomy. J Urol 161:1585–1586

Kupelian PA, Klein EA, Witte JS, Kupelian VA, Suh JH (1997a) Familial prostate cancer: a different disease? J Urol 158:2197–2201

Kupelian PA, Kupelian VA, Witte JS, Macklis R, Klein EA (1997b) Family history of prostate cancer in patients with localized prostate cancer: an independent predictor of treatment outcome. J Clin Oncol 15:1478–1480

Kupelian PA, Reddy CA, Reuther AM, Mahadevan A, Ciezki JP, Klein EA (2006) Aggressiveness of familial prostate cancer. J Clin Oncol 24:3445–3450

Lange EM, Ho LA, Beebe-Dimmer JL, Wang Y, Gillanders EM, Trent JM, Lange LA et al (2006) Genome-wide linkage scan for prostate cancer susceptibility genes in men with aggressive disease: significant evidence for linkage at chromosome 15q12. Hum Genet 119:400–407

Lange EM, Robbins CM, Gillanders EM, Zheng SL, Xu J, Wang Y, White KA et al (2007) Fine-mapping the putative chromosome 17q21–22 prostate cancer susceptibility gene to a 10 cm region based on linkage analysis. Hum Genet 121:49–55

Lange EM, Gillanders EM, Davis CC, Brown WM, Campbell JK, Jones M, Gildea D et al (2003) Genome-wide scan for prostate cancer susceptibility genes using families from the University of Michigan prostate cancer genetics project finds evidence for linkage on chromosome 17 near BRCA1. Prostate 57:326–334

Li C, Dong J, Guan W (2001) CAG microsatellite polymorphisms of androgen receptor gene and the stage and grade of prostate cancer. Zhonghua Zhong Liu Za Zhi 23:217–219

Li H, Stampfer MJ, Hollis JB, Mucci LA, Gaziano JM, Hunter D, Giovannucci EL et al (2007) A prospective study of plasma vitamin D metabolites, vitamin D receptor polymorphisms, and prostate cancer. PLoS Med 4:e103

Liu X, Cicek MS, Plummer SJ, Jorgenson E, Casey G, Witte JS (2007) Association of testis derived transcript gene variants and prostate cancer risk. J Urol 177:894–898

Loman N, Bladstrom A, Johannsson O, Borg A, Olsson H (2003) Cancer incidence in relatives of a population-based set of cases of early-onset breast cancer with a known BRCA1 and BRCA2 mutation status. Breast Cancer Res 5:R175–R186

Loukola A, Chadha M, Penn SG, Rank D, Conti DV, Thompson D, Cicek M et al (2004) Comprehensive evaluation of the association between prostate cancer and genotypes/haplotypes in CYP17A1, CYP3A4, and SRD5A2. Eur J Hum Genet 12:321–332

Lutchman M, Pack S, Kim AC, Azim A, Emmert-Buck M, van Huffel C, Zhuang Z et al (1999) Loss of heterozygosity on 8p in prostate cancer implicates a role for dematin in tumor progression. Cancer Genet Cytogenet 115:65–69

MacGrogan D, Levy A, Bostwick D, Wagner M, Wells D, Bookstein R (1994) Loss of chromosome arm 8p loci in prostate cancer: mapping by quantitative allelic imbalance. Genes Chromosomes Cancer 10:151–159

Maistro S, Snitcovsky I, Sarkis AS, da Silva IA, Brentani MM (2004) Vitamin D receptor polymorphisms and prostate cancer risk in Brazilian men. Int J Biol Markers 19:245–249

Matsuyama H, Pan Y, Oba K, Yoshihiro S, Matsuda K, Hagarth L, Kudren D et al (2001) Deletions on chromosome 8p22 may predict disease progression as well as pathological staging in prostate cancer. Clin Cancer Res 7:3139–3143

Menon M (1997) Predicting biological aggressiveness in prostate cancer – desperately seeking a marker. J Urol 157:228–229

Mikhak B, Hunter DJ, Spiegelman D, Platz EA, Hollis BW, Giovannucci E (2007) Vitamin D receptor (VDR) gene polymorphisms and haplotypes, interactions with plasma 25-hydroxyvitamin D and 1, 25-dihydroxyvitamin D, and prostate cancer risk. Prostate 67:911–923

Mir K, Edwards J, Paterson PJ, Hehir M, Underwood MA, Bartlett JM (2002) The CAG trinucleotide repeat length in the androgen receptor does not predict the early onset of prostate cancer. BJU Int 90:573–578

Mishra DK, Bid HK, Srivastava DS, Mandhani A, Mittal RD (2005) Association of vitamin D receptor gene polymorphism and risk of prostate cancer in India. Urol Int 74:315–318

Molitierno J, Evans A, Mohler JL, Wallen E, Moore D, Pruthi RS (2006) Characterization of biochemical recurrence after radical prostatectomy. Urol Int 77:130–134

Mononen N, Ikonen T, Syrjakoski K, Matikainen M, Schleutker J, Tammela TL, Koivisto PA et al (2001) A missense substitution A49T in the steroid 5-alpha-reductase gene (SRD5A2) is not associated with prostate cancer in Finland. Br J Cancer 84:1344–1347

Montironi R, Mazzuccheli R, Scarpelli M, Lopez-Beltran A, Fellegara G, Algaba F (2005) Gleason grading of prostate cancer in needle biopsies or radical prostatectomy specimens: contemporary approach, current clinical significance and sources of pathology discrepancies. BJU Int 95:1146–1152

Nastiuk KL, Mansukhani M, Terry MB, Kularatne P, Rubin MA, Melamed J, Gammon MD et al (1999) Common mutations in BRCA1 and BRCA2 do not contribute to early prostate cancer in Jewish men. Prostate 40:172–177

Neuhouser ML, Barnett MJ, Kristal AR, Ambrosone CB, King I, Thornquist M, Goodman G (2007) (n-6) PUFA increase and dairy foods decrease prostate cancer risk in heavy smokers. J Nutr 137:1821–1827

Neville PJ, Conti DV, Krumroy LM, Catalona WJ, Suarez BK, Witte JS, Casey G (2003) Prostate cancer aggressiveness locus on chromosome segment 19q12–q13.1 identified by linkage and allelic imbalance studies. Genes Chromosomes Cancer 36:332–339

Neville PJ, Conti DV, Paris PL, Levin H, Catalona WJ, Suarez BK, Witte JS et al (2002) Prostate cancer aggressiveness locus on chromosome 7q32–q33 identified by linkage and allelic imbalance studies. Neoplasia 4:424–431

Nilsen TI, Vatten LJ (1999) Anthropometry and prostate cancer risk: a prospective study of 22, 248 Norwegian men. Cancer Causes Control 10:269–275

Nilsen TI, Romundstad PR, Vatten LJ (2006) Recreational physical activity and risk of prostate cancer: a prospective population-based study in Norway (the HUNT study). Int J Cancer 119:2943–2947

Nock NL, Cicek MS, Li L, Liu X, Rybicki BA, Moreira A, Plummer SJ et al (2006) Polymorphisms in estrogen bioactivation, detoxification and oxidative DNA base excision repair genes and prostate cancer risk. Carcinogenesis 27:1842–1848

Noe M, Schroy P, Demierre MF, Babayan R, Geller AC (2007) Increased cancer risk for individuals with a family history of prostate cancer, colorectal cancer, and melanoma and their associated screening recommendations and practices. Cancer Causes Control 19(1):1–12

Onen IH, Ekmekci A, Eroglu M, Polat F, Biri H (2007) The association of 5alpha-reductase II (SRD5A2) and 17 hydroxylase (CYP17) gene polymorphisms with prostate cancer patients in the Turkish population. DNA Cell Biol 26:100–107

Oyama T, Allsbrook WC Jr, Kurokawa K, Matsuda H, Segawa A, Sano T, Suzuki K et al (2005) A comparison of interobserver reproducibility of Gleason grading of prostatic carcinoma in Japan and the United States. Arch Pathol Lab Med 129:1004–1010

Paiss T, Worner S, Kurtz F, Haeussler J, Hautmann RE, Gschwend JE, Herkommer K et al (2003) Linkage of aggressive prostate cancer to chromosome 7q31–33 in German prostate cancer families. Eur J Hum Genet 11:17–22

Pakkanen S, Baffoe-Bonnie AB, Matikainen MP, Koivisto PA, Tammela TL, Deshmukh S, Ou L et al (2007) Segregation analysis of 1, 546 prostate cancer families in Finland shows recessive inheritance. Hum Genet 121:257–267

Paris PL, Kupelian PA, Hall JM, Williams TL, Levin H, Klein EA, Casey G et al (1999) Association between a CYP3A4 genetic variant and clinical presentation in African-American prostate cancer patients. Cancer Epidemiol Biomarkers Prev 8:901–905

Patel AV, Rodriguez C, Jacobs EJ, Solomon L, Thun MJ, Calle EE (2005) Recreational physical activity and risk of prostate cancer in a large cohort of U.S. men. Cancer Epidemiol Biomarkers Prev 14:275–279

Perinchery G, Bukurov N, Nakajima K, Chang J, Hooda M, Oh BR, Dahiya R (1999) Loss of two new loci on chromosome 8 (8p23 and 8q12–13) in human prostate cancer. Int J Oncol 14:495–500

Peters MA, Janer M, Kolb S, Jarvik GP, Ostrander EA, Stanford JL (2001) Germline mutations in the p73 gene do not predispose to familial prostate-brain cancer. Prostate 48:292–296

Plaskon LA, Penson DF, Vaughan TL, Stanford JL (2003) Cigarette smoking and risk of prostate cancer in middle-aged men. Cancer Epidemiol Biomarkers Prev 12:604–609

Plummer SJ, Conti DV, Paris PL, Curran AP, Casey G, Witte JS (2003) CYP3A4 and CYP3A5 genotypes, haplotypes, and risk of prostate cancer. Cancer Epidemiol Biomarkers Prev 12:928–932

Pound CR, Partin AW, Eisenberger MA, Chan DW, Pearson JD, Walsh PC (1999) Natural history of progression after PSA elevation following radical prostatectomy. Jama 281:1591–1597

Powell IJ (2007) Epidemiology and pathophysiology of prostate cancer in African-American men. J Urol 177:444–449

Powell IJ, Zhou J, Sun Y, Sakr WA, Patel NP, Heilbrun LK, Everson RB (2004) CYP3A4 genetic variant and disease-free survival among white and black men after radical prostatectomy. J Urol 172:1848–1852

Rebbeck TR, Jaffe JM, Walker AH, Wein AJ, Malkowicz SB (1998) Modification of clinical presentation of prostate tumors by a novel genetic variant in CYP3A4. J Natl Cancer Inst 90:1225–1229

Risch N, Merikangas K (1996) The future of genetic studies of complex human diseases. Science 273:1516–1517

Roach M 3rd, De Silvio M, Rebbick T, Grignon D, Rotman M, Wolkov H, Fisher B et al (2007) Racial differences in CYP3A4 genotype and survival among men treated on radiation therapy oncology group (RTOG) 9202: a phase III randomized trial. Int J Radiat Oncol Biol Phys 69(1):79–87

Rodriguez C, Tatham LM, Thun MJ, Calle EE, Heath CW Jr (1997a) Smoking and fatal prostate cancer in a large cohort of adult men. Am J Epidemiol 145:466–475

Rodriguez C, Patel AV, Calle EE, Jacobs EJ, Chao A, Thun MJ (2001) Body mass index, height, and prostate cancer mortality in two large cohorts of adult men in the United States. Cancer Epidemiol Biomarkers Prev 10:345–353

Rodriguez C, Calle EE, Miracle-McMahill HL, Tatham LM, Wingo PA, Thun MJ, Heath CW Jr (1997b) Family history and risk of fatal prostate cancer. Epidemiology 8:653–657

Rodriguez C, Calle EE, Tatham LM, Wingo PA, Miracle-McMahill HL, Thun MJ, Heath CW Jr (1998) Family history of breast cancer as a predictor for fatal prostate cancer. Epidemiology 9:525–529

Roemeling S, Roobol MJ, de Vries SH, Gosselaar C, van der Kwast TH, Schroder FH (2006) Prevalence, treatment modalities and prognosis of familial prostate cancer in a screened population. J Urol 175:1332–1336

Rohrmann S, Genkinger JM, Burke A, Helzlsouer KJ, Comstock GW, Alberg AJ, Platz EA (2007) Smoking and risk of fatal prostate cancer in a prospective U.S. study. Urology 69:721–725

Rouprêt M, Fromont G, Bitker MO, Gattegno B, Vallancien G, Cussenot O (2006) Outcome after radical prostatectomy in young men with or without a family history of prostate cancer. Urology 67:1028–1032

Rukin NJ, Luscombe CJ, Strange RC (2007) Re: A systematic review of vitamin D receptor gene polymorphisms and prostate cancer risk. S. I. Berndt, J. L. Dodson, W. Y. Huang and K. K. Nicodemus, J Urol 2006; 175: 1613–1623. J Urol 177:404

Sacco E, Prayer-Galetti T, Pinto F, Ciaccia M, Fracalanza S, Betto G, Pagano F (2005) Familial and hereditary prostate cancer by definition in an italian surgical series: clinical features and outcome. Eur Urol 47:761–768

Sato K, Qian J, Slezak JM, Lieber MM, Bostwick DG, Bergstralh EJ, Jenkins RB (1999) Clinical significance of alterations of chromosome 8 in high-grade, advanced, nonmetastatic prostate carcinoma. J Natl Cancer Inst 91:1574–1580

Schaid DJ (2006) Pooled genome linkage scan of aggressive prostate cancer: results from the International Consortium for Prostate Cancer Genetics. Hum Genet 120:471–485

Schaid DJ, McDonnell SK, Blute ML, Thibodeau SN (1998) Evidence for autosomal dominant inheritance of prostate cancer. Am J Hum Genet 62:1425–1438

Schaid DJ, Stanford JL, McDonnell SK, Suuriniemi M, McIntosh L, Karyadi DM, Carlson EE et al (2007) Genome-wide linkage scan of prostate cancer Gleason score and confirmation of chromosome 19q. Hum Genet 121(6):729–735

Schaid DJ, McDonnell SK, Zarfas KE, Cunningham JM, Hebbring S, Thibodeau SN, Eeles RA et al (2006) Pooled genome linkage scan of aggressive prostate cancer: results from the International Consortium for Prostate Cancer Genetics. Hum Genet 120:471–485

Schumacher FR, Feigelson HS, Cox DG, Haiman CA, Albanes D, Buring J, Calle EE et al (2007) A common 8q24 variant in prostate and breast cancer from a large nested case-control study. Cancer Res 67:2951–2956

Schuurman AG, Goldbohm RA, Dorant E, van den Brandt PA (2000) Anthropometry in relation to prostate cancer risk in the Netherlands Cohort Study. Am J Epidemiol 151:541–549

SEER Cancer Statistics Review, 1975-2004 (2007) Ries LAG, Melbert D, Krapcho M, Mariotto A, Miller BA, Feuer EJ, Clegg L, Horner MJ, Howlader N, Eisner MP, Reichman M, Edwards BK (eds) National Cancer Institute. Bethesda, MD, http://seer.cancer.gov/csr/1975_2004/, based on November 2006 SEER data submission, posted to the SEER web site, 2007

Severi G, Hayes VM, Padilla EJ, English DR, Southey MC, Sutherland RL, Hopper JL et al (2007) The common variant rs1447295 on chromosome 8q24 and prostate cancer risk: results from an Australian population-based case-control study. Cancer Epidemiol Biomarkers Prev 16:610–612

Sfar S, Hassen E, Saad H, Mosbah F, Chouchane L (2006) Association of VEGF genetic polymorphisms with prostate carcinoma risk and clinical outcome. Cytokine 35:21–28

Sfar S, Saad H, Mosbah F, Gabbouj S, Chouchane L (2007) TSP1 and MMP9 genetic variants in sporadic prostate cancer. Cancer Genet Cytogenet 172:38–44

Siddiqui SA, Sengupta S, Slezak JM, Bergstralh EJ, Zincke H, Blute ML (2006) Impact of familial and hereditary prostate cancer on cancer specific survival after radical retropubic prostatectomy. J Urol 176:1118–1121

Sigurdsson S, Thorlacius S, Tomasson J, Tryggvadottir L, Benediktsdottir K, Eyfjord JE, Jonsson E (1997) BRCA2 mutation in Icelandic prostate cancer patients. J Mol Med 75:758–761

Singh R (2000) No evidence of linkage to chromosome 1q42.2–43 in 131 prostate cancer families from the ACTANE consortium. Anglo, Canada, Texas, Australia, Norway, EU Biomed. Br J Cancer 83:1654–1658

Slager SL, Zarfas KE, Brown WM, Lange EM, McDonnell SK, Wojno KJ, Cooney KA (2006) Genome-wide linkage scan for prostate cancer aggressiveness loci using families from the University of Michigan Prostate Cancer Genetics Project. Prostate 66:173–179

Slager SL, Schaid DJ, Cunningham JM, McDonnell SK, Marks AF, Peterson BJ, Hebbring SJ et al (2003) Confirmation of linkage of prostate cancer aggressiveness with chromosome 19q. Am J Hum Genet 72:759–762

Slattery ML, Schumacher MC, West DW, Robison LM, French TK (1990) Food-consumption trends between adolescent and adult years and subsequent risk of prostate cancer. Am J Clin Nutr 52:752–757

Smith JR, Freije D, Carpten JD, Gronberg H, Xu J, Isaacs SD, Brownstein MJ et al (1996) Major susceptibility locus for prostate cancer on chromosome 1 suggested by a genome-wide search. Science 274:1371–1374

Snowdon DA, Phillips RL, Choi W (1984) Diet, obesity, and risk of fatal prostate cancer. Am J Epidemiol 120:244–250

Spangler E, Zeigler-Johnson CM, Malkowicz SB, Wein AJ, Rebbeck TR (2005) Association of prostate cancer family history with histopathological and clinical characteristics of prostate tumors. Int J Cancer 113:471–474

Stanford JL, McDonnell SK, Friedrichsen DM, Carlson EE, Kolb S, Deutsch K, Janer M et al (2006) Prostate cancer and genetic susceptibility: a genome scan incorporating disease aggressiveness. Prostate 66:317–325

Steinberg GD, Carter BS, Beaty TH, Childs B, Walsh PC (1990) Family history and the risk of prostate cancer. Prostate 17:337–347

Struewing JP, Hartge P, Wacholder S, Baker SM, Berlin M, McAdams M, Timmerman MM et al (1997) The risk of cancer associated with specific mutations of BRCA1 and BRCA2 among Ashkenazi Jews. N Engl J Med 336:1401–1408

Suarez BK, Lin J, Witte JS, Conti DV, Resnick MI, Klein EA, Burmester JK et al (2000) Replication linkage study for prostate cancer susceptibility genes. Prostate 45: 106–114

Suuriniemi M, Agalliu I, Schaid DJ, Johanneson B, McDonnell SK, Iwasaki L, Stanford JL et al (2007) Confirmation of a positive association between prostate cancer risk and a locus at chromosome 8q24. Cancer Epidemiol Biomarkers Prev 16:809–814

Tayeb MT, Clark C, Haites NE, Sharp L, Murray GI, McLeod HL (2003) CYP3A4 and VDR gene polymorphisms and the risk of prostate cancer in men with benign prostate hyperplasia. Br J Cancer 88:928–932

Tayeb MT, Clark C, Murray GI, Sharp L, Haites NE, McLeod HL (2004) Length and somatic mosaicism of CAG and GGN repeats in the androgen receptor gene and the risk of prostate cancer in men with benign prostatic hyperplasia. Ann Saudi Med 24:21–26

Tayeb MT, Clark C, Sharp L, Haites NE, Rooney PH, Murray GI, Payne SN et al (2002) CYP3A4 promoter variant is associated with prostate cancer risk in men with benign prostate hyperplasia. Oncol Rep 9:653–655

Tollefson MK, Leibovich BC, Slezak JM, Zincke H, Blute ML (2006) Long-term prognostic significance of primary Gleason pattern in patients with Gleason score 7 prostate cancer: impact on prostate cancer specific survival. J Urol 175:547–551

Tryggvadottir L, Vidarsdottir L, Thorgeirsson T, Jonasson JG, Olafsdottir EJ, Olafsdottir GH, Rafnar T et al (2007) Prostate cancer progression and survival in BRCA2 mutation carriers. J Natl Cancer Inst 99:929–935

Tulinius H, Egilsson V, Olafsdottir GH, Sigvaldason H (1992) Risk of prostate, ovarian, and endometrial cancer among relatives of women with breast cancer. BMJ 305:855–857

Tulinius H, Olafsdottir GH, Sigvaldason H, Arason A, Barkardottir RB, Egilsson V, Ogmundsdottir HM et al (2002) The effect of a single BRCA2 mutation on cancer in Iceland. J Med Genet 39:457–462

Valeri A, Briollais L, Azzouzi R, Fournier G, Mangin P, Berthon P, Cussenot O et al (2003) Segregation analysis of prostate cancer in France: evidence for autosomal dominant inheritance and residual brother-brother dependence. Ann Hum Genet 67:125–137

Vazina A, Baniel J, Yaacobi Y, Shtriker A, Engelstein D, Leibovitz I, Zehavi M et al (2000) The rate of the founder Jewish mutations in BRCA1 and BRCA2 in prostate cancer patients in Israel. Br J Cancer 83:463–466

Verhage BA, Aben KK, Witjes JA, Straatman H, Schalken JA, Kiemeney LA (2004) Site-specific familial aggregation of prostate cancer. Int J Cancer 109:611–617

Verhage BA, Baffoe-Bonnie AB, Baglietto L, Smith DS, Bailey-Wilson JE, Beaty TH, Catalona WJ et al (2001) Autosomal dominant inheritance of prostate cancer: a confirmatory study. Urology 57:97–101

Villeneuve PJ, Johnson KC, Kreiger N, Mao Y (1999) Risk factors for prostate cancer: results from the Canadian National Enhanced Cancer Surveillance System. The Canadian Cancer Registries Epidemiology Research Group. Cancer Causes Control 10:355–367

Wang L, McDonnell SK, Slusser JP, Hebbring SJ, Cunningham JM, Jacobsen SJ, Cerhan JR et al (2007) Two common chromosome 8q24 variants are associated with increased risk for prostate cancer. Cancer Res 67:2944–50

West DW, Slattery ML, Robison LM, French TK, Mahoney AW (1991) Adult dietary intake and prostate cancer risk in Utah: a case-control study with special emphasis on aggressive tumors. Cancer Causes Control 2:85–94

Whittemore AS, Halpern J (2006) Nonparametric linkage analysis using person-specific covariates. Genet Epidemiol 30:369–379

Whittemore AS, Lin IG, Oakley-Girvan I, Gallagher RP, Halpern J, Kolonel LN, Wu AH et al (1999) No evidence of linkage for chromosome 1q42.2–43 in prostate cancer. Am J Hum Genet 65:254–256

Wiklund F, Jonsson BA, Goransson I, Bergh A, Gronberg H (2003) Linkage analysis of prostate cancer susceptibility: confirmation of linkage at 8p22–23. Hum Genet 112:414–418

Wilkens EP, Freije D, Xu J, Nusskern DR, Suzuki H, Isaacs SD, Wiley K et al (1999) No evidence for a role of BRCA1 or BRCA2 mutations in Ashkenazi Jewish families with hereditary prostate cancer. Prostate 39:280–284

Williams H, Powell IJ, Land SJ, Sakr WA, Hughes MR, Patel NP, Heilbrun LK et al (2004) Vitamin D receptor gene polymorphisms and disease free survival after radical prostatectomy. Prostate 61:267–275

Witte JS, Suarez BK, Thiel B, Lin J, Yu A, Banerjee TK, Burmester JK et al (2003) Genome-wide scan of brothers: replication and fine mapping of prostate cancer susceptibility and aggressiveness loci. Prostate 57:298–308

Witte JS, Goddard KA, Conti DV, Elston RC, Lin J, Suarez BK, Broman KW et al (2000) Genomewide scan for prostate cancer-aggressiveness loci. Am J Hum Genet 67:92–99

Xu J (2000) Combined analysis of hereditary prostate cancer linkage to 1q24–25: results from 772 hereditary prostate cancer families from the International Consortium for Prostate Cancer Genetics. Am J Hum Genet 66:945–957

Xu J, Zheng SL, Chang B, Smith JR, Carpten JD, Stine OC, Isaacs SD et al (2001a) Linkage of prostate cancer susceptibility loci to chromosome 1. Hum Genet 108:335–345

Xu J, Zheng SL, Hawkins GA, Faith DA, Kelly B, Isaacs SD, Wiley KE et al (2001b) Linkage and association studies of prostate cancer susceptibility: evidence for linkage at 8p22–23. Am J Hum Genet 69:341–350

Xu J, Gillanders EM, Isaacs SD, Chang BL, Wiley KE, Zheng SL, Jones M et al (2003) Genome-wide scan for prostate cancer susceptibility genes in the Johns Hopkins hereditary prostate cancer families. Prostate 57:320–325

Xu J, Dimitrov L, Chang BL, Adams TS, Turner AR, Meyers DA, Eeles RA et al (2005) A combined genomewide linkage scan of 1, 233 families for prostate cancer-susceptibility genes conducted by the international consortium for prostate cancer genetics. Am J Hum Genet 77:219–229

Yang G, Addai J, Ittmann M, Wheeler TM, Thompson TC (2000) Elevated caveolin-1 levels in African-American versus white-American prostate cancer. Clin Cancer Res 6:3430–3433

Yeager M, Orr N, Hayes RB, Jacobs KB, Kraft P, Wacholder S, Minichiello MJ et al (2007) Genome-wide association study of prostate cancer identifies a second risk locus at 8q24. Nat Genet 39:645–9

Zeigler-Johnson C, Friebel T, Walker AH, Wang Y, Spangler E, Panossian S, Patacsil M et al (2004) CYP3A4, CYP3A5, and CYP3A43 genotypes and haplotypes in the etiology and severity of prostate cancer. Cancer Res 64:8461–8467

Chapter 11
Susceptibility Alleles for Testicular Germ Cell Tumor

Elizabeth A. Rapley

11.1 Introduction

A family history of Testicular Germ Cell Tumor (TGCT) is among the strongest and most well-documented risk factors for TGCT (Forman et al. 1992; Westergaard et al. 1996; Heimdal et al. 1996; Sonneveld et al. 1999; Hemminki and Li 2004). In a proportion of cases (~2%), a first-degree family member is also affected with the disease (Forman et al. 1992). The relative risk to a brother of a TGCT case is 8–10 and between fathers and sons is 4–6 (Forman et al. 1992; Heimdal et al. 1996; Hemminki and Li 2004). This relative risk is higher than for most other cancer types, which are commonly 2 and rarely exceed 4 (Dong and Hemminki 2001). The high relative risk suggests that susceptibility genes are involved in the etiology of TGCT, which cannot be accounted for solely by shared environmental factors.

To account for a relative risk greater than 3 without some form of genetic predisposition requires that the environmental risk factor(s) be extremely strong (Khoury et al. 1988). Such potent risk factors have not been identified for TGCT (Richiardi et al. 2007). In addition, the causal factors for TGCT are thought to occur in utero or in very early childhood. While some of the relative risk to brothers could be accounted for by a shared maternal environment, this is not true for fathers and sons who cannot share a maternal environment and are less likely to share early childhood environmental factors. Moreover studies examining possible pre- and post-natal environmental exposures have largely been inconclusive and no environmental causes have been definitively identified (Richiardi et al. 2007). For a detailed discussion of the epidemiology of testicular cancer, see the chapter by McGlynn and Cook.

E.A. Rapley
Institute of Cancer Research, Cancer Genetics Unit, Brookes-Lawley Building, Sutton, Section of Cancer Genetics, 15 Cotswold Road, Belmont, Sutton, Surrey, SM6 8RW, UK
e-mail: liz.rapley@icr.ac.uk

W.D. Foulkes and K.A. Cooney (eds.), *Male Reproductive Cancers:*
Epidemiology, Pathology and Genetics, Cancer Genetics,
DOI 10.1007/978-1-4419-0449-2_11, © Springer Science+Business Media, LLC 2010

11.2   Evidence for TGCT Susceptibility Alleles

Support for a genetic component to TGCT is provided by several well-documented observations, in addition to the high relative risk.

Bilateral involvement of paired organs, that is, breast, retina, and kidney, has proven to be a clinical marker of hereditary cancer, with bilateral cases more often associated with a positive family history. Similarly for TGCT it has been demonstrated that patients with a family history of TGCT have a higher incidence of bilateral TGCT (9.8%) than patients without a family history (2.8%) (Heimdal et al. 1996).

Twin studies can be utilized to determine if there is a heritable component to cancer. If a heritable component exists, one would expect the relative risk in monozygotic twins to be greater than that in dizygotic twins or siblings. Twin studies for TGCT, while very small and to be viewed with caution, have demonstrated that monozygotic twins have a greater concordance for TGCT than dizygotic twins or siblings (Swerdlow et al. 1997; Lichtenstein et al. 2000). In a study by Swerdlow et al., six pairs of concordant (i.e., both affected) twins were identified. The risk of TGCT was raised in twin brothers of patients with TGCT (RR 37.5; 95% CI 12.3–115.6), and this risk was greater in MZ (RR 76.5) than DZ (RR 35.7) twins which would be expected if there is a heritable aspect to TGCT (Swerdlow et al. 1997).

A segregation analysis provides further evidence for TGCT susceptibility alleles. The analysis, which determines if familial clustering is best described by shared genetic or shared environmental factors, demonstrated that shared genetics most likely explained the familial clustering observed in the series of Scandinavian cases. The analysis predicted that TGCT susceptibility is likely to be due to a single major gene with a recessive mode of inheritance, an estimated gene frequency of 3.8%, and a life-time risk of developing TGCT of 43% among homozygous men (Heimdal et al. 1997). While clearly showing a shared genetic rather than a shared environmental cause, the analysis did not allow for an X-linked component to TGCT susceptibility and dominant mode of inheritance could not be completely ruled out.

A recessive mode of inheritance was also suggested by an analysis based on the age at onset of TGCT and the frequency of bilateral disease (Nicholson and Harland 1995). This model, which made the assumption that all cases of bilateral disease were due to inherited susceptibility, predicted that the relative risk to a brother of a bilateral TGCT case would be four to five times that of a brother of a unilateral case. This prediction was confirmed with 4.7-fold greater risk to brothers of bilateral TGCT cases than to brothers of unilateral TGCT cases. Interestingly, they also showed that fathers of patients with bilateral TGCT had a 3.9-fold greater risk than fathers of unilateral cases (Harland et al. 2006). While the greater risk observed in fathers of bilateral cases was not statistically significant due to small numbers, the trend would support a genetic component rather than a shared environmental component to TGCT susceptibility.

Geographical clustering of TGCT and racial differences in the incidence of TGCT also support a genetic component in the etiology of the disease. The highest incidence is observed in Caucasians of Northern European descent, whereas people of African or Asian descent seem to have a universally low incidence of TGCT (Bosl and Motzer 1997; Heimdal and Fossa 1994; Forman et al. 1990; Senturia 1987). African-Americans have only one quarter of the incidence observed in their white fellow countrymen (Gajendran et al. 2005; McGlynn et al. 2005). Moreover, the incidence in African-Americans is similar to that of native African populations, thus there has been little change in this population's incidence with migration to the USA, arguing in favor of genetic rather than exogenous risk factors. This mainte-nance is in sharp contrast to the situation with breast, stomach, colon, and ovarian cancers, for which the incidence in immigrant populations tends rapidly (within one or two generations) toward that of the host population.

11.3   Familial TGCT

Families with two or more members affected with TGCT are widely reported. Approximately 2% of TGCT patients report a first-degree relative also affected with TGCT, usually a brother or a father, and up to 6% of TGCT patients report a more distant relative (Forman et al. 1992). The relative risk to a brother of a TGCT case is 8–10 and between fathers and sons is 4–6 (Forman et al. 1992; Heimdal et al. 1996; Hemminki and Li 2004). The majority of TGCT pedigrees reported in the literature are sibling or father–son pairs (Forman et al. 1992; Crockford et al. 2006), although larger pedigrees have been rarely described (Goss and Bulbul 1990; Gedde-Dahl et al. 1985).

At the Royal Marsden Hospital (RMH), Sutton, England, we have been system-atically identifying and collecting families with two or more cases of TGCT since 1992, and this represents one of the larger series of pedigrees collected from a single institution. Currently we have identified 78 pedigrees, containing 160 cases and 170 TGCTs (Coffey et al. 2006). In the period 1994–2003, 6% of all cases attending the RMH clinic reported a family history of TGCT. The series contains 37 (47.4%) sib pairs, 12 (15.4%) father–son pairs, 12 (15.4%) uncle–nephew pairs, 10 (12.8%) cousin pairs, 2 (2.6%) grandfather–grandson pairs, a pair (1.3%) of monozygotic twins, and 4 (5.1%) pedigrees with >3 cases of TGCT. The median age at diagnosis was 33 years (range 17–87). The median difference in age at diagnosis between the cases in each pedigree was 6 years (0–58). Histology was concordant between family members in 22 of the 53 (41.5%) 2-case pedigrees, reflecting a similar observation in other family series and also patients with bilateral disease. Eleven pedigrees contained a case with bilateral TGCTs (6.9% of all cases, com-pared to 1.1% in the sporadic patient population from the RMH clinic, $p < 0.001$) with 50% histological concordance. In the series of pedigrees collected via the RMH testicular cancer clinic, we see a higher number of TGCT cases with a family history reporting a previous history of undescended testes (UDT) than would be expected for TGCT cases in general (15% vs. 10%; $p = 0.045$).

The International Testicular Cancer Linkage Consortium (ITCLC) (Table 11.1, Fig. 11.1a) was established in 1994 to collect pedigrees with TGCT for genetic linkage studies. Many of the features documented in the RMH pedigree series are reflected in this global collection of TGCT pedigrees. Within the ITCLC pedigree set, almost half of the families identified are sib pairs, with large pedigrees of three or more cases contributing just 9% of the total (Fig. 11.1b).

There are a few reports that examine known risk factors for TGCT in relatives of TGCT patients and from these there is a suggestion that TGCT risk factors may be more common in male relatives of patients than men without any family history.

Fertility is a known risk factor for TGCT. TGCT patients often present with abnormal semen characteristics beyond those that can easily be explained by localized or systemic effects of the tumor, and TGCT is found at increased frequency among men with abnormal semen analysis (Petersen et al. 1998; Jacobsen et al. 2000). TGCT patients have been documented to have lower fecundity compared to healthy controls. Fertility, as measured by the number of offspring and frequency of dizygotic twinning, has been shown to be reduced in brothers of TGCT patients but not sisters (Richiardi and Akre 2005). In a small series of families, Tollerud suggested that the frequency of urogenital abnormalities (another TGCT risk factor) was higher in male relatives of TGCT cases than would be expected by chance (Tollerud et al. 1985).

We performed testicular ultrasounds on 328 men as part of a larger study investigating testicular abnormalities in TGCT patients, their unaffected male relatives, and healthy male controls (Coffey et al. 2007). Testicular microlithiasis (TM) is characterized by small intratesticular calcifications which can be visualized by ultrasound. Men with testicular germ cell tumor (TGCT) have a higher frequency of TM than men without TGCT. To clarify the association between TGCT and TM and to investigate the relationship between TGCT susceptibility and TM, we recruited TGCT patients with and without family history of TGCT, unaffected male relatives, and healthy male controls from the UK. TM was more frequent in TGCT cases than controls (36.7% vs. 17.8%, age-adjusted $p < 0.0001$) and in unaffected male relatives than controls (34.5% vs. 17.8%, age-adjusted $p = 0.02$). TGCT case and matched relative pairs showed greater concordance for TM than would be expected by chance ($p = 0.05$). We showed that TM is present at a higher frequency in relatives of TGCT cases than expected by chance indicating that TM is a familial risk factor for TGCT. Although the familiality of TM could be due to shared exposures, it is likely that there exists a genetic susceptibility to TM that also predisposes to TGCT. We suggest that TM is an alternative manifestation of a TGCT susceptibility allele.

Further phenotypic studies of TGCT patients and male relatives may bring to light additional phenotypes which represent alternative phenotypes of TGCT susceptibility alleles and assist in identifying these genes.

Table 11.1 The International Testicular Cancer Linkage Consortium (ITCLC) groups by country. Number in right-hand column corresponds to numbers in Fig. 11.1

Authors	Institutions	Figure 11.1
	Australia	
Kathy Tucker, Michael Friedlander	Department of Medical Oncology, Division of Medicine, University of New South Wales and Prince of Wales Hospital Randwick, Sydney, Australia	4
Kelly-Anne Phillips	Department of Hematology and Medical Oncology, Peter MacCallum Cancer Centre, East Melbourne, Victoria, Australia	5
	Canada	
David Hogg, Michael A.S. Jewett	Princess Margaret Hospital and University of Toronto, Toronto, ON, Canada	6
	Czech Republic	
Radka Lohynska	University Hospital, Department of Radiotherapy and Oncology, Prague, Czech Republic	7
	Denmark	
Gedske Daugaard	Department of Oncology, Rigshospitalet, Copenhagen, Denmark	8
	France	
Stéphane Richard	Génétique Oncologique EPHE-UMR 8125 Faculté de Médecine Paris-Sud and Service d'Urologie, CHU, Le Kremlin-Bicêtre, France	9
Agnes Chompret	Génétique Oncologique, Institut Gustave Roussy, Villejuif, France	10
Catherine Bonaïti-Pellié	INSERM U 535, Villejuif, F-94817 France and Univ Paris-Sud, IFR 69, UMR-S535, Villejuif, F-94817 France	11
	Germany	
Axel Heidenreich	Department of Urology, Division of Oncological Urology, University of Köln, Germany	12
Peter Albers	Department of Urology, Klinikum Kassel GmbH, Moenchebergstr. 41-43, D-34125 Kassel, Germany	13
	Hungary	
Edith Olah, Lajos Geczi, Istvan Bodrogi	Department of Molecular Genetics and Department of Chemotherapy, National Institute of Oncology, Budapest, Hungary	14
	Ireland	
Peter A. Daly	Department of Medical Oncology, St James's Hospital, Dublin, Ireland	15
	New Zealand	
Parry Guilford	Cancer Genetics Laboratory, University of Otago, Dunedin, New Zealand	16
	Norway	
Sophie D. Fosså, Ketil Heimdal	Departments of Clinical Cancer Research and Medical Genetics, Rikshospitalet-Radiumhospitalet, Oslo, Norway	17

(continued)

Table 11.1 (continued)

Authors	Institutions	Figure 11.1
	Russian Federation	
Sergei A.Tjulandin, Ludmila Liubchenko	Laboratory of Clinical Genetics, Institute of Clinical Oncology, N.N.Blokhin Russian Cancer Research Center, Moscow, Russian Federation	18
	Switzerland	
Hans Stoll, Walter Weber	Medical Oncology, University Hospital, Basel, Switzerland	19
United Kingdom		
Gillian P. Crockford & D. Timothy Bishop	Genetic Epidemiology Division, Cancer Research UK Clinical Centre, St. James's University Hospital, Leeds, UK	1
Robert Huddart, Rachel Linger, Darshna Dudakia, Michael R. Stratton, Elizabeth A. Rapley	Academic Radiotherapy Unit and the Section of Cancer Genetics, Institute of Cancer Research, Sutton, Surrey, UK	2 & 3
David Forman	Cancer Epidemiology, University of Leeds, Cookridge Hospital, Leeds, LS16 6QB, UK	20
Timothy Oliver	Department of Medical Oncology, Barts and The London Queen Mary's School of Medicine, London, UK	21
Douglas F. Easton	Cancer Research U.K. Genetic Epidemiology Unit, Strangeways Research Laboratory, Cambridge, UK	26
	United States of America	
Lawrence Einhorn	Department of Medicine, Indiana University School of Medicine, Indianapolis, USA	22
Mary McMaster, Larissa Korde, Mark H. Greene	Clinical Genetics Branch, Division of Cancer Epidemiology & Genetics, National Cancer Institute National Institutes of Health, Rockville, MD, USA	23
Katherine L. Nathanson	Departments of Medicine and Biostatistics and Epidemiology, Abramson Family Cancer Research Institute, University of Pennsylvania School of Medicine, Philadelphia, PA, USA	24
Victoria Cortessis	Department of Preventive Medicine, Keck School of Medicine, USC/Norris Comprehensive Cancer Center, Los Angeles, California, USA	25

11.4   Identifying TGCT Susceptibility Alleles – Genetic Linkage Analysis

Genetic linkage analysis has been highly successful in isolating cancer susceptibility genes. However, the search for TGCT susceptibility genes has proven difficult. Large multiple generation pedigrees with many affected individuals of the type

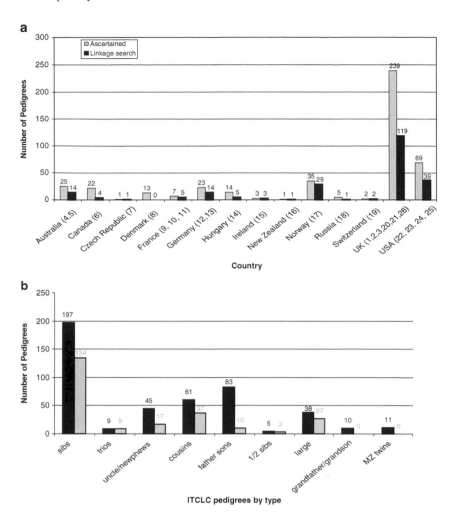

Fig. 11.1 (**a**) The ITCLC pedigree set by country, numbers beside country correspond to center and author affiliation in Table 11.1 (Crockford et al. 2006). (**b**) The ITCLC set by pedigree. *Shaded* show pedigrees ascertained by the ITCLC for which a DNA sample from at least one affected case has been collected and submitted to the ITCLC for genetic studies. *Black solid bars* indicate pedigrees examined in the linkage search

which have been critical to identifying the genes underlying hereditary breast, ovarian, and colorectal cancer are unknown for TGCT. The majority of TGCT pedigrees are relative pairs, predominantly siblings, which provide relatively weak linkage information and therefore large numbers of pedigrees are required to achieve adequate power.

11.4.1   Linkage to a Region at Xq27

In 2000, using 134 pedigrees with two or more cases of TGCT, 99 of which were compatible with X linkage, the ITCLC published evidence of linkage of TGCT susceptibility to a locus at Xq27 (Rapley et al. 2000). Among families with a disease distribution compatible with X linkage, the HLOD was 2.01, rising to 4.7 among kindreds containing at least one bilateral TGCT case.

This region was evaluated further in 66 previously untyped pedigrees (Crockford et al. 2006). There was no evidence for this locus among this new pedigree set (HLOD = 0.02). In the previous analysis, the locus at Xq27 was associated with a subset of families with bilateral disease. Of the new pedigrees, 16 had a case with a history of bilateral disease but there was no evidence for a TGCT locus in these new families. Overall, 163 pedigrees in the entire data set were compatible with X linkage (no male-to-male transmission) and the maximum HLOD was 1.07. The maximum HLOD in the 29 pedigrees with a history of bilateral disease from the entire set was 1.82. The linkage evidence supporting a TGCT susceptibility locus at Xq27 weakened considerably in the expanded family set.

The analysis of the entire pedigree set compatible with X linkage demonstrates a positive HLOD score > 1 for Xq27, so a gene in this region cannot be completely excluded. However, these data suggest that if such a gene in this region does predispose to TGCT, it would account for only a small proportion of TGCT susceptibility.

11.4.2   Genome-Wide Linkage Analysis

In 2006, the ITCLC published the results of a genome-wide analysis on 237 TGCT pedigrees. The data were examined by parametric linkage models including both a dominant and a recessive model of inheritance and by non-parametric analysis. All analyses were conducted under the assumption of genetic heterogeneity. The study demonstrated six regions of interest with heterogeneity LOD scores (HLOD) greater than 1.0 on chromosomes 2p23, 3p12, 3q26, 12p13-q21, 18q21-q23, and Xq27 (Crockford et al. 2006). None of the regions demonstrated significant evidence for linkage or exceeded a maximum HLOD of 2. Simulation analysis suggested that the number of LOD score peaks was not greater than that expected by chance.

An important observation from the exclusion analyses performed in this study is that no locus is likely to explain a sibling relative risk of 4. The study showed that susceptibility to TGCT could not be accounted for by a single major gene or even two major genes (like for example *BRCA1* or *BRCA2* in breast cancer). Thus results of these analyses suggest that several loci must contribute to TGCT susceptibility, and that no one locus explains a large fraction of the familial risk.

11.5   The Y Chromosome

The Y chromosome carries a number of testis- and germ cell-specific genes. The ampliconic element of the male-specific Y (MSY) region of the human Y chromosome contains a high density of genes from nine gene families, each gene existing in multiple (2 to 35) near identical copies (Skaletsky et al. 2003). Genes within the MSY region are expressed predominantly or exclusively in the testis and are believed to contribute to the development and proliferation of germ cells. As such, alterations in these genes could impact male reproductive health and germ cell neoplasia.

Microdeletions of the Y chromosome are the most common known cause of infertility caused by spermatogenic failure and account for ~10% of patients (Vogt et al. 1996, Kuroda-Kawaguchi et al. 2001). Male infertility has been associated with specific deletions of Yq11: AZFa, b, and c [MIM 415000]. The AZF deletions are due to recombination between large palindromic sequences that have >99.9% identity and are composed of long direct and indirect repeats called amplicons (Vogt et al. 1996; Kuroda-Kawaguchi et al. 2001; Skaletsky et al. 2003). Deletions in the AZF regions remove some or all copies of the male-specific genes (Vogt et al. 1996; Skaletsky et al. 2003). The majority of the AZF deletions result in azoospermia and complete infertility. Complete AZF deletions have not been identified in TGCT patients (Frydelund-Larsen et al. 2003; Lutke Holzik et al. 2005; Linger et al. 2007b).

11.5.1   gr/gr as a Low-Penetrance Susceptibility Allele

A novel Y chromosome 1.6 Mb deletion, designated "gr/gr," has been found to be associated with spermatogenic failure in some (Repping et al. 2003; Machev et al. 2004; de Llanos et al. 2005; Hucklenbroich et al. 2005; Ferlin et al. 2005; Lynch et al. 2005) but not all studies (de Carvalho et al. 2006; Carvalho et al. 2006; Zhang et al. 2006). Since father-to-son transmission is observed, the "gr/gr" deletion likely results in subfertility rather than complete infertility. The deletion was observed in association with numerous Y haplotypes, suggesting multiple independent recombination events give rise to the deletion (Repping et al. 2003).

We demonstrated that the "gr/gr" deletion on the Y chromosome is associated with susceptibility to TGCT (Nathanson et al. 2005). The study was conducted in 4,441 males including 431 TGCT cases with a family history of the disease and 1,376 non-familial TGCT cases compared to 2,599 controls. The "gr/gr" deletion was present in 3.0% (13/431) of TGCT cases with a family history, 2% (28/1,376) of TGCT cases without a family history, and 1.3% (33/2,599) of unaffected males. The presence of the "gr/gr" deletion was associated with a twofold increased risk of TGCT (adjusted odds ratio or aOR 2.1; 95% confidence interval [CI] 1.3–3.6; $p=0.005$) and a threefold increased risk of TGCT among patients with a positive family history (aOR 3.2; 95% CI 1.5–6.7, $p = 0.0027$). The association between the "gr/gr" deletion and TGCT was seen within each study center from which cases and unaffected males were genotyped, but because of the rarity of both the disease and the "gr/gr" deletion, the association was most significant when the sample populations were combined. The association between gr/gr and TGCT was stronger for cases of seminoma than for non-seminoma (aOR3.0; 95% CI 1.6–5.4; $p = 0.0004$). The data indicate that the "gr/gr" microdeletion is a rare, low-penetrance allele that is associated with susceptibility to TGCT. Given the results of the genome-wide linkage search the "gr/gr" deletion may represent one possible TGCT susceptibility allele (Crockford et al. 2006).

The "gr/gr" deletion as detected by the absence of the marker sY1291 can be generated by a number of different Y rearrangements (Fig. 11.2). Eight UK patients with deletions of the "gr/gr" region as characterized by the absence of the marker sY1291 were further investigated with additional Y STS markers (Linger et al. 2007b). Three TGCT cases demonstrated deletions in both the STS markers sY1291 and Y-DAZ3, which might suggest that these variants arose via the recombination mechanism known as r1/r4 mechanism (Fig. 11.2). The other five cases with "gr/gr" deletions did not have an accompanying deletion of Y-DAZ3, which could implicate that these have arisen via the g1/g2 or r1/r3 recombination mechanisms (Fig. 11.2). This observation suggests that further characterization of the "gr/gr" deletion region may be valuable in providing information on the gene(s) in this region that are critical for TGCT susceptibility.

11.5.2   Other Y Regions?

While entire deletions of AZF regions of the Y chromosome have not been identified in TGCT patients (Frydelund-Larsen et al. 2003; Lutke Holzik et al. 2005), other smaller Y deletions like "gr/gr" that could account for TGCT susceptibility have been investigated. Two studies have examined the AZF regions in a series of TGCT patients in constitutional and tumor material and reported a high frequency of deletions of single STSs within the AZF regions in normal and tumor samples. In a series of 17 Finnish men, 76.4% showed deletions of between 1 and 8 STS markers and in 40 TGCT cases from Norway and Argentina, 25% of cases showed a deletion of at least one STS marker. Interestingly, none of these deletions showed a contiguous pattern with more than two STS markers deleted, indicating that perhaps only a part of the AZF regions was deleted. Furthermore, the deletions or absence of an STS marker in constitutional DNA was shown to be present in the corresponding tumor material. It is difficult therefore to conclude if these are real Y microdeletions or if the deletions are due to some form of mosaicism as the authors suggest (Bianchi et al. 2002, 2006; Richard et al. 2004).

A series of 271 UK TGCT cases was investigated with a fine STS marker map of the Y chromosome. From the NCBI database (http://www.ncbi.nlm.nih.gov/),

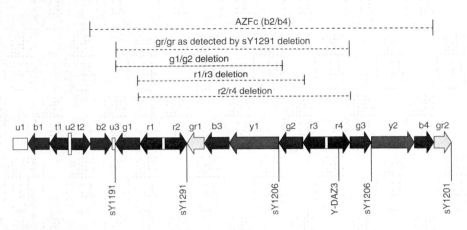

Fig. 11.2 Schematic of the AZFc deletion region showing gr/gr deletion and mechanisms whereby this deletion can arise (Linger et al. 2007b)

192 single copy Y STS markers with known location on the Y chromosome sequence map (Homo sapiens build 35.1) were evaluated for deletions. The average marker spacing of the STS markers was 128 kb. Excluding the possibility of small deletions existing between the STS markers used or very rare deletions of Y that may not have been detected in this series, the study showed that other than the previously characterized "gr/gr" deletion, Y chromosome deletions do not make a significant contribution to TGCT susceptibility (Linger et al. 2007b).

11.6 Evaluation of Candidate Genes for TGCT

One approach to identifying TGCT susceptibility alleles is to select candidate genes from a biological clue or from genes giving rise to the disease in appropriate animal models and conducting a mutational search of the gene in a series of patients. Few candidates for TGCT are described. Two genes, however, have been examined by this approach.

11.6.1 The Androgen Receptor Gene

Patients with androgen insensitivity syndrome (AIS) or testicular feminization syndrome (MIM 300068) are reported to have a high risk of malignancy, primarily of germ cell tumors. AIS is usually due to mutations in the androgen receptor gene (*AR*) on Xq11-q22. *AR* has eight exons and codes for a protein with three functional domains, an N-terminal domain, a DNA binding domain, and an androgen binding domain. The mutations most commonly observed in AIS are missense. The phenotypes associated with these mutations range from phenotypic females with complete AIS, characterized by normal breast development and female external genitalia, to phenotypic males with subtle undervirilization or infertility. There are at least seven reported cases of *AR* mutations where the only clinical phenotype is infertility (Levin 2000). All types of GCT have been recognized in patients with AIS and the tumors have a similar prognosis to that of patients without AIS. Germ cell tumors are largely reported in phenotypic females with *AR* mutations (Chen et al. 1999; Sakai et al. 2000).

The *AR* gene was investigated in a series of 116 TGCT patients and 7 patients with other non-germ cell testicular tumors (Garolla et al. 2005). Three TGCT patients (2.6%) were reported to have putative disease causing variants in this gene. This report of rare variants that potentially change AR function in 2.6% of TGCT patients needs to be validated in a significantly larger series, to further test whether this gene plays a role in TGCT susceptibility. We have examined a series of 771 TGCT patients from the UK and detected only one non-synonymous variant; however, the variant also appears to be present in controls. Our data would suggest that variants in the gene do not substantially contribute to TGCT susceptibility.

11.6.2 *Dnd1*

Animal models can provide leads to possible candidate genes that may cause disease in humans. For example, the *Ter* mutation is a strong modifier of TGCT risk in mice. Homozygosity for *Ter* causes complete germ cell deficiency in adult males and females, regardless of the genetic background (Sakurai et al. 1995). A homozygous *Ter* mutation on the background of the 129 mouse strain is a strong modifier of spontaneous germ cell tumor susceptibility and markedly increases the incidence of TGCT in 129-Ter/Ter males (Stevens 1973). The *Ter* gene was mapped to mouse chromosome 18, syntenic to human chromosome 5 (Asada et al. 1994), and the gene has been isolated (Youngren et al. 2005). The Ter phenotype is due to a single point mutation which introduces a stop codon (R178X) in the mouse orthologue (*Dnd1*) of the zebrafish dead-end (*dnd*) gene (Youngren et al. 2005). Dnd1 is expressed in the fetal testis during the critical period when TGCT are believed to develop in mice. The likely functional inactivation of the *Dnd1* gene in mice leads to both severe germ cell depletion and TGCT. Comparative sequence analysis of proteins showed that Dnd1 is closely related to apobec complementation factor (APF), which is involved in RNA editing, suggesting a similar role for the Dnd1 protein (Matin and Nadeau 2005).

Human *DND1* is located on chromosome 5q31.3 and consists of four exons (NM_194249). *DND1* was examined in 263 patients with TGCT and a rare heterozygous variant, c. a301c; p. Glu86Ala, was identified in a single case. The variant was not present in control chromosomes (0/4132). Analysis of the variant in an additional 842 index TGCT cases did not reveal any additional p.Glu86Ala alleles. p. Glu86Ala is within a known functional domain of *DND1* and is highly conserved through evolution. Although the variant may be a rare polymorphism, a change at a highly conserved residue is characteristic of a disease-causing variant. Whether it is disease-causing or not, mutations in *DND1* make, at most, a very small contribution to TGCT susceptibility (Linger et al. 2007a).

11.7 Association Studies

Traditionally, association studies aim to find statistical evidence of a difference in allele frequency between cases and controls at polymorphic loci on, or closely linked to, candidate genes [e.g., genes involved in the metabolism of mutagenic agents, known tumor suppressor genes or oncogenes and a particular phenotype (e.g., TGCT)].

Few association studies have been performed on TGCT possibility reflecting the difficulty in choosing a "suitable" candidate gene or genes. The Human leukocyte antigen (HLA) region has been extensively studied [for review see Holzik et al. (2004)], with mainly inconclusive results. More recently, the length of the androgen receptor "CAG" repeat has been evaluated in TGCT patients again with inconclusive and conflicting results (Giwercman et al. 2004; Rajpert-De Meyts et al. 2002). Other association-based studies include: (1) an evaluation of the Wilms tumor locus (*WT1*) on chromosome 11 (Heimdal et al. 1994) which demonstrated no association between the locus and TGCT; (2) an evaluation of cytochrome P450 genes in estrogen metabolism which suggests that genetic variation in maternal and or offspring catechol estrogen activity may influence a sons' risk of TGCT (Starr et al. 2005); (3) an evaluation of immune function gene polymorphisms which, although not robust when adjusted for multiple testing, suggest that genetic variants in *TGFB1*, *LTA/TNK*, *IL2*, *IFNGR2*, and *IL1D* may influence susceptibility to TGCT (Purdue et al. 2007).

It is important that the findings of the last two studies be replicated in additional cases and controls before meaningful inferences about their causal relevance can be drawn.

11.8 Identifying TGCT Susceptibility Alleles

The consistently reported high relative risks of TGCT coupled with the evidence for multiple predisposing alleles of modest effects indicate that additional approaches to the detection of TGCT susceptibility genes are required. Substantially larger pedigree sets would be required to identify such genes via linkage analysis. Since TCGT is a rare tumor and only 2–6% of patients report an affected relative, it will take a very long time to acquire sufficiently large pedigree collections. Furthermore, father/son pedigrees, which contribute to almost a third of pedigrees collected, are not useful for linkage analysis. Effectively 50% of the pedigrees identified in the global ITCLC collection are not usable in the linkage search due to family structure or inability to collect DNA samples from pedigree members. (Fig. 11.1).

Association studies are generally better powered for the detection of low-penetrance disease loci. Moreover all pedigree types can be examined and since only one case per family is needed, incomplete pedigrees can be utilized in the search. Most association studies conducted have been based on a candidate gene approach. This strategy is limited, as the selection criteria for genes of interest is based on an "educated guess," usually derived from a biological hypothesis or a previously determined region of interest. Without a clear understanding of the pathophysiology of TGCT and without convincing evidence of linkage, definition of "suitable" candidate genes for TGCT is problematic. Moreover, the large majority of studies based on a candidate gene hypothesis have ultimately proven negative.

Following the sequencing of the human genome, large-scale harvests of single nucleotide polymorphisms have been conducted. Over 10 million single nucleotide polymorphisms (SNPs) have now been identified (http://www.dbsnp.org), with smaller numbers of small insertion/deletion and copy number polymorphisms. Patterns of linkage disequilibrium (LD) between SNPs, and the physical distances they extend over, have been characterized in detail. The HapMap project has explored the extent of LD across the genome in multiple populations testing over 5 million SNPs (2003). With the data of the second phase of HapMap released and its analysis underway, it is now possible to select subsets of the 3 million typed SNPs that, through LD with other variants, inform on a large proportion of the common sequence variation in the human genome (Hirschhorn and Daly 2005).

The advent of large numbers of SNPs has driven the development of several technology platforms which are designed to analyze hundreds of thousands of variants in thousands of samples. The current availability of high-resolution LD maps and hence comprehensive sets of tag SNPs that capture most of the common sequence variation (minor allele frequency > 5%) coupled with the new technology platforms now allows whole genome studies for disease associations (Hirschhorn and Daly 2005; Houlston and Peto 2003). This approach is unbiased and does not depend upon understanding the biology of the disease.

Increasing numbers of genome-wide association studies are now being reported (The Wellcome Trust Case Control Consortium 2007; Easton et al. 2007). The Wellcome trust study of seven major common diseases represents a proof of principle that the genome-wide association approach can identify susceptibility alleles. Furthermore, on the basis of replication studies thus far completed, almost all of the signals identified in the initial phases reflect true susceptibility alleles.

A genome-wide association study is now underway for TGCT utilizing 2,000 cases from the UK, including patients with and without a family history of disease, and a similar number of UK controls. Based on the results of the Wellcome Trusts analyses and other genome-wide association studies this approach should yield TGCT susceptibility alleles. The initial signals from this search will need to be replicated in larger series of TGCT cases requiring an international collaboration like the ITCLC. While the association signals can define regions of interest, it is important to recognize that they cannot provide unambiguous identification of causal genes. Extensive re-sequencing and fine mapping followed by functional studies will be required before robust statements can be made about the molecular and physiological mechanisms of the susceptibility genes identified.

11.9   Conclusion

The search for TGCT susceptibility alleles has been challenging. The high relative risk and other evidence support the notion that these genes are important in the etiology of TGCT. The largest genome-wide linkage study has demonstrated that a single major gene cannot account for a substantial proportion of the familial risk and that many genes with modest or small effects are likely to contribute to disease susceptibility. One such gene is likely to exist in the "gr/gr" deletion region on the Y chromosome. The data suggest that "gr/gr" is a low-penetrance susceptibility allele. However, confirmatory studies of additional large case-control series are required. Genome-wide SNP association studies are now technically and financially feasible, and we are embarking on such a study for TGCT. Association studies are generally better powered for the detection of lower penetrance disease loci such as those believed to contribute to TGCT susceptibility. Any genome-wide association study will require an international collaboration such as the ITCLC to allow the evaluation of putative loci in large series of both cases and controls to confirm regions of association to a genome-wide significance level of $p < 10^{-7}$ and to identify and characterize TGCT susceptibility genes.

Note

Since the prepration of this chapter the results of the first genome wide association studies for TGCT are now published and have implicated several loci in TGCT susceptibility (Rapley et al, 2009; Kanetsky et al, 2009)

References

Asada Y, Varnum DS, Frankel WN, Nadeau JH (1994) A mutation in the Ter gene causing increased susceptibility to testicular teratomas maps to mouse chromosome 18. Nat Genet 6:363–368

Bianchi NO, Richard SM, Pavicic W (2006) Y chromosome instability in testicular cancer. Mutat Res 612:172–188

Bianchi NO, Richard SM, Peltomaki P, Bianchi MS (2002) Mosaic AZF deletions and susceptibility to testicular tumors. Mutat Res 503:51–62

Bosl GJ, Motzer RJ (1997) Testicular germ-cell cancer. N Engl J Med 337:242–253

Carvalho CM, Zuccherato LW, Bastos-Rodrigues L, Santos FR, Pena SD (2006) No association found between gr/gr deletions and infertility in Brazilian males. Mol Hum Reprod 12:269–273

Chen CP, Chern SR, Wang TY, Wang W, Wang KL, Jeng CJ (1999) Androgen receptor gene mutations in 46, XY females with germ cell tumours. Hum Reprod 14:664–670

Coffey J, Huddart R, Elliott F, Sohaib AS, Parker E, Dudakia D, Pugh J, Easton DF, Bishop DT, Stratton MR, Rapley EA (2007) Testicular microlithiasis as a familial risk factor for testicular germ cell tumour. BJC. Br J Cancer. 97:1701–6

Coffey J, Huddart RA, Norman AR, Dudakia D, Stratton M, Rapley EA (2006) Characteristics of a single-centre series of familial testicular germ cell tumours. ASCO Annual Meeting Proceedings. J Clin Oncol 24 (Abst. no. 10039)

Crockford GP, Linger R, Hockley S, Dudakia D, Johnson L, Huddart R, Tucker K, Friedlander M, Phillips KA, Hogg D, Jewett MA, Lohynska R, Daugaard G, Richard S, Chompret A, Bonaiti-Pellie C, Heidenreich A, Albers P, Olah E, Geczi L, Bodrogi I, Ormiston WJ, Daly PA, Guilford P, Fossa SD, Heimdal K, Tjulandin SA, Liubchenko L, Stoll H, Weber W, Forman D, Oliver T, Einhorn L, McMaster M, Kramer J, Greene MH, Weber BL, Nathanson KL, Cortessis V, Easton DF, Bishop DT, Stratton MR, Rapley EA (2006) Genome-wide linkage screen for testicular germ cell tumour susceptibility loci. Hum Mol Genet 15:443–451

de Carvalho CM, Zuccherato LW, Fujisawa M, Shirakawa T, Ribeiro-dos-Santos AK, Santos SE, Pena SD, Santos FR (2006) Study of AZFc partial deletion gr/gr in fertile and infertile Japanese males. J Hum Genet 51:794–799

de Llanos M, Ballesca JL, Gazquez C, Margarit E, Oliva R (2005) High frequency of gr/gr chromosome Y deletions in consecutive oligospermic ICSI candidates. Hum Reprod 20:216–220

Dong C, Hemminki K (2001) Modification of cancer risks in offspring by sibling and parental cancers from 2, 112, 616 nuclear families. Int J Cancer 92:144–150

Easton DF, Pooley KA, Dunning AM, Pharoah PD, Thompson D, Ballinger DG, Struewing JP, Morrison J, Field H, Luben R, Wareham N, Ahmed S, Healey CS, Bowman R, Luccarini C, Conroy D, Shah M, Munday H, Jordan C, Perkins B, West J, Redman K, Meyer KB, Haiman CA, Kolonel LK, Henderson BE, Le Marchand L, Brennan P, Sangrajrang S, Gaborieau V, Odefrey F, Shen CY, Wu PE, Wang HC, Eccles D, Evans DG, Peto J, Fletcher O, Johnson N, Seal S, Stratton MR, Rahman N, Chenevix-Trench G, Bojesen SE, Nordestgaard BG, Axelsson CK, Garcia-Closas M, Brinton L, Chanock S, Lissowska J, Peplonska B, Nevanlinna H, Fagerholm R, Eerola H, Kang D, Yoo KY, Noh DY, Ahn SH, Hunter DJ, Hankinson SE, Cox DG, Hall P, Wedren S, Liu J, Low YL, Bogdanova N, Schurmann P, Dork T, Tollenaar RA, Jacobi CE, Devilee P, Klijn JG, Sigurdson AJ, Doody MM, Alexander BH, Zhang J, Cox A, Brock IW, Macpherson G, Reed MW, Couch FJ, Goode EL, Olson JE, Meijers-Heijboer H, van den OA, Uitterlinden A, Rivadeneira F, Milne RL, Ribas G, Gonzalez-Neira A, Benitez J, Hopper JL, McCredie M, Southey M, Giles GG, Schroen C, Justenhoven C, Brauch H, Hamann U, Ko YD, Spurdle AB, Beesley J, Chen X, Aghmesheh M, Amor D, Andrews L, Antill Y, Armes J, Armitage S, Arnold L, Balleine R, Begley G, Beilby J, Bennett I, Bennett B, Berry G, Blackburn A, Brennan M, Brown M, Buckley M, Burke J, Butow P, Byron K, Callen D, Campbell I, Chenevix-Trench G, Clarke C, Colley A, Cotton D, Cui J, Culling B, Cummings M, Dawson SJ, Dixon J, Dobrovic A, Dudding T, Edkins T, Eisenbruch M, Farshid G, Fawcett S, Field M, Firgaira F, Fleming J, Forbes J, Friedlander M, Gaff C, Gardner M, Gattas M, George P, Giles G, Gill G, Goldblatt J, Greening S, Grist S, Haan E, Harris M, Hart S, Hayward N, Hopper J, Humphrey E, Jenkins M, Jones A, Kefford R, Kirk J, Kollias J, Kovalenko S, Lakhani S, Leary J, Lim J, Lindeman G, Lipton L, Lobb L, Maclurcan M, Mann G, Marsh D, McCredie M, McKay M, Anne MS, Meiser B, Milne R, Mitchell G, Newman B, O'loughlin I, Osborne R, Peters L, Phillips K, Price M, Reeve J, Reeve T, Richards R, Rinehart G, Robinson B, Rudzki B, Salisbury E, Sambrook J, Saunders C, Scott C, Scott E, Scott R, Seshadri R, Shelling A, Southey M, Spurdle A, Suthers G, Taylor D, Tennant C, Thorne H, Townshend S, Tucker K, Tyler J, Venter D, Visvader J, Walpole I, Ward R, Waring P, Warner B, Warren G, Watson E, Williams R, Wilson J, Winship I, Young MA, Bowtell D, Green A, Defazio A, Chenevix-Trench G, Gertig D, Webb P, Mannermaa A, Kosma VM, Kataja V, Hartikainen J, Day NE, Cox DR, Ponder BA (2007) Genome-wide association study identifies novel breast cancer susceptibility loci. Nature 447(7148):1087–1093

Ferlin A, Tessari A, Ganz F, Marchina E, Barlati S, Garolla A, Engl B, Foresta C (2005) Association of partial AZFc region deletions with spermatogenic impairment and male infertility. J Med Genet 42:209–213

Forman D, Gallagher R, Moller H, Swerdlow TJ (1990) Aetiology and epidemiology of testicular cancer: report of consensus group. Prog Clin Biol Res 357:245–253

Forman D, Oliver RT, Brett AR, Marsh SG, Moses JH, Bodmer JG, Chilvers CE, Pike MC (1992) Familial testicular cancer: a report of the UK family register, estimation of risk and an HLA class 1 sib-pair analysis. Br J Cancer 65:255–262

Frydelund-Larsen L, Vogt PH, Leffers H, Schadwinkel A, Daugaard G, Skakkebaek NE, Rajpert-De Meyts E (2003) No AZF deletion in 160 patients with testicular germ cell neoplasia. Mol Hum Reprod 9:517–521

Gajendran VK, Nguyen M, Ellison LM (2005) Testicular cancer patterns in African-American men. Urology 66:602–605

Garolla A, Ferlin A, Vinanzi C, Roverato A, Sotti G, Artibani W, Foresta C (2005) Molecular analysis of the androgen receptor gene in testicular cancer. Endocr Relat Cancer 12:645–655

Gedde-Dahl TJ, Hannisdal E, Klepp OH, Grottum KA, Waksvik H, Fossa SD, Stenwig AE, Broogger A (1985) Testicular neoplasms occurring in four brothers. A search for a genetic predisposition. Cancer 55:2005–2009

Giwercman A, Lundin KB, Eberhard J, Stahl O, Cwikiel M, Cavallin-Stahl E, Giwercman YL (2004) Linkage between androgen receptor gene CAG trinucleotide repeat length and testicular germ cell cancer histological type and clinical stage. Eur J Cancer 40:2152–2158

Goss PE, Bulbul MA (1990) Familial testicular cancer in five members of a cancer-prone kindred. Cancer 66:2044–2046

Harland SJ, Daugaard G, Horwich A, Mead GM, Fossa S, Sokal M, Morgenstern D, Oliver R, Cook P, Stenning SP (2006) The familial influence on bilateral testicular germ cell cancer: medical research council study TER2. Annual Meeting Proceedings. J Clin Oncol 24:239s (Abst. no. 4590)

Heimdal K, Fossa SD (1994) Genetic factors in malignant germ-cell tumors. World J Urol 12:178–181

Heimdal K, Olsson H, Tretli S, Flodgren P, Borresen AL, Fossa SD (1996) Familial testicular cancer in Norway and southern Sweden. Br J Cancer 73:964–969

Heimdal K, Olsson H, Tretli S, Fossa SD, Borresen AL, Bishop DT (1997) A segregation analysis of testicular cancer based on Norwegian and Swedish families. Br J Cancer 75:1084–1087

Heimdal KR, Lothe RA, Fossa SD, Borresen AL (1994) Association studies of a polymorphism in the Wilms' tumor 1 locus in Norwegian patients with testicular cancer. Int J Cancer 58:523–526

Hemminki K, Li X (2004) Familial risk in testicular cancer as a clue to a heritable and environmental aetiology. Br J Cancer 90:1765–1770

Hirschhorn JN, Daly MJ (2005) Genome-wide association studies for common diseases and complex traits. Nat Rev Genet 6:95–108

Holzik MF, Rapley EA, Hoekstra HJ, Sleijfer DT, Nolte IM, Sijmons RH (2004) Genetic predisposition to testicular germ-cell tumours. Lancet Oncol 5:363–371

Houlston RS, Peto J (2003) The future of association studies of common cancers. Hum Genet 112:434–435

Hucklenbroich K, Gromoll J, Heinrich M, Hohoff C, Nieschlag E, Simoni M (2005) Partial deletions in the AZFc region of the Y chromosome occur in men with impaired as well as normal spermatogenesis. Hum Reprod 20:191–197

Jacobsen R, Bostofte E, Engholm G, Hansen J, Olsen JH, Skakkebaek NE, Moller H (2000) Risk of testicular cancer in men with abnormal semen characteristics: cohort study. BMJ 321:789–792

Kanetsky PA, Mitra N, Vardhanabhuti S, Li M, Vaughn DJ, Letrero R, Ciosek SL, Doody DR, Smith LM, Weaver J, Albano A, Chen C, Starr JR, Rader DJ, Godwin AK, Reilly MP, Hakonarson H, Schwartz SM, Nathanson KL. (2009) Common variation in KITLG and at 5q31.3 predisposes to testicular germ cell cancer. Nat Genet. 41:811–5.

Khoury MJ, Beaty TH, Liang KY (1988) Can familial aggregation of disease be explained by familial aggregation of environmental risk factors? Am J Epidemiol 127:674–683

Kuroda-Kawaguchi T, Skaletsky H, Brown LG, Minx PJ, Cordum HS, Waterston RH, Wilson RK, Silber S, Oates R, Rozen S, Page DC (2001) The AZFc region of the Y chromosome features massive palindromes and uniform recurrent deletions in infertile men. Nat Genet 29:279–286

Levin HS (2000) Tumors of the testis in intersex syndromes. Urol Clin North Am 27:543–551, x

Lichtenstein P, Holm NV, Verkasalo PK, Iliadou A, Kaprio J, Koskenvuo M, Pukkala E, Skytthe A, Hemminki K (2000) Environmental and heritable factors in the causation of cancer – analyses of cohorts of twins from Sweden, Denmark, and Finland. N Engl J Med 343:78–85

Linger R, Dudakia D, Huddart R, Tucker K, Friedlander M, Phillips K-A, Hogg D, Jewett MAS, Lohynska R, Daugaard G, Richard S, Chompret A, Stoppa-Lyonnet D, Bonaiti-Pellie C, Heidenreich A, Albers P, Olah E, Geczi L, Bodrogi I, Daly PA, Guildford P, Fossa S, Heimdal K, Tjulandin SA, Liubchenko L, Stoll H, Weber W, Einhorn L, McMaster M, Korde L, Greene MH, Nathanson KL, Cortessis V, Easton DF, Bishop DT, Stratton MR, Rapley EA (2007a) Analysis of the DND1 gene in men with sporadic and familial testicular germ cell tumours. Genes Chromosomes Cancer. 2008 47:247–52.

Linger R, Dudakia D, Huddart R, Easton D, Bishop DT, Stratton MR, Rapley EA (2007b) A physical analysis of the Y chromosome shows no additional deletions, other than Gr/Gr, associated with testicular germ cell tumour. Br J Cancer 96:357–361

Lutke Holzik MF, Storm K, Sijmons RH, D'hollander M, Arts EG, Verstraaten ML, Sleijfer DT, Hoekstra HJ (2005) Absence of constitutional Y chromosome AZF deletions in patients with testicular germ cell tumors. Urology 65:196–201

Lynch M, Cram DS, Reilly A, O'Bryan MK, Baker HW, de Kretser DM, McLachlan RI (2005) The Y chromosome gr/gr subdeletion is associated with male infertility. Mol Hum Reprod 11:507–512

Machev N, Saut N, Longepied G, Terriou P, Navarro A, Levy N, Guichaoua M, Metzler-Guillemain C, Collignon P, Frances AM, Belougne J, Clemente E, Chiaroni J, Chevillard C, Durand C, Ducourneau A, Pech N, McElreavey K, Mattei MG, Mitchell MJ (2004) Sequence family variant loss from the AZFc interval of the human Y chromosome, but not gene copy loss, is strongly associated with male infertility. J Med Genet 41:814–825

Matin A, Nadeau JH (2005) Search for testicular cancer gene hits dead-end. Cell Cycle 4:1136–1138

McGlynn KA, Devesa SS, Graubard BI, Castle PE (2005) Increasing incidence of testicular germ cell tumors among black men in the United States. J Clin Oncol 23:5757–5761

Nathanson KL, Kanetsky PA, Hawes R, Vaughn DJ, Letrero R, Tucker K, Friedlander M, Phillips KA, Hogg D, Jewett MA, Lohynska R, Daugaard G, Richard S, Chompret A, Bonaiti-Pellie C, Heidenreich A, Olah E, Geczi L, Bodrogi I, Ormiston WJ, Daly PA, Oosterhuis JW, Gillis AJ, Looijenga LH, Guilford P, Fossa SD, Heimdal K, Tjulandin SA, Liubchenko L, Stoll H, Weber W, Rudd M, Huddart R, Crockford GP, Forman D, Oliver DT, Einhorn L, Weber BL, Kramer J, McMaster M, Greene MH, Pike M, Cortessis V, Chen C, Schwartz SM, Bishop DT, Easton DF, Stratton MR, Rapley EA (2005) The Y deletion gr/gr and susceptibility to testicular germ cell tumor. Am J Hum Genet 77:1034–1043

Nicholson PW, Harland SJ (1995) Inheritance and testicular cancer. Br J Cancer 71:421–426

Petersen PM, Skakkebaek NE, Giwercman A (1998) Gonadal function in men with testicular cancer: biological and clinical aspects. APMIS 106:24–34

Purdue MP, Sakoda LC, Graubard BI, Welch R, Chanock SJ, Sesterhenn IA, Rubertone MV, Erickson RL, McGlynn KA (2007) A case-control investigation of immune function gene polymorphisms and risk of testicular germ cell tumors. Cancer Epidemiol Biomarkers Prev 16:77–83

Rajpert-De Meyts E, Leffers H, Daugaard G, Andersen CB, Petersen PM, Hinrichsen J, Pedersen LG, Skakkebaek NE (2002) Analysis of the polymorphic CAG repeat length in the androgen receptor gene in patients with testicular germ cell cancer. Int J Cancer 102:201–204

Rapley EA, Crockford GP, Teare D, Biggs P, Seal S, Barfoot R, Edwards S, Hamoudi R, Heimdal K, Fossa SD, Tucker K, Donald J, Collins F, Friedlander M, Hogg D, Goss P, Heidenreich A, Ormiston W, Daly PA, Forman D, Oliver TD, Leahy M, Huddart R, Cooper CS, Bodmer JG (2000) Localization to Xq27 of a susceptibility gene for testicular germ-cell tumours. Nat Genet 24(2):197–200

Rapley EA, Turnbull C, Al Olama AA, Dermitzakis ET, Linger R, Huddart RA, Renwick A, Hughes D, Hines S, Seal S, Morrison J, Nsengimana J, Deloukas P; UK Testicular Cancer

Collaboration, Rahman N, Bishop DT, Easton DF, Stratton MR. (2009) A genome-wide association study of testicular germ cell tumor. Nat Genet. 41:807–10.

Repping S, Skaletsky H, Brown L, van Daalen SK, Korver CM, Pyntikova T, Kuroda-Kawaguchi T, de Vries JW, Oates RD, Silber S, van der Veen F, Page DC, Rozen S (2003) Polymorphism for a 1.6-Mb deletion of the human Y chromosome persists through balance between recurrent mutation and haploid selection. Nat Genet 35:247–251

Richard SM, Bianchi NO, Bianchi MS, Peltomaki P, Lothe RA, Pavicic W (2004) Ethnic variation in the prevalence of AZF deletions in testicular cancer. Mutat Res 554:45–51

Richiardi L, Akre O (2005) Fertility among brothers of patients with testicular cancer. Cancer Epidemiol Biomarkers Prev 14:2557–2562

Richiardi L, Pettersson A, Akre O (2007) Genetic and environmental risk factors for testicular cancer. Int J Androl 30(4):230–240

Sakai N, Yamada T, Asao T, Baba M, Yoshida M, Murayama T (2000) Bilateral testicular tumors in androgen insensitivity syndrome. Int J Urol 7:390–392

Sakurai T, Iguchi T, Moriwaki K, Noguchi M (1995) The ter mutation first causes primordial germ cell deficiency in ter/ter mouse embryos at 8 days of gestation. Dev Growth Differ 37:293–302

Senturia YD (1987) The epidemiology of testicular cancer. Br J Urol 60:285–291

Skaletsky H, Kuroda-Kawaguchi T, Minx PJ, Cordum HS, Hillier L, Brown LG, Repping S, Pyntikova T, Ali J, Bieri T, Chinwalla A, Delehaunty A, Delehaunty K, Du H, Fewell G, Fulton L, Fulton R, Graves T, Hou SF, Latrielle P, Leonard S, Mardis E, Maupin R, McPherson J, Miner T, Nash W, Nguyen C, Ozersky P, Pepin K, Rock S, Rohlfing T, Scott K, Schultz B, Strong C, Tin-Wollam A, Yang SP, Waterston RH, Wilson RK, Rozen S, Page DC (2003) The male-specific region of the human Y chromosome is a mosaic of discrete sequence classes. Nature 423:825–837

Sonneveld DJ, Sleijfer DT, Schrafford KH, Sijmons RH, van der Graaf WT, Sluiter WJ, Hoekstra HJ (1999) Familial testicular cancer in a single-centre population. Eur J Cancer 35:1368–1373

Starr JR, Chen C, Doody DR, Hsu L, Ricks S, Weiss NS, Schwartz SM (2005) Risk of testicular germ cell cancer in relation to variation in maternal and offspring cytochrome p450 genes involved in catechol estrogen metabolism. Cancer Epidemiol Biomarkers Prev 14:2183–2190

Stevens LC (1973) A new inbred subline of mice (129-terSv) with a high incidence of spontaneous congenital testicular teratomas. J Natl Cancer Inst 50:235–242

Swerdlow AJ, De Stavola BL, Swanwick MA, Maconochie NE (1997) Risks of breast and testicular cancers in young adult twins in England and Wales: evidence on prenatal and genetic aetiology. Lancet 350:1723–1728

Tollerud DJ, Blattner WA, Fraser MC, Brown LM, Pottern L, Shapiro E, Kirkemo A, Shawker TH, Javadpour N, O'Connell K (1985) Familial testicular cancer and urogenital developmental anomalies. Cancer 55:1849–1854

The International HapMap Project (2003) Nature 426:789–796

The Wellcome Trust Case Control Consortium (2007) Genome-wide association study of 14,000 cases of seven common diseases and 3,000 shared controls. Nature 447:661–678

Vogt PH, Edelmann A, Kirsch S, Henegariu O, Hirschmann P, Kiesewetter F, Kohn FM, Schill WB, Farah S, Ramos C, Hartmann M, Hartschuh W, Meschede D, Behre HM, Castel A, Nieschlag E, Weidner W, Grone HJ, Jung A, Engel W, Haidl G (1996) Human Y chromosome azoospermia factors (AZF) mapped to different subregions in Yq11. Hum Mol Genet 5:933–943

Westergaard T, Olsen JH, Frisch M, Kroman N, Nielsen JW, Melbye M (1996) Cancer risk in fathers and brothers of testicular cancer patients in Denmark. A population-based study. Int J Cancer 66:627–631

Youngren KK, Coveney D, Peng X, Bhattacharya C, Schmidt LS, Nickerson ML, Lamb BT, Deng JM, Behringer RR, Capel B, Rubin EM, Nadeau JH, Matin A (2005) The Ter mutation in the dead end gene causes germ cell loss and testicular germ cell tumours. Nature 435:360–364

Zhang F, Li Z, Wen B, Jiang J, Shao M, Zhao Y, He Y, Song X, Qian J, Lu D, Jin L (2006) A frequent partial AZFc deletion does not render an increased risk of spermatogenic impairment in East Asians. Ann Hum Genet 70:304–313

Summary and Future Directions

This book has focused on the etiology and pathology of cancers that exclusively affect men. What common themes emerge? On the basis of twin and family studies, both cancers are likely to have a strong genetic component. Nevertheless, it is notable that specific, strongly acting dominant susceptibility genes have not been identified for testicular cancer or prostate cancer. This is unlike the situation in most other solid tumors of adulthood, where up to 5% of all cases of cancer are explained by five or ten "high-risk" genes, such as *BRCA1*, *BRCA2*, *TP53*, *APC* and *MLH1*. Family history is a surrogate for the presence or absence of cancer susceptibility alleles. However, based on today's knowledge, a strong family history of prostate or testicular cancer may not be due to recognized high-risk genes. This fact has complicated genetic counseling for those at increased risk for prostate and testicular cancer. Few men are currently offered advice based on genetic status. For many adult cancers, numerous low penetrance alleles have been identified. Whereas these alleles individually are of no real clinical significance, they could be important if used collectively for risk assessment. More two dozen loci have been identified that slightly increase the risk (less than 1.5 fold) for prostate cancer. These findings point toward new serum markers for early detection, new targets for therapy, and possibly, when used in combination, new models of risk. Improving the performance of panels of alleles in predicting risk, and more especially risk of clinically serious disease, is the major challenge facing the prostate cancer genetics community. There may be individual familial prostate cancer pedigrees that will yield important new information, but this has not so far been a fruitful avenue of research. Two recent genome-wide association studies of testicular cancer have just been completed, and several important novel loci have been discovered.

There is a large amount of knowledge regarding the epidemiology of prostate and testicular cancers, but it is notable that, as for genetics, much of the data for both cancers do not point to a small number of key risk factors. For this reason, it is unlikely that additional epidemiological research of a traditional kind will alone yield important new etiological insights. Key questions of great clinical importance remain unanswered and are currently under investigation. For example, the role of PSA in screening for prostate cancer, while in widespread use in the USA, remains unclear, and until large-scale clinical trials report, skepticism, and a substantial transatlantic division of opinion will remain. For testicular cancer, one key question seems to be whether or not *in utero* factors are a major contributor to testicular cancer risk. This is especially important as some of the risk factors may be modifiable. Another interesting etiological issue is the question of testicular microlithiasis and testicular cancer, especially as carcinoma *in situ* of the testes, a precursor lesion for testicular germ cell tumors, is also associated with microlithiasis. Testicular microlithiasis is also associated with cryptorchidism and subfertility, and recent family studies have shown that relatives of men with testicular germ cell tumors are more likely to have testicular microlithiasis than are controls. Perhaps, are there common etiologic factors for both conditions? Combined efforts in genetics, epidemiology, and pathology should help.

Over the past few years, research into the pathology of prostate and testicular cancer has yielded important insights, especially at the nexus between epidemiology, pathology, and genetics. For example, based on risk factor analysis, which men are likely to develop aggressive prostate cancers, and can the future behavior of these cancers be reliably predicted from traditional and molecular pathological findings on initial biopsy? The emerging role of fusion proteins involving TMPRSS2 is an example of this – are some men (e.g., *BRCA2* mutation carriers) more likely to develop prostate cancers which express oncogenic fusion proteins? For testicular cancers, the seemingly inherent curability of these cancers has always been a fascinating (and welcome) aspect of their biology. The significance of the lack of *TP53* alterations in these cancers remains uncertain, but seems to be a contributor to the good prognosis of most testicular germ cell tumors. As efforts to devise less toxic treatments continue, using molecular pathology to establish which tumors really do need the most aggressive chemotherapy, and which ones can be treated with less intensive regimens will be an important development in the coming years.

William D. Foulkes, MB, PhD
Kathleen A. Cooney, MD

Index